McGraw-Hill Clinical Care Plans

Medical-Surgical Nursing

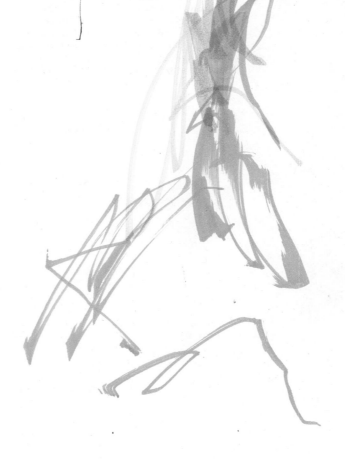

Notice

Medicine is an ever-changing science. As new research and clinical experience broaden our knowledge, changes in treatment and drug therapy are required. The authors, editor, and publisher of this work have checked with sources believed to be reliable in their efforts to provide information that is complete and generally in accord with the standards accepted at the time of publication. However, in view of the possibility of human error or changes in medical sciences, neither the editors nor the publisher nor any other party who has been involved in the preparation or publication of this work warrants that the information contained herein is in every respect accurate or complete, and they are not responsible for any errors or omissions or for the results obtained from the use of such information. Readers are encouraged to confirm the information contained herein with other sources. For example and in particular, readers are advised to check the product information sheet included in the package of each drug they plan to administer to be certain that the information contained in this book is accurate and that changes have not been made in the recommended dose or in the contraindications for administration. This recommendation is of particular importance in connection with new or infrequently used drugs.

McGraw-Hill Clinical Care Plans

Medical-Surgical Nursing

Marlene Mayers, RN, MS
Series Editor

Consultant, Nursing Practice / Administration

Carol Pankratz, RN, MSN
Associate Editor

Medical-Surgical Clinical Nurse Specialist

Preceptor, Regional RN / BS Program
Oregon Health Sciences University, Portland

McGraw-Hill, Inc.
Health Professions Division

New York St. Louis San Francisco Auckland Bogotá Caracas
Lisbon London Madrid Mexico City Milan Montreal New Delhi
San Juan Singapore Sydney Tokyo Toronto

McGraw-Hill Clinical Care Plans: Medical-Surgical Nursing

1234567890 MALMAL 9987654

ISBN: 0-07-105464-2
ISSN: 1074-4231

The editors were Gail Gavert and Mariapaz Ramos Englis; the production supervisor was Gyl Favours; the text design and production was by Beneda Design. Malloy Lithographing was printer and binder.

This book is printed on acid-free paper.

To—

My husband Jim who said "You really get to know a person when you write a book with them."

Mom, Jim Jr., Marie, and Charlotte, who were close to me to begin with;

Marlene, her staff, and Annette, who made this book possible;

My close professional colleagues, the clinical editors, whose names are listed in this book;

The medical/surgical nurses who created these care plans, whose names are listed in this book;

And to all present and future medical/surgical nurses who will make these plans happen.

CONTENTS

CONTENTS

REVIEWERS AND CONTRIBUTORS

CLINICAL REVIEWERS

Jeffrey R. Baumgart, RN, MS, BSN
Nursing Supervisor
Hospital Home Care/Hospice

Constance M. Dahlin, RN, MSN, OCNS
Hospice Coordinator
Hospital Home Care/Hospice

Michele J. Harvey, RN, MS, ET
Clinical Nurse Specialist-ET
Home Health Services

Janet Pipitone RN, CS, MN, OCN
Nurse Manager
Oncology and Neurology

Lynn Radford, RN, MSN, CCRN
Clinical Nurse Specialist
Critical Care/Immunology

Denise Butler Sharp, RN, CS, MN
Clinical Nurse Specialist
PACU and Anesthesia Support

Bonnie C. Thomas, RN, BSN
Nurse Educator
Clinical Education

Bob Upward, RN, MSN, RNFA(C)
Clinical Specialist
Surgical Services

CONTRIBUTORS

Dale Abendroth-Lenski, RN, MN
Assistant Professor, Nursing
Gonzaga University
Spokane, Washington

Doreen M. Ahern, RN
Nursing Coordinator
Maimonides Medical Center
Brooklyn, New York

Jan M. Bailey, RN, MSN
Clinical Nurse Specialist
Memorial Mission Medical Center
Asheville, North Carolina

Sandra Irene Bakke, RN, C, MN
CNS, Hematology/Oncology
Cedars Sinai Medical Center
Assistant Clinical Professor
University of California
Los Angeles, California

Robin Rago Bankhead, RN, MS, CNSN
CNS, Nutrition Support Team
Cooper Hospital/University Medical Center
Camden, New Jersey

Jeffrey R. Baumgart, RN, MS, BSN
Nursing Supervisor
Home Care/Hospice
McKenzie-Willamette Hospital
Springfield, Oregon

Doris Bennett, RN
Director, Oncology
Good Samaritan Hospital
Lexington, Kentucky

Madelaine L. Binner, RN, BSN, MBA
Educator, Staff Development
Women's Christian Association Hospital
Jamestown, New York

Portia A. Botchway, RN, MSN
Lecturer, Nursing
Clemson University
Clemson, South Carolina

Patricia T. Campbell, RN, C, MSN
RN Instructor
Maimonides Medical Center
Brooklyn, New York

Shirley Cantrell, RN, MSN
Nursing Faculty
Valdosta State University
Valdosta, Georgia

Olivia Catolico, RN, C, MS
Associate Chief Nursing Service Education
Jerry L. Pettis Memorial VA Medical Center
Loma Linda, California

Ramona L. Cheek, RN, CS, MS
CNS, Medical/Surgical
Spartanburg Regional Medical Center
Spartanburg, South Carolina

DeLana Childress, RN, CS, MSN
CNS Critical Care
St. Josephs Regional Health Center
Hot Springs, Arkansas

Christine McDonald Clarkin, RN, CDE, MPA
Program Coordinator
Diabetes Learning Center
Stormont Vail Regional Medical Center
Topeka, Kansas

Deborah Coates, RN, MSN, CETN
Clinical Specialist, Surgical
Memorial Mission Medical Center
Asheville, North Carolina

Christine Lind Colella, RN, CS, MSN
Clinical Education Specialist
Medical-Surgical Nursing
Deaconess Hospital
Cincinnati, Ohio

Janice C. Colwell, RN, MS, CETN
CNS, Enterostomal Therapy
University of Chicago Hospitals
Chicago, Illinois

Margaret R. Colyar, RN, MSN
Assistant Professor
Valdosta State University
Valdosta, Georgia

Teresita E. Corvera, RN, MN, CCRN
CNS, Cardiology
Cedars Sinai Medical Center
Los Angeles, California

Constance M. Dahlin, RN, MSN, OCNS
Coordinator, Hospice
Home Care/Hospice
McKenzie-Willamette Hospital
Springfield, Oregon

Nadine K. Dexter, RN, MSN, ARNP
Director, Gerontology
Stormont-Vail Medical Center
Topeka, Kansas

Betty J. Ducharme, RN, BSN, MAEd
Director, Nursing Education
Appalachian Regional Healthcare
Lexington, Kentucky

Ginny Eaker, RN, CCRN
Staff Nurse, ICU
Kalispell Regional Hospital
Kalispell, Montana

Nenette M. Ebalo, RN, MPA, CCRN
Nurse Manager, Surgical Unit
Kaiser Permanente Medical Center
Hayward, California

Phyllis J. Ellena-McCluskey, RN, CS, MSN
Clinical Specialist, Psychiatric
Jerry L. Petttis Memorial VA Medical Center
Loma Linda, California

Kathleen Ellstrom, RN, CS, MS
CNS, Critical Care
Irvine Medical Center
University of California
Orange, California

CONTRIBUTORS

Steven W. Evans, RN, BSN
Director, Surgical Cardiac
and Telemetry Department
St. John's Regional Medical Center
Joplin, Missouri

Marlene A.S. Foreman RN, CS, MN,
BSN
Associate Professor, Nursing
Louisiana State University
Eunice, Louisiana

Linda M. Gorman, RN, CS, MN, OCN
CNS, Hospice Program
Cedar Sinai Medical Center
Los Angeles, California

Joanne P. Gucciardo, RN, C, MS
Administrative Coordinator, Special
Projects
Maimonides Medical Center
Brooklyn, New York

Nancy C. Hamm, RN
Staff Nurse, Radiology Nursing
Durham Regional Hospital
Durham, North Carolina

Brenda B. Harton, RN, C, BS
Staff Development Educator,
Medical-Surgical
Memorial Mission Medical Center
Asheville, North Carolina

Michele J. Harvey, RN, MS, ET
CNS-ET, Home Health Services
Sacred Heart General Hospital
Eugene, Oregon

Annette Beebe Hayman, RN, MSN, CCRN
Education Coordinator, Professional
Development
Saint Joseph's Hospital
Savannah, Georgia

Cathy Hebert, RN, MS
Clinical Nurse Specialist
Memorial Mission Medical Center
Asheville, North Carolina

Karen A. Hogan, RN, MSN, ARNP
CNS, University Medical Center
Clinical Instructor, Nursing
University of Florida
Jacksonville, Florida

Karen Jeans, RN, MSN, CCRN
CNS, Medical Center
University of Arkansas Medical Sciences
Campus
Little Rock, Arkansas

Jo Ann Jenkins, RN, MSN, CCRN
Assistant Professor, Nursing
Central Missouri State University
Warrensburg, Missouri

Lynne Jett, RN, BSN, PHN
Nurse Educator
Tri City Medical Center
Oceanside, California

Rhonda Johnston, RN, MS
Assistant Professor
University of Southern Colorado
Pueblo, Colorado

Drexel Jordan, RNP, MSN, OCN
CNS, Medical Center
University of Arkansas
Medical Sciences Campus
Little Rock, Arkansas

Rena Kaiser, RN, C, MN
Nurse Educator, Medical/Surgical
Irvine Medical Center
University of California
Orange, California

Deborah L. Kark, RN, MS, CCRN
Assistant Professor, Nursing
Purdue University Calumet
Hammond, Indiana

Kathleen Ann Kick, RN, MS
Assistant Professor, Nursing
Purdue University Calumet
Hammond, Indiana

Merritt E. Knox, RN, PhD
Associate Professor, Nursing
University of Wisconsin
Oshkosh, Wisconsin

Nancy Korchek, RN, MSN
Associate Professor, Nursing
Purdue University Calumet
Hammond, Indiana

Marilee Kuhrik, RN, MSN
Assistant Professor
Barnes College
St. Louis, Missouri

Nancy Kuhrik, RN, MSN
Assistant Professor, Nursing
and Allied Health
Jewish Hospital College
St. Louis, Missouri

Jane McCausland Kurz, RN, MSN
Assistant Professor
Delaware State College
Dover, Delaware

Cdr. Mary M. Leemhuis, RN, BS
Assistant Chief Nurse/Nurse Educator
US Public Health Service
Carl Albert Indian Health Facility
Ada, Oklahoma

Susan M. Leininger, RN, MSN
Assistant Professor
Kent State University
East Liverpool, Ohio

Virginia L. Levin, RN, MS
Assistant Director, Nursing
Kaiser Permanente
Panorama City, California

Delores A. Lorentzen, RN
Assistant Director, Nursing
Sehome Park Care Center
Bellingham, Washington

Suzanne E. Malloy, RN, MSN, EdD
Assistant Professor, Nursing
San Jose State University
San Jose, California

Maria Fe Mangila, RN, MSN, CCRN
Clinical Nurse Specialist
Surgical Intensive Care Unit
Los Angeles, California

Susan L. Mansell, RN, BSN, CCRN
Charge Nurse, MICU
Columbia Regional Hospital
Columbia, Missouri

Margaret Maron, RN, CS, MSN
CNS, Surgical Nursing Department
Maimonides Medical Center
Brooklyn, New York

Victoria Maryatt, RN, MSN
Acting Executive Head, Nursing
De Anza College
Cupertino, California

Regina M. Matera, RN, C, MS
Assistant Director, Nursing
Staff Development & Continuing Education
Maimonides Medical Center
Brooklyn, New York

Anita A. Matito, RN, MA
Nurse Educator, Medical/Surgical Services
Queen of Angels-Hollywood
Presbyterian Medical Center
Los Angeles, California

Sharyn L. Mills, CCC, MS
Director, Speech Pathology/Audiology
Baptist Medical Center
Kansas City, Missouri

Joyce Torline Mitchell, RN, ADN, BS
Supervisor, 3-11 Shift
Saint Luke East
Fort Thomas, Kentucky

Virginia Konkoly Mulack, RN, MS
Clinical Nurse Specialist
University of Chicago Hospitals
Chicago, Illinois

Nancy Mure, RN, BS, MA
Director of Nursing
Maimonides Medical Center
Brooklyn, New York

Jean Nelson, RN, MSN, MeD
Assistant Professor
Barnes Hospital
St. Louis, Missouri

Patricia A. O'Neill, RN, MSN, CCRN
Instructor
De Anza College
Cupertino, California

Ethel T. Patterson, RN, CS, MA
Clinical Nurse Specialist
Spartanburg Regional Medical Center
Spartanburg, South Carolina

Jan Perun, RN, BSN, OCN
Educational Coordinator
Orlando Regional HealthCare System
Orlando, Florida

Janet Pipitone, RN, CS, MN, OCN
Nurse Manager, Oncology and Neurology
Sacred Heart General Hospital
Eugene, Oregon

Lynn Radford, RN, MSN, CCRN
Clinical Nurse Specialist
McKenzie Willamette Hospital
Springfield, Oregon

Mary Ann Reale, RN, CS, MS
Clinical Assistant Professor, Nursing
University of Wisconsin
Nurse Practitioner
Wm. S. Middleton Memorial Veterans'
Hospital
Madison, Wisconsin

Monica Redekopp, RN, MN
Clinical Nurse Specialist
Charleston Area Medical Center
Charleston, West Virginia

Christina A. Sakomoto, RN, MS, CCRN
Clinical Nurse Specialist
Straub Hospital
Honolulu, Hawaii

Carol A. Salkind, RN, C, BSN,
Staff Development Instructor,
Medical/Surgical
University of Mississippi Medical Center
Jackson, Mississippi

Anna Marie Schmidt, RN, ADN
Nursing Administrative Supervisor
HealthEast Bethesda Lutheran
Hospital & Rehabilitation Center
St. Paul, Minnesota

Denise Butler Sharp, RN, CS, MN
CNS, PACU and Anesthesia Support
Sacred Heart General Hospital
Eugene, Oregon

Sylvia J. Sheffler, RN, DNS
Assistant Professor, Nursing
Delaware State University
Dover, Delaware

Laurie A. Sienkiewicz, RN, C, BSN, OCN
Nurse Educator
Irvine Medical Center
University of California
Orange, California

Pamela B. Simmons, RN, C, MSN
Director, Staff Support & Development
Louisiana State University Medical Center
Shreveport, Louisiana

Margaret E. Sosnowski, RN, C, MS
Instructor
Staff Development and Continuing
Education
Maimonides Medical Center
Brooklyn, New York

Pat Spiller, RN, BSN
Coordinator, Nursing Inservice
Walker Regional Medical Center
Jasper, Alabama

Cynthia Mills Spiro, RN, MSN
Instructor, Barnes College
Staff Nurse, Emergency Department
Saint Mary's Health Center
St. Louis, Missouri

Annette S. Stacy, RN, CS, MSN
Assistant Professor, Nursing
Arkansas State University
Jonesboro, Arkansas

Karen L. Stanley, RN, CS, MSN
CNS, Surgical Services
Charleston Area Medical Center
Charleston, West Virginia

Marilyn Seyb Thies, RN, C, BS
Educator, Nursing Staff Development
Midwest City Regional Hospital
Midwest City, Oklahoma

Bonnie C. Thomas, RN, BSN
Nurse Educator
Sacred Heart General Hospital
Eugene, Oregon

Eugenia H. Tickle, RN, MS, EdD
Associate Professor
Midwestern State University
Wichita Falls, Texas

Judith E. Tivnan, RN, BA, CRNI
Educator, Medical-Surgical
HCA Central Florida Regional Hospital
Sanford, Florida

Renee Samples Twibell, RN, DNS
Assistant Professor
Ball State University
Muncie, Indiana

Amy E. Uhler, RN, C, BSN
Nurse Educator
Northwest Medical Center
Franklin, Pennsylvania

Bob Upward, RN, MSN, RNFA(C)
Clinical Specialist, Surgical Services
Sacred Heart General Hospital
Eugene, Oregon

Katherine F. Watts, RN, MN, BSN
Instructor, Staff Development
University of Mississippi Medical Center
Jackson, Mississippi

Michael L. Williams, RN, MSN, CCRN
CNS, Thoracic Nursing Services
University of Michigan Medical Center
Ann Arbor, Michigan

Rebecca F. Wiseman, RN, PhD
Hospital Professor
Spartanburg Regional Med Center
Adjunct Faculty, Nursing
University of South Carolina
Spartanburg, South Carolina

Sharon M. Wisneski, RN, MSN
Instructor, Nursing
Delaware State University
Dover, Delaware

Lt. Col. Sarah A. Wright, RN
USAF, NC
Minot, North Dakota

PREFACE

THE McGRAW-HILL CLINICAL CARE PLAN SERIES

This book and its companions in the McGraw-Hill Clinical Care Plan series are the most current editions of the now "classic" Standard Nursing Care Plans that were first published by Mayers/El Camino in the mid-seventies. These books, in frequently updated versions, have been published continuously since that time. In those early years, as the first of their kind, they did much to stimulate nursing's early development of formalized, systematic care planning/evaluation systems in hospitals throughout most English-speaking countries. Today they continue to be a part of nursing's continuing effort to articulate and advance the knowledge base of nursing. In addition, metric conversions have been given as appropriate to facilitate global audiences.

These new editions, now published by McGraw-Hill, preserve all of the most preferred features of previous editions. They also contain many enhancements in format and style which make them even easier to use than ever before. The content has benefited from the contributions of a greater number, and wider range, of nurse caregivers, specialists, and educators than before.

These books maintain continuity with previous editions through oversight by the same Series Editor, Marlene Mayers. In addition, a new Associate Editor, Carol Pankratz has been added to the editorial team for this book, *Medical-Surgical Nursing*. She is a clinical nurse specialist and clinical educator for the medical-surgical departments of a large regional medical center.

This editorial team, in close collaboration with panels of clinical reviewers, have combined their talents to produce these definitive books of nursing care plans for the acute care setting.

The books in the McGraw-Hill Clinical Care Plan series are: *Perinatal/Neonatal Nursing, Pediatric Nursing,* and *Medical-Surgical Nursing.* They are specifically designed to be used by nurses in the hospital setting. The three books address the acute problems that are experienced by many people at some time during their lives: from before birth, through childhood, and into adulthood. These problems frequently result in hospitalization where nurses, as the predominant caregivers, provide the moment-by-moment care that assesses, nurtures, and guides them through their acute crises.

Guides for Care Planning in the Hospital Setting

These books are entitled "Clinical Care Plans" because they are carefully written in the succinct style associated with the clinical setting. They help nurses and students visualize how a functional care plan might be phrased. Some of these plans contain more items of information than a nurse might normally need for a specific patient, but they offer groups or combinations of activities from which to select the most relevant items. By referring to these already carefully crafted documents, and by adding the necessary qualifying words and phrases, a nurse can thereby efficiently produce care plans that contain both standardized and carefully individualized elements.

The plans' format is the familiar three-column design. Terminology is consistent with what is actually written in charts and on care plans in the clinical setting. Terms are succinct enough so that, with only minor modification, they can be entered into a critical pathway, a flow sheet, or into computerized information systems.

Each book includes the most commonly occurring medical diagnoses (or topics of concern) that are experienced by patients admitted to that clinical area.

Familiar Phraseology

Phraseology tends to conform to generally familiar hospital nursing form and style practices. (1) Nursing Diagnoses are those developed by NANDA; (2) Outcome Criteria include action verbs that direct attention to those measurable/observable phenomena (subjective and objective) which make evaluation possible; (3) Interventions (groups/combinations of nursing activities) are phrased as directives.

Because these plans are meant to be used in the acute care setting, their terms are those of hospital nurses. Brief and succinct phrases are used rather than sentences. Outcome criteria are written in the present tense, active voice. Symbols and abbreviations common to the hospital setting are used.

Easy to Individualize

These care plans are easy to individualize because they are carefully crafted to apply to specific clinical situations. For example, the management of "Fluid Volume Deficit" (a NANDA diagnosis) for a child with leukemia will differ from fluid volume management for an adult or child with an eating disorder. Or, for example, "Altered Nutrition: Less than body requirements" is treated differently in the care plan for diabetes mellitus than it is in that for a child with biliary atresia or for an infant with cleft palate.

It is also within the individualization process that the patient's collaboration becomes vital. Involvement empowers people to become competent and knowledgeable about their health and, thus, to become effective on their own behalf. Including the patient and family in reviewing, understanding, and amending the plan of care can make a significant difference in the outcomes of that care. It can also influence patients' long-term healthcare practices.

Excellent Reference Tools

The books are designed to be used on a daily basis. They provide easy to find information about clinical nursing care. When kept near at hand, for instance on the nursing unit as well as in school and hospital libraries, they serve as reminder systems – as do other reference texts and manuals. They are excellent references to use when nurses are reviewing literature as part of the periodic updates of their own standard nursing care plans.

A Clinical Care Plan prompts a nurse to address all of the relevant issues for a patient's care. It is difficult, when under the pressures of an acute care setting, to rely on human memory to recall each and every one of the variables to be addressed in a patient's situation. A responsible professional in any field uses "lists and prompts" to bolster human memory. Every caregiver, too, needs various kinds of reference and reminder systems to provide safe and effective care. Clinical Care Plans are among the best of them.

Excellent Learning Tools

The clearly organized format and graphic nonlinear design makes these books excellent learning tools for hospital or school instruction. Each care plan illuminates the logic that underlies nursing practice. Nursing Diagnoses and etiologies along with their outcome criteria are specified. These, in turn, trigger groups or combinations of nursing activities that are understood to prevent, ameliorate, or resolve the underlying problems. The graphic format structures and organizes these units of information. Their relationships are made clear.

This logical framework helps students to more easily understand and to integrate the detailed information found in their major nursing texts.

Outcome Criteria for Quality Assurance/Improvement

Included are many outcome criteria that are directly linked to care assessment for quality enhancement. Clinical Care Plans typically offer several outcome criteria for each nursing diagnosis. Criteria are phrased in specific, measurable terms.

These care plans express commonly understood outcome and process criteria and thereby provide an excellent device for measuring quality and identifying accountability. With only minor modification they can be utilized as the source of outcome and process criteria for patient care evaluation tools such as those used in Total Quality Management (TQM), chart reviews, concurrent reviews, patient surveys, etc.

Practice-Based Development

These books are the result of a process of collaboration among nurse clinicians, caregivers, and educators from across the country. Through this process standards and practices have become integrated into a carefully organized, inductively developed, practice-based whole. Yet, each book also clearly reflects the differing nursing cultures and voices that are unique to each clinical area.

Our goal has been to provide care plans that specifically address the needs of hospitalized patients. And we respectfully acknowledge the extraordinary commitment and skill of their caregivers, today's hospital nurses.

Acknowledgments

We wish to thank the following individuals for their extraordinary contributions to manuscript development: Christine Beneda, Keith Albin, Sandra Irene Bakke, Regina M. Matera, Barbara Land, Penny Allmett, Cheryl Hunt, Carol Roth, and Peggy Pickens. A special note of appreciation goes to Shasta Hatter, our manuscript coordinator.

Marlene Mayers, RN, MS
Series Editor

Carol Pankratz, RN, MSN
Associate Editor

McGraw-Hill Clinical Care Plans

Medical-Surgical Nursing

CONTENTS   Instructions

INSTRUCTIONS

HOW TO USE McGRAW-HILL CLINICAL CARE PLANS

This definitive, easy-to-use reference book provides the hospital nurse or nursing student, with a fast-track approach to patient care planning. The design is easy to read, well-indexed, and gives the reader a jump start in developing an individualized plan of care.

THE FORMAT

The care plans are divided into six categories: Nursing Diagnoses, Outcome Criteria, Interventions, Rationale, Other Less Common Nursing Diagnoses, and Essential Discharge Criteria. Take each category and review the specific components contained within.

Nursing Diagnoses

NANDA nursing diagnoses are used as the standard nomenclature for these care plans. They are listed in the first, or left-hand, column of the care plan as noted below.

		EDUCATION FOR DISCHARGE
URSING DIAGNOSIS	**OUTCOME CRITERIA**	**INTERVENTIONS**
1 Knowledge Deficit (relevant healthcare needs) *r.t. lack of recall, cognitive limitation, impaired communication, depression, illiteracy, lack of exposure, withdrawal*	• Verbalizes understanding of instructions	• Describe how to use new skills, behaviors in daily living • Use open-ended questions to derive information regarding learning • Simplify information to meet the patient's/family's level of understanding or developmental age

Our example is "Knowledge Deficit" as it appears in our *Education for Discharge* care plan.

Because of shortened lengths of stay in the hospital, all relevant nursing diagnoses likely will be addressed upon admission. Otherwise, the diagnoses may be prioritized according to patient need and nurse judgment. The diagnostic *hunch* can be confirmed by reviewing those diagnoses listed under the topic, since they are most likely to characterize patient problems associated with that particular topic or medical diagnosis. Sometimes, the reader is referred to other care plans in the book that may help develop a particular plan or address a specific issue, such as *pain* or *education for discharge*.

The last part of the diagnostic statement is the etiology, or list of risk factors, that follows the "related to" phrase as shown. We have chosen to abbreviate the "related to" statement to *r.t.* within each care plan. A variety of potential etiology statements are listed to get you going. You will want to select the specific etiology for your patient as you begin to develop an individualized plan of care.

For example, Knowledge Deficit might be related to "lack of recall" for one patient, to "cognitive limitation" for another, to "illiteracy" for a third patient.

Clearly, the different etiologies would require different teaching-learning interventions.

EDUCATION FOR DISCHARGE

NURSING DIAGNOSIS	OUTCOME CRITERIA	INTERVENTIONS
1 Knowledge Deficit (relevant healthcare needs) *r.t. lack of recall, cognitive limitation, impaired communication, depression, illiteracy, lack of exposure, withdrawal*	• Verbalizes understanding of instructions	• Describe how to use new skills, behaviors in daily living • Use open-ended questions to derive information regarding learning • Simplify information to meet the patient's/family's level of understanding or developmental age

Outcome Criteria

The next column addresses *Outcome Criteria* which is the term chosen to reflect the goals for the patient. Here you will find the patient outcomes anticipated for the certain nursing diagnoses. The outcome, which is written in specific terms, may address the patient and/or family.

These objective and subjective criteria are written in terms of measurable patient behaviors, and each criterion identifies the patient's goals by the time of discharge. Similarly, outcome criteria include objective and subjective parameters that describe successful resolution of the nursing diagnoses.

Because the length of stay in today's acute care setting is compressed, all outcome criteria should be met during the patient's hospital stay. For clarity and simplicity, outcomes have not been separated into short- or long-term phrases. However, care plans can be used as guides for critical pathways or care maps by assigning daily goals, determined by institutional preferences and regional population needs.

You will find that the term *within normal limits* (WNL) has been used to allow for the variation of normal. That variation may be normal for that patient, i.e., return to baseline, or preadmission status. Or normal may reflect the variation within the literature. And it can reflect the variation between institutions or physician preferences for monitoring response to treatment.

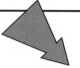

EDUCATION FOR DISCHARGE

NURSING DIAGNOSIS	OUTCOME CRITERIA	INTERVENTIONS
1 Knowledge Deficit (relevant healthcare needs) *r.t. lack of recall, cognitive limitation, impaired communication, depression, illiteracy, lack of exposure, withdrawal*	• Verbalizes understanding of instructions	• Describe how to use new behaviors in daily living • Use open-ended questions to derive information regarding learning • Simplify information to meet the patient's/family's level of understanding or developmental age

Interventions

Nursing actions are listed in the third column. *Interventions* identify independent and interdependent strategies designed to facilitate or accomplish the outcome criteria. Interventions are specific enough to ensure that established standards of clinical practice are met, yet general enough to allow for institutional preferences. Monitoring and assessment strategies are listed to guide the nurse in ascertaining that outcomes have been met.

Actions listed are both independent and interdependent. Suggestions for referrals are stated when the plan of care may require the expertise of another healthcare discipline. The care plan format can be easily adapted to document which interventions were provided by each discipline. For instance, the nurse can reinforce the plans set forth by the social worker, while saving time in redundant efforts.

In this column you may find the term *within parameters*. This term was chosen to address those assessments that a physician or other primary care provider may state as an acceptable range of normal, such as in blood gases or blood glucose levels. (You may want to refer to the appendixes for normative data.)

Many plans include specific teaching content to correct knowledge deficits and enhance important self-care strategies. You may want to refer to the *Education for Discharge* care plan to supplement this section.

Rationale

Listed at the end of the *Intervention* column you will find *Rationale* for the interventions as they relate to the nursing diagnosis and etiologies. These statements are simple, concise, and offer key concepts to use in researching these concepts further.

EDUCATION FOR DISCHARGE

NURSING DIAGNOSIS	OUTCOME CRITERIA	INTERVENTIONS
	• Participates in care activities	• Establish an environment that enables patient/family to gain control
		• Build on patient's developmental and learning level; consult with expert as indicated

RATIONALE: *Learning activities that are geared to the patient's/family's level of prior experience, knowledge, and developmental level are likely to produce positive cognitive behavior changes that are relevant to healthcare needs. Repetition, participation, and graphic/written cues and lists foster learning and recall.*

Other Less Common Nursing Diagnoses

Next you will find that we have included a listing of other diagnoses that tend to be associated with the medical diagnosis or problem. These diagnoses may also reflect other potential problems that patients with this medical condition present in the acute care setting.

You will see that etiologies have been omitted from the diagnostic statement, allowing for individual variations in patient assessment by the nurse. These additional nursing diagnoses, supported by a particular patient's characteristics and etiology, can be developed through the nursing process.

We refer to these diagnoses as "less common" because they are less likely to be addressed during a brief hospital stay. However, these nursing diagnoses may be commonly addressed with complications or in the outpatient or home care setting.

Essential Discharge Criteria

The final section in each care plan is the *Essential Discharge Criteria*. Here you will find that we have broadly summarized the Outcome Criteria contained within the care plan. The outcome criteria have been collapsed into essential aspects that

EDUCATION FOR DISCHARGE

OTHER LESS COMMON NURSING DIAGNOSES: Anxiety; Ineffective Individual Coping; Noncompliance; Social Isolation; Self-Esteem Disturbance

ESSENTIAL DISCHARGE CRITERIA

- Patient/family verbalize and/or demonstrate specific knowledge, behavior, skills relevant to condition

- Demonstrates knowledge relevant to condition: pathophysiology, prognosis, expected course of recovery

- Verbalizes, discusses specific knowledge relevant to healthcare needs: treatment plans and their rationale, potential complications and s/s to report

- Demonstrates competence in use of required equipment, assistive devices

- Verbalizes/demonstrates safe and effective use of prescribed medications

- Identifies potential drug or food interactions to be avoided

- Verbalizes realistic plans to integrate required dietary modifications into normal family diet

- Possesses follow-up appointments for required treatments and healthcare supervision

must be present to allow for a safe and effective discharge from the acute care setting.

For example, you will notice that we have assumed that basic physiologic function is present but we will speak to the need for "resolution of respiratory compromise" for the patient who was admitted with pneumonia. You won't necessarily find discussion of HR WNL, BP WNL, or bowel function WNL, since these are only indirectly related to the presenting problem. And maybe that patient has a superimposed cardiac abnormality that will not be ameliorated by the care provided during the bout with pneumonia.

Additionally, we incorporated JCAHO requirements regarding discharge. You will find strategies to ensure compliance in the *Education for Discharge* plan, which addresses Knowledge Deficit.

GETTING STARTED

Now that you have an understanding of the layout and content, it's time to get started developing your individualized care plan.

- Select the medical diagnoses you are interested in and turn to the standard care plan.
- Identify the nursing diagnosis relevant to your patient based on your assessment. Remember to review the *Other Less Common Nursing Diagnoses* section for other potential diagnoses.

- Select the appropriate etiology for each nursing diagnosis.
- Identify outcome criteria specific to the etiology demonstrated by the patient.
- Review the essential discharge criteria to ensure inclusion of essential aspects.
- List interventions necessary to facilitate achieving the identified outcomes as they relate to the patient.
- Review the plan of care with the patient and family and revise as needed.
- Implement the plan of care, communicating with other healthcare providers.
- Evaluate the patient's progress toward attaining the outcome criteria; revise the plan as needed.
- Identify variances for developing Improvement of Organizational Program (quality assurance).

HELPFUL HINTS

A successful plan begins with a solid nursing admission data base. Objective and subjective information is clustered to determine whether or not defining characteristics support a particular nursing diagnosis.

You will not find *exact* wording from care plan to care plan concerning a specific nursing diagnoses, e.g., impaired skin integrity. This is intentional, providing the reader with a variety of phrasing options. (It's also less boring that way!)

You will find the term *family* is used broadly to describe persons significant to the patient. These persons may be mother, brother, father, aunt, neighbor, friend, or any other "significant other."

For diagnoses that tend to span age groups, such as meningitis, the reader needs to incorporate developmental considerations as indicated. Additionally, the diagnosis may occur across the life span, and these developmental "passages" should be considered as well.

Achievement of Essential Discharge Criteria should be addressed and documented as part of the discharge notation. The behaviors listed are those that the patient must demonstrate before safely leaving the hospital. The nurse obtains data from ongoing patient assessment, return demonstrations, and the patient record to evaluate whether outcome criteria have been met. If the criteria are not met, appropriate referrals should be made and documented to ensure care continuity after discharge.

Appendixes may be helpful to you when looking for abbreviations, normal lab values, listing of NANDA nursing diagnoses, definitions of medical problems, or defining characteristics of NANDA diagnoses.

GENERAL

CASTING

NURSING DIAGNOSES	OUTCOME CRITERIA	INTERVENTIONS
1 Pain *r.t. injury, surgery, immobilization*	• Verbalizes/displays sustained comfort - identifies medication or activity that reduces or aggravates discomfort - reports comfort following analgesia	• Assess location, duration, severity of pain, identifying precipitating or relieving factors • Reposition for comfort, in proper alignment • Provide an orthopedic bedpan as indicated • Routinely administer narcotic and NSAIDs as prescribed; progress to PO analgesics, using equianalgesic scale
2 Impaired Tissue Integrity *r.t. possible constriction from cast*	• Is able to move and feel affected extremity/extremities	• Inspect above and below cast for circulation (cyanosis, pallor, swelling, coldness, capillary filling, numbness) and assess mobility qh for 48h, q4h for 72h, then q8h • Keep cast cutter available for emergency cast removal
	• Displays dry, intact skin - has no musty odor under cast	• Dry cast; keep it exposed to air the first 48 h; may use hair dryer, heat cradle, or sunlight
	• Has no complaint of burning pressure under cast	• Elevate to avoid flattening around bony prominences • Turn q2h • When dried, pull stockinette out over the edges; secure with adhesive for smooth edges • If spica or body cast, protect groin edges with plastic

RATIONALE: *Frequent inspection produces early detection and management of compartment syndrome. Proper cast drying and lining prevent pressure sores and skin breakdown.*

NURSING DIAGNOSES	OUTCOME CRITERIA	INTERVENTIONS
3 High Risk for Infection *r.t. bleeding, drainage from compound fracture*	• Has no drainage or foul, musty odor from cast	• Examine for odor under cast
	• Shows VS, WBC count WNL	• Monitor VS, WBC count q4h
	• Has no foreign objects in cast	• Instruct not to put foreign object under cast • Report any large cast stain accompanied by tachycardia and low BP
		RATIONALE: *Frequent inspection produces early detection and management of infection.*
4 High Risk for Injury *r.t. decalcification of bones, atrophy of muscles*	• Experiences no fractures, falls, muscle strain when cast is removed	• Provide support for all casted joints when removed • Assist when using extremity for the first time • Encourage isometric exercises to affected muscles q2h during the day; reinforce physical therapy
		RATIONALE: *Support and muscle toning help to prevent complications such as fractures and muscle injury.*
5 Impaired Physical Mobility *r.t. casting*	• Describes restricted, modified, and acceptable activities	• Teach ADL in cast: plastic to protect cast to bathe, shower, blow dry small areas of dampened cast • Obtain required assistive device
	• Demonstrates exercises to joints above and below cast; demonstrates full ROM for all unaffected joints	• Teach active ROM for all unaffected joints
	• Describes how and when to do isometric exercises	• Teach isometric exercises to affected muscles
		RATIONALE: *Knowledge of how to do ADL despite restriction fosters independence.*

GENERAL

NURSING DIAGNOSES	OUTCOME CRITERIA	INTERVENTIONS
6 Body Image Disturbance *r.t. cast and altered functioning*	• Verbalizes fear and concerns • Asks questions and expresses optimism	• Encourage expression of feelings
	• Participates in ADL	• Initiate discussion of lifestyle adaptation • Encourage self-care, grooming • Give positive feedback for progress
		RATIONALE: *Helps patient cope with illness and prevent loss of self-esteem.*
7 Knowledge Deficit *r.t. complications, limited mobility when home*	• Correctly describes cast care	• Teach and obtain return demonstration of cast care
	• Lists reportable s/s	• Instruct about reportable s/s: odor, pain, burning, pallor, numbness, tingling, coldness, swelling, throbbing, loss of movement
	• Participates in ADL; describes plans for ADL at home	• Remind of need to continue isometric exercises • Encourage innovation to maintain ADL
		RATIONALE: *Effective coping and rehabilitation require knowledge and understanding of condition.*

OTHER LESS COMMON NURSING DIAGNOSES: *Altered Peripheral Tissue Perfusion; Altered Urinary Elimination; Self-Care Deficit*

ESSENTIAL DISCHARGE CRITERIA

- Is afebrile
- Shows no skin breakdown or contractures
- Controls pain with oral analgesia
- Performs ADL

- Verbalizes understanding of cast care and reportable s/s
- Has follow-up appointment

CONFUSION

NURSING DIAGNOSES	OUTCOME CRITERIA	INTERVENTIONS

1 Altered Thought Processes
 	
r.t. maturational dementia, nervous system disorder, metabolic alteration, unfamiliar environment
	• Shows serum electrolytes, H&H, ABGs WNL	• Assess for possible metabolic causes
		  - monitor serum electrolytes, H&H, ABGs as ordered
		  - provide O$_2$ as ordered prn

	• Demonstrates improvement in (or adaptation to) altered thought process	• Decrease environmental stress
		  - approach patient in a calm, unhurried manner
		  - provide consistency by having same staff care for patient
		  - keep decision-making simple; offer limited choices
		  - explain procedures, changes from routine in advance
		  - keep direction, explanations simple
		
		• Promote orientation by providing sensory input that is sufficient, meaningful
		  - introduce self
		  - provide clocks, calendars
		  - assist with functioning hearing aid, eyeglasses, as indicated
		  - reorient to time and place prn

		RATIONALE: *Electrolyte imbalances and hypoxia can contribute to confusion. Decreasing unnecessary stimuli reduces stress and promotes reorientation.*

2 High Risk for Injury (trauma)
 	
r.t. cognitive impairment: disorientation, impaired judgment
	• Is free of s/s of injury related to cognitive impairment	• Maintain environmental safety
		  - keep room uncluttered and free of hazards
		  - keep small light on in room at night
		  - keep bed in low position, side rails up
		
		• Discourage use of restraints; explore other alternatives (sitter, family, or friends)

		RATIONALE: *Protection and prevention of agitation and further confusion lessen risk of injury.*

NURSING DIAGNOSES	OUTCOME CRITERIA	INTERVENTIONS
3 Feeding, Bathing/Hygiene Self-Care Deficit *r.t. cognitive impairment, altered state of wellness*	• Participates in self-care activities at expected optimal level	• Provide a consistent time for self-care routines • Avoid distractions during performance of ADL • Assist with those ADL patient cannot perform • Encourage participation to the extent possible • Supervise ADL until they can be safely performed unassisted
		RATIONALE: *Reorientation is promoted by involvement in purposeful activity.*
4 Sleep Pattern Disturbance *r.t. age-related changes, environmental changes (hospitalization), pathophysiological disturbances*	• Sleeps uninterrupted for up to 6 h	• Monitor daytime activities; discourage excessive daytime napping • Assess usual bedtime routine, time, hygiene practices, rituals • Reduce environmental distractions at night (i.e., noise or light) • Organize care to provide fewest disturbances during sleep • Evaluate medication regimen for medications that may interfere with sleep and mentation
		RATIONALE: *These measures promote normal sleep-wake cycle, eliminates barriers to sleep/rest.*
5 Impaired Social Interaction *r.t. cognitive impairment, impaired communication*	• Engages in meaningful social interaction	• Provide an individual, supportive relationship - call patient by name - introduce self - establish climate of mutual respect, trust
	• Demonstrates an improved ability to communicate	• Encourage visits by family, friends • Provide nonrushed environment - use normal loudness - encourage patient to take time talking and enunciating words

NURSING DIAGNOSES	OUTCOME CRITERIA	INTERVENTIONS
		• Teach techniques to significant others and need for repetitive approaches
		RATIONALE: *Supporting relationships decrease isolation and improve orientation.*
6 High Risk for Violence (directed at others) *r.t. cognitive impairment, decreased impulse control*	• Experiences control of behavior	• Use touch with caution • Control sensory overload; decrease stimulation • Make environmental changes slowly • Make requests simple, nondemanding • Use restraints only when necessary to prevent injury to self/others
		RATIONALE: *Rapid environmental changes or excessive stimuli can provoke violent outbursts.*
7 Knowledge Deficit *r.t. home care plan*	• Patient/family verbalize understanding of patient's illness and coping strategies • Patient/family or caregiver verbalize understanding of medication regime	• Review s/s of recurrent illness that indicate impending maladjustment
	• Patient/family verbalize understanding of s/s to report to physician	• Discuss concerns about returning to community and elicit family reaction to individual's discharge • Refer to other professionals or social agencies
		RATIONALE: *Knowledgeable, competent caregivers are likely to succeed with healthcare regimen.*

GENERAL

> **OTHER LESS COMMON NURSING DIAGNOSES:** *Sensory/Perceptual Alterations; Relocation Stress Syndrome; Self-Esteem Disturbance; Ineffective Individual Coping; Social Isolation*

ESSENTIAL DISCHARGE CRITERIA

- Experiences diagnosis and treatment of cognitive impairment

- Is free of injuries

- Has attained optimal level of cognitive functioning as evidenced by control of behavior, improved ability to communicate, and participation in self-care activities at expected level

NURSING DIAGNOSES	OUTCOME CRITERIA	INTERVENTIONS
1 Chronic Pain *r.t. terminal disease process*	• Manifests reduced or minimal pain	• Assess for verbal and nonverbal indices of pain: crying, moaning, guarding, muscle tension, restlessness, alterations in VS, BP
	• Reports/displays comfort following analgesia	• Administer narcotic and NSAID analgesics and adjuncts *regularly*; monitor response
	• Patient/family identify medication or activity that reduces or aggravates discomfort	• Position for comfort • Provide music therapy, imagery, counterstimulations, or touch • Encourage family participation in the elimination of pain; keep trying to relieve pain • Consult with physician to achieve optimal pain relief
		RATIONALE: *Freedom from pain is a human right of dying patients, even if the effective dose of analgesic hastens death. Nonpharmacologic interventions are effective as adjuncts to pharmacologic ones, but not alone.*
2 Spiritual Distress *r.t. unresolved feelings about death*	• Expresses acceptance of death; discusses death without severe anxiety	• Assess symptoms of spiritual distress: struggling with meaning, depression • Be open, present, and empathetic to feelings about death, using touch and therapeutic use of self • Be there for patient/family during pain, suffering, and death • Assure patient/family of nurse's presence during these times • Support patient's beliefs of afterlife/diety • Prepare patient for religious and cultural rituals of choice • Facilitate personal reflection, meditation, prayer • Assist patient to find ways to express and relieve anger • Offer to pray with patient

GENERAL

NURSING DIAGNOSES	OUTCOME CRITERIA	INTERVENTIONS
		• Refer to clergy as indicated
		RATIONALE: *Interventions that enhance clarification of and contact with patient's religion or culture help alleviate feelings of isolation, separation, and spiritual distress. Anger is an important part of grieving that must be relieved.*
3 Body Image Disturbance *r.t. weight loss or gain, facial edema, hirsutism or loss of hair, mutilating surgery*	• Develops a realistic, accepting and positive self-concept of body image	• Provide information about affected body parts • Suggest ways and support efforts to improve body image, such as grooming and posture • Encourage and facilitate use of support, cosmetic, and rehabilitative services prescribed by the physician
		RATIONALE: *Everyone needs to identify and integrate feelings about changes in body structure and/or function.*
4 Constipation *r.t. decreased activity, decreased food and fluid intake, narcotic intake*	• Demonstrates no abdominal discomfort or bloated feelings; has bowel movements on consistent basis	• Assess bowels status in regard to activity level, nutrition, and medications • Institute daily bowel regimen using patient preference for natural laxatives, fruit, and fiber if possible • Administer enema as necessary • Check for impaction and disimpact as ordered, if attempts fail • Increase stool softeners and laxative doses as narcotic dosages increase • Encourage fluids as tolerated
		RATIONALE: *Reduced activity, dietary intake, and some medications have a constipating effect. Natural laxatives, fruit and fiber, fluids, and a scheduled elimination routine will enhance regular bowel movements.*

NURSING DIAGNOSES	OUTCOME CRITERIA	INTERVENTIONS
5 Ineffective Airway Clearance *r.t. inability to eliminate secretions, semicomatose/comatose state*	• Maintains patent airway	• Auscultate lungs for rhonchi, crackles, wheezes
	• Shows no s/s of dehydration - maintains balanced I&O	• Assess hydration status: skin turgor, mucous membranes, I&O • Assist with suctioning, oral hygiene as needed • Administer corticosteroids and anti-infective agents as ordered
		RATIONALE: *Respiratory status is assessed to determine extent of airway obstruction. Monitoring hydration status helps determine need for fluids. Medications and suctioning decrease the production and facilitate removal of secretions, promoting comfort and ease of breathing.*
6 Ineffective Family Coping: Compromised *r.t. family disorganization and role changes, imminent death of loved one*	• Family member(s) develop sufficient understanding of death/dying process	• Evaluate the family system: identify the members and their relationships; assess family equilibrium, their degree of openness, and their coping capacity • Provide adequate and correct information to family • Discuss loss of significant other with family • Encourage realistic perception based on accurate information • Discuss grieving process and usual reactions to death/dying
	• Demonstrate decreased levels of anxiety	• Maintain patient/family privacy; provide alternative to patient's room for family discussions • Encourage family members to verbalize feelings of guilt, loss, anger, and relief • Acknowledge acceptance of feelings
	• Begin to verbalize concerns about changes in family structure	• Assist family to identify changes in relationships needed to maintain family integrity

GENERAL

NURSING DIAGNOSES	OUTCOME CRITERIA	INTERVENTIONS

- Involve family members in care of patient as much as possible; reassure family that they are doing a good job and that their feelings are okay

- Encourage family members to seek support of others: friends, clergy, other health professionals

- Consult with mental health specialist as indicated

RATIONALE: *Interventions will vary according to the needs of the family. Providing accurate information about patient status in relation to the dying process will assist the family to cope with grief and changing family roles.*

OTHER LESS COMMON NURSING DIAGNOSES: *Altered Nutrition: Less than body requirements; Impaired Physical Mobility; Fluid Volume Deficit/Excess; Sleep Pattern Disturbance; Hopelessness; Powerlessness; Knowledge Deficit; Social Isolation; Anticipatory Grieving*

ESSENTIAL DISCHARGE CRITERIA

- Experiences a peaceful, comfortable death

- Family member(s) grieve appropriately in response to patient's death and begin to cope with resulting changes

EDUCATION FOR DISCHARGE

NURSING DIAGNOSES	OUTCOME CRITERIA	INTERVENTIONS
1 Knowledge Deficit (relevant healthcare needs) *r.t. lack of recall, cognitive limitation, impaired communication, illiteracy, lack of exposure, withdrawal, depression*	• Verbalizes understanding of instructions	• Describe how to use new skills, behaviors in daily living • Use open-ended questions to derive information regarding learning • Simplify information to meet the patient's/family's level of understanding or developmental age
	• Demonstrates appropriate decision-making	• Discuss healthcare needs and methods to achieve success • Teach use of cues to remember health actions • Assess knowledge deficit at every interaction • Consult as needed to develop appropriate teaching plan for patient/family with neurologic learning deficits
	• Assumes responsibility for own learning	• Contact patient/family to provide support; evaluate learning
	• Participates in care activities	• Establish an environment that enables patient/family to gain control • Build on patient's developmental and learning level; consult with expert as indicated
	• Possesses phone numbers for emergency medical help	• Provide opportunities for patient/family to be actively involved in learning • Assess satisfaction with education plan • Provide written materials to reinforce teaching
		RATIONALE: *Learning activities that are geared to the patient's/family's level of prior experience, knowledge, and developmental level are likely to produce positive cognitive behavior changes that are relevant to healthcare needs. Repetition, participation, and graphic/written cues and lists foster learning and recall.*

NURSING DIAGNOSES	OUTCOME CRITERIA	INTERVENTIONS
2 Knowledge Deficit (specific knowledge, skills, behaviors) *r.t. lack of future orientation, impaired communication, anger, insufficient maturation to comprehend, refusal to listen*	• Demonstrates skills, behaviors correctly	• Provide information at level of learner's understanding • Utilize self-care protocols and/or instructional packets (as available)
	• Demonstrates ability to perform care	• Set clear learning goals • Utilize motivational techniques to assist patient/family to self-identify necessity of skill
	• Asks questions; seeks clarification	• Provide opportunity to review process or concepts related to skills, behaviors • Discuss realistic expectations to assist in guiding learning
	• Makes realistic statements about expected course, recovery, prognosis	• Offer peer support network or opportunity to observe others successfully mastering care skills and symptom control • Facilitate sense of mastery of skills, behaviors, attitudes
		RATIONALE: *Mutual goal-setting, positive feedback, and return demonstrations motivate the learner to gain desired competencies. The support of significant others also fosters motivation.*
3 Knowledge Deficit (medications) *r.t. lack of exposure, irrational beliefs, need to make sense of life-threatening disease, inability to recall*	• Acquires knowledge of medication administration - lists medications - discusses dosages, effects, side effects	• Provide opportunity to gain sense of control - provide instruction in several modalities • Anticipate and provide assists when sensory or psychomotor limitations are present
	• Verbalizes knowledge of complications	• Provide written and/or audiovisual materials to enable review by patient/family as needed
	• Lists reportable s/s	• Assess patient's/family's acceptance of diagnosis • If available, help patient/family to learn computerized monitoring systems, e.g., OneTouch, Accucheck

NURSING DIAGNOSES	OUTCOME CRITERIA	INTERVENTIONS
		• Discuss sign of decrease in symptoms and/or improvement in health state
	• Discusses rationale for treatment	• Use patient's/family's ideas about illness as a starting point for education and/or training
		RATIONALE: *Use of various teaching-learning modalities that stimulate cognitive, affective, and motor abilities reinforces new and accurate information. Clear, specific information, accompanied by cues and lists, fosters recall of important information.*
4 Knowledge Deficit (diet) *r.t. lack of interest in learning, lack of belief in efficacy of treatment, decreased motivation to learn, misinterpretation of information*	• Demonstrates prescribed diet planning - selects indicated foods from list - recognizes contraindicated foods	• Describe problem-solving process to assist patient/family to integrate diet plan • Discuss with other healthcare providers the need to actively involve patient/family in decision-making • Establish an environment conducive to learning - free of distraction - with visual aids and diet lists • Teach how to provide rewards for maintenance of positive health behaviors
	• Verbalizes knowledge of follow-up appointments	• Reinforce utilization of information gained - include support persons in integration of information • Teach patient/family how to find, use, and evaluate community resources - education - support - treatment

GENERAL

21

NURSING DIAGNOSES	OUTCOME CRITERIA	INTERVENTIONS
	• Copes adequately	• Discuss plans for patient/family to include health behaviors identified as valuable to self • Set clear, mutually agreed-upon learning goals • Be accessible to patient/family to reinforce teaching
		RATIONALE: *Involvement in anticipatory problem-solving and planning raises likelihood of effective problem-solving after discharge. Discussion by patient and family of coping strengths and healthcare goals raises the likelihood of a continuation of this kind of support network. Discussion and support foster effective behavior changes.*
5 Knowledge Deficit (equipment) *r.t. excessive anxiety, need to follow new and/or complex treatment, unfamiliarity with information*	• Demonstrates competence in equipment use	• Teach how to mentally and physically rehearse skill • Describe how mastery meets patient's/family's own standard for adequate coping
	• Possesses phone numbers for equipment and supplies	• Demonstrate to patient/family how to use equipment and obtain services • Discuss where to access supplies and/or equipment; provide written information
	• Demonstrates required skills related to supplies required	• Assist with practice of skill until performance shows mastery and confidence
	• Verbalizes understanding of instructions	• Check with patient/family often during teaching to elicit and evaluate understanding
		RATIONALE: *Demonstration and return demonstration with positive, supportive feedback enhance motor skill mastery.*

> *OTHER LESS COMMON NURSING DIAGNOSES:* Anxiety; Ineffective Individual Coping; Noncompliance; Social Isolation; Self-Esteem Disturbance

ESSENTIAL DISCHARGE CRITERIA

- Patient/family verbalize and/or demonstrate specific knowledge, behavior, skills relevant to condition

- Demonstrates knowledge relevant to condition: pathophysiology, prognosis, expected course of recovery

- Verbalizes, discusses specific knowledge relevant to healthcare needs: treatment plans and their rationale; potential complications and s/s to report

- Demonstrates competence in use of required equipment, assistive devices

- Verbalizes/demonstrates safe and effective use of prescribed medications

- Identifies potential drug or food interactions to be avoided

- Verbalizes realistic plans to integrate required dietary modifications into normal family diet

- Possesses follow-up appointments for required treatments and healthcare supervision

GENERAL

GERIATRIC PATIENT, HOSPITALIZED

NURSING DIAGNOSES	OUTCOME CRITERIA	INTERVENTIONS
1 Altered Thought Processes *r.t. maturational dementia*	• Has basic physical needs met	• Assess physical needs, i.e., elimination q2h
	• Is free from injury/harm	• Orient to person, time, place as necessary • Maintain a safe, accepting environment
	• Participates in decision-making to maximum ability • Communicates effectively	• Include in all decision-making activities as appropriate
		RATIONALE: *Altered thought processes may create unmet needs due to inability to adequately express oneself. The risk of harm or injury is also increased. Altered thought processes do not diminish the need to be treated as an adult at all times.*
2 Relocation Stress Syndrome *r.t. change in environment, impaired psychosocial health status*	• Freely expresses feelings of concern, anxiety, and anger	• Encourage to express feelings about changes in the environment
	• Participates to the fullest extent possible in decision-making related to the new environment	• Include in all decision-making activities as appropriate
	• Exhibits positive adaptation to the new environment	• Eliminate environmental changes or keep to a minimum • Orient to surroundings in a calm, nonthreatening manner, repeat as necessary • Allow, within space and regulation limits, for familiar items from home to be brought into the environment
		RATIONALE: *Orientation to new surroundings helps to decrease anxiety and the feelings of loss of control. Including the individual, as much as possible, in decision-making helps to reduce anxiety. Familiar items can be brought into the new environment to assist in reduction of anxiety and allow the person to feel more in control.*

NURSING DIAGNOSES	OUTCOME CRITERIA	INTERVENTIONS
3 Altered Nutrition: Less than body requirements *r.t. edentulous, financial limitations, social alteration*	• Maintains oral intake adequate to meet daily nutritional requirements	• Provide for the appropriate consistency of food, i.e., regular, soft • Allow adequate time for food intake; provide for snacks/supplements as necessary • Initiate appropriate referrals as necessary, i.e., social services, dentist, nutritionist
		RATIONALE: *Providing for the proper consistency of food allows the person with chewing difficulties to eat more easily. Elderly individuals often need a longer time period to eat, and many are accustomed to eating smaller portions. Referrals may be appropriate if the person has chewing difficulty and/or may have difficulty in buying or cooking meals when discharged.*
4 Impaired Physical Mobility *r.t. decreased activity tolerance, pain, musculoskeletal/ neuromuscular impairment*	• Reports an increase in activity tolerance • Uses assistive devices, as appropriate, to aid in physical mobility	• Encourage and assist in physical activities
	• Describes safety measures that minimize injury potential	• Teach safety procedures when involved in any physical activity • Reinforce safety procedures during each physical activity
	• Verbalizes/displays freedom from pain	• Give pain medication as ordered
	• Demonstrates safe use of assistive devices	• Refer to appropriate health professionals, i.e., physical therapy, occupational therapy
		RATIONALE: *Physical mobility is essential for the person's physical, mental, and emotional well-being. Adaptive devices can increase mobility while helping to reduce physical discomfort.*

GENERAL

NURSING DIAGNOSES	OUTCOME CRITERIA	INTERVENTIONS
5 Sleep Pattern Disturbance *r.t. age-related changes, boredom, inactivity, impaired elimination*	• Reports feeling adequately rested • Exhibits signs of having adequate rest	• Monitor and manage rest/sleep regimen - assess normal rest patterns - provide, as possible, a relaxing environment - encourage stimulating activities when awake - provide for elimination needs - offer relaxation therapies to assist in obtaining rest, i.e., back rubs
		RATIONALE: *The elderly person may have a different pattern of rest than many other patients. A person who is not stimulated when awake may nap frequently, thus making it difficult to obtain adequate sleep for feeling rested.*
6 Social Isolation *r.t. alteration in physical appearance, state of wellness, death/disability of peers*	• Participates in activities	• Assess past patterns of social interaction
	• Expresses self about current social circumstances	• Provide, as needed, adaptive devices, i.e., incontinence briefs
	• Identifies appropriate future activities	• Discuss strategies for decreasing future social isolation • Refer, as necessary, to appropriate health professionals
		RATIONALE: *Knowing a person's past social interaction status is necessary before suggesting new activities. An elderly person who has a life-long history of little interaction is not likely to respond well to many new group activities. Some individuals may not be participating in activities because of some physical condition such as incontinence. Providing adaptive devices may assist that person in becoming more active. Providing information about available community resources may also help in reducing isolation.*

NURSING DIAGNOSES	OUTCOME CRITERIA	INTERVENTIONS
7 Spiritual Distress *r.t. separation from religious/cultural ties, loss of sense of life's meaning*	• Affirms satisfaction of spiritual/cultural needs	• Assess spiritual/cultural needs • Make provision for meeting any special spiritual/cultural needs • Take time to listen to expressions of loneliness and spiritual distress • Provide time for personal reflection, prayer, etc., as indicated • Assist with value clarification • Assure patient that nurse will be available in times of suffering • Be present and open to patient's feelings of guilt, isolation, fear of death • Consult with clergy

RATIONALE: *An individual may want to have spiritual/cultural needs met in a specific way. Provision for an individual's special needs should be provided as much as possible, i.e., privacy, religious personnel, native healers.*

OTHER LESS COMMON NURSING DIAGNOSES: Altered Urinary Elimination; Powerlessness; Self-Care Deficit; Constipation; High Risk for Disuse Syndrome; Self-Esteem Disturbance

---

ESSENTIAL DISCHARGE CRITERIA

- Is able to have basic needs met
- Is aware of community resources to meet physical, emotional, and mental needs
- Adjusts to new environment without complications
- Verbalizes knowledge of safety measures to reduce risk of accidental injury

- Is adequately rested
- Achieves optimal level of mobility, using assistive devices as needed
- Experiences sense of meaning and purpose in life, illness, and suffering

GENERAL

IMMOBILITY

NURSING DIAGNOSES	OUTCOME CRITERIA	INTERVENTIONS
1 **High Risk for Impaired Skin Integrity** *r.t. musculoskeletal inactivity*	• Skin remains intact and free of pressure ulcers	• Assist with repositioning q30 min to 2 h or instruct person to turn/reposition self at this frequency • When turning patient to side, use a pillow, foam, or blanket to pad between bony prominences (e.g., between knees) • Use pillows, foam, or suspension to elevate heels off of bed; make sure support is beneath calf, not heel or Achilles tendon • Limit Fowler's position if sacrum is at risk • Use elbow and heel protectors to prevent friction over these areas • When assisting person to move up in bed, have patient lift or have personnel assist with lifting in order to prevent shearing with movement • If possible, leave bed flat to prevent sliding down in bed and shearing • If in traction, make sure there is sufficient countertraction to keep patient from sliding down in bed • Encourage ROM to promote blood flow • Inspect skin q8h for blanching, redness, or breakdown • Palpate high risk areas for warmth or bogginess; high risk areas include occiput, heels, sacrum, elbows, ischia, scrotum, and scapulae • Instruct patient to report burning sensation and/or pain of high risk areas

RATIONALE: *Unrelieved pressure, shearing, and friction contribute to development of skin breakdown in persons who are immobile.*

NURSING DIAGNOSES	OUTCOME CRITERIA	INTERVENTIONS
2 **Ineffective Airway Clearance** *r.t. musculoskeletal inactivity*	• Shows no s/s of atelectasis/pneumonia - VS and temperature WNL - lungs clear to auscultation - respirations even and unlabored (rate of 12-20 breaths/min for adult) - SaO_2 WNL	• Monitor respiratory parameters q4h • Encourage activity as consistent with medical plan of care • Assist with repositioning or encourage patient to change position if able, so that patient turns side to side q1-2h • Encourage/assist patient with deep breathing and coughing exercises 5 times every hour
	• Performs use of incentive spirometer, coughing, and deep breathing exercises	• Auscultate lung fields q8h, more frequently if alteration noted • Encourage/assist patient to use incentive spirometer or blow bottle hourly while awake
		RATIONALE: *Bed rest, i.e., lying flat, causes a shift of abdominal organs toward the chest, which makes it more difficult to fully expand the lungs with inspiration. Decreasing the demands of physical activity may decrease the body's O_2 demands temporarily and result in more shallow respirations. Immobility may lead to pooling of pulmonary secretions. Because these three factors contribute to the development of atelectasis/pneumonia, interventions are designed to help mobilize secretions and encourage lung expansion.*
3 **Colonic Constipation** *r.t. effects of immobility on peristalsis*	• Maintains usual pattern of bowel elimination	• Teach which foods are high in bulk (fresh unpeeled fruits, bran, nuts, whole grain bread and cereal, fruit juices, vegetables) • Encourage intake of 2 L (8-10 glasses) of fluid per day unless contraindicated • Determine patient's usual elimination routine and help to re-establish pattern • Assist to identify effective stimulus for bowel movement, such as coffee, prune juice, post-meal peristalsis • Provide for privacy during elimination

GENERAL

NURSING DIAGNOSES	OUTCOME CRITERIA	INTERVENTIONS
		• If possible, assist to bedside commode or bathroom rather than using a bedpan
		• Encourage increased activity if medical condition allows
		RATIONALE: *Decreased peristalsis, fluid intake, inactivity, and psychosocial factors can all contribute to the development of constipation.*
4 High Risk for Activity Intolerance *r.t. bed rest deconditioning*	• Demonstrates strength and energy sufficient to participate in necessary or desired activities	• Assess adequacy of nutritional intake; contact dietitian if inadequate intake noted or suspected
		• Encourage active, passive ROM
		• Position in correct anatomical alignment
		• Coordinate physical therapy consult for individualized strengthening exercise regimen
		• Assist with prescribed activity progression; monitor response
		RATIONALE: *With immobility, muscle strength decreases about 3 percent per day, and without ROM, joint contractures can develop within 3 days.*

OTHER LESS COMMON NURSING DIAGNOSES: *Altered Tissue Perfusion; High Risk for Infection; High Risk for Injury; Sensory/Perceptual Alterations; Powerlessness*

ESSENTIAL DISCHARGE CRITERIA

• Shows temperature and VS WNL

• Maintains usual pattern of bowel elimination

• Shows sufficient strength and energy to participate in ADL as needed or provisions for assistance arranged

• Skin is intact or arrangements for wound management are made

PAIN MANAGEMENT

NURSING DIAGNOSES	OUTCOME CRITERIA	INTERVENTIONS
1 Pain (acute) *r.t. injury, illness, surgery, unknown cause*	• Verbalizes/displays sustained freedom from pain	• Obtain history of onset of pain and characteristics of pain • Validate patient's pain experience • Recognize cultural and psychological components of pain • Assess pain regularly - use self-rating scale (scale of 0-10), if possible • Recognize age-related differences in pain expression between younger, old, and older people • Use relaxation techniques, music therapy, imagery, TENS to help reduce pain • Position for comfort
	• Reports comfort following analgesia	• Administer analgesics (narcotic and non-narcotic) regularly to prevent pain, as well as antidepressants that may be used for specific types of pain • Base dosages and schedules on individual responses rather than assumptions of expected pain control • Use equianalgesic conversion scale when changing one drug/route to another • Consult with physician regarding route, such as epidural, intrathecal, dermal
	• Identifies medication or activity that reduces or aggravates discomfort	• Encourage patient to participate in pain management

GENERAL

RATIONALE: *Pain is an individual experience. A trusting relationship between nurse and patient increases success of pain control. Nonverbal patients and the elderly are often under-treated because of differing ways of communicating pain. Some patients benefit from a regular dosing schedule rather than prn, and others need higher doses based on individual pain thresholds.*

NURSING DIAGNOSES	OUTCOME CRITERIA	INTERVENTIONS
2 Activity Intolerance *r.t. pain*	• Participates in ADL; initiates strategies for increasing activity	• Assess current activity status and desired activity level • Include patient in planning schedule of activities (include rest periods and premedication before painful activities) • Encourage to increase activity as tolerated • Instruct to use distraction to help increase activity tolerance • Teach family about medication scheduling and importance of premedicating prior to painful activities
		RATIONALE: *Learning about pain helps the patient set realistic expectations. Both behavioral and pharmacological measures combine to increase the patient's activity level.*
3 Sleep Pattern Disturbance *r.t. pain*	• Reports/displays sense of feeling rested 　- relaxed body posture, facial expressions 　- sleeps, naps at near-normal intervals 　- willingly participates in care activities	• Assess patient's sleep and rest patterns • Assess effectiveness of pain control measures • Schedule control measures to cause little disruption of sleep and rest (continuous narcotic infusion during the night) • Instruct patient/family of importance of consistency in medication schedule • Encourage rest in between activities; identify other rest strategies per patient preference
		RATIONALE: *Sleep/rest affects pain tolerance and ability to function normally.*

NURSING DIAGNOSES	OUTCOME CRITERIA	INTERVENTIONS
4 Knowledge Deficit *r.t. pain and medication administration*	• Discusses physiology of disease process/pain; rationale for treatment	• Foster the patient's understanding of his own pain and its management • Describe different types of pain, along with behavioral and pharmacological interventions for that type of pain
	• Patient/family express concerns, questions	• Give appropriate written materials such as ACS/NCI booklet on pain questions; review as needed
	• Patient/family verbalize knowledge of pain medications: dosages, effects, side effects	• Encourage decision-making process regarding dosing schedule, including their side effects which may affect dosing schedule • Encourage patient to verbalize understanding of pain and medications • Explore cultural and personal feelings about pain, medications, fear of addiction, fear of narcotics
	• Patient/family participate in care activities	• Explain pain principles to patient/family • Encourage use of individually preferred pain control measures • Remind to use nonpharmacologic interventions, such as distraction, relaxation, heat/cold

RATIONALE: *Since there are many myths about pain, it is important to provide valid information that puts the patient in control of his pain.*

GENERAL

OTHER LESS COMMON NURSING DIAGNOSES: *Anxiety; Ineffective Individual Coping; Noncompliance; Powerlessness; Sexual Dysfunction; Spiritual Distress*

ESSENTIAL DISCHARGE CRITERIA

- Reports, displays sustained comfort
- Identifies side effects of pain medications
- Describes interventions that reduce pain

- Performs ADL independently
- Experiences satisfactory sleep patterns
- Participates in self-care

PARENTERAL NUTRITION, TOTAL (HYPERALIMENTATION)

NURSING DIAGNOSES	OUTCOME CRITERIA	INTERVENTIONS
1 Altered Nutrition: Less than body requirements *r.t. inability to ingest and absorb nutrients via GI tract*	• Achieves/maintains adequate nutritional status - balanced I&O	• Assess status • Monitor I&O closely • Administer parenteral nutrition as ordered
	• Shows normal serum electrolytes, glucose levels	• Monitor lab studies • Monitor for hyper/hypoglycemia
	• Maintains recommended body weight	• Weigh daily
		RATIONALE: *The human body requires enough protein for tissue repair and growth, enough calories in the form of carbohydrates and fats for energy, and enough vitamins, minerals, electrolytes, and trace elements for normal body functions.*
2 High Risk for Injury (internal) *r.t. infusion of total parenteral nutrition via central line (i.e., air embolism, glucose imbalance, impaired catheter integrity)*	• Maintains serum glucose and electrolytes WNL	• Monitor electrolytes and finger stick glucose q4-6h during therapy

	• Is free of complications associated with parenteral nutrition
	  - no chest pain, SOB
	  - no s/s of hyperglycemia
	  - no s/s of hypoglycemia
		• Monitor VS q8h
		• Monitor for signs of hyperglycemia (polyuria, headache, thirst, nausea, weakness)
		• Monitor for signs of hypoglycemia (blurred vision, pallor, palpitations, hunger, headache, shakiness)
		• Assess catheter insertion site and length of external catheter q4h and prn for kinks, twisting, tension to maintain patency
		• Administer insulin as ordered
		• Tape all catheter connections securely to avoid disconnections
		• To discontinue therapy, taper down rate and concentration to prevent hypoglycemia

		RATIONALE: *Initial TPN therapy, changes in solution, coupled with inaccurate doses of insulin may lead to hypo/hyperglycemia. Inadvertent catheter/IV tubing absence may result in air embolism. Kinking, twisting, inordinate amounts of tension may cause damage or movement of catheter leading to disruption of infusion.*

GENERAL

> **OTHER LESS COMMON NURSING DIAGNOSES:** *High Risk for Fluid Volume Deficit;*
> *High Risk for Fluid Volume Excess; Ineffective Management of Therapeutic Regimen;*
> *Altered Health Maintenance; Knowledge Deficit*

ESSENTIAL DISCHARGE CRITERIA

- Maintains goal weight
- Demonstrates appropriate catheter care and administration of parenteral nutrition
- Verbalizes knowledge of s/s of complications and management of TPN within lifestyle

- Verbalizes which s/s to report to healthcare team
- Verbalizes understanding of use of community resources

NURSING DIAGNOSES	OUTCOME CRITERIA	INTERVENTIONS
1 Pain *r.t. tissue trauma, edema, pressure*	• Verbalizes/displays freedom from pain	• Assess pain level q2-4h • Use a flow sheet to monitor and document pain location, type, and intensity • Encourage patient to describe pain and response to interventions on 1-10 scale
	• Reports comfort following analgesia	• Administer prescribed analgesics and assess VS prior to medicine administration • Evaluate and document response to medicine 30-60 min after medication • Instruct patient on the importance of regular pain medication dosing

	• Identifies medication or activity that reduces or aggravates discomfort
	  - identifies source of comfort
	  - alternates periods of activity and rest
		• Medicate prior to activity
		• Determine realistic pain control goals with patient
		• Instruct patient in noninvasive pain relief measures (diversion, relaxation, music, position changes, etc.)
		• Intervene at the onset of pain
		• Instruct patient to move gradually and avoid sudden movements
		• Splint incision with pillow
		• Position for comfort

		RATIONALE: *Pain is a combination of sensory and perceptual components. A preventative approach to pain is to establish a regular schedule for medication administration to treat the pain before it becomes severe.*
2 Impaired Skin Integrity *r.t. surgical intervention*	• Incision clean and dry and wound edges well approximated	• Change position frequently • Maintain sterile technique when caring for wounds • Cover surgical incisions with dressings, ointments, etc. • Provide balanced diet or nutritional supplementation as ordered

GENERAL

NURSING DIAGNOSES	OUTCOME CRITERIA	INTERVENTIONS
		• Monitor wound drainage and lab values for signs of infection
		RATIONALE: *Blocking pressure points and entry of microorganisms prevents further injury. Adequate nutritional status promotes healing.*
3 Ineffective Breathing Pattern *r.t. anesthesia, pain, cognitive/perception impairment*	• Takes at least 12-20 deep, regular respirations per min	• Assess respiratory depth and rate status with vital signs
	• Exhibits improving respiratory status - SaO$_2$ WNL - lungs clear bilaterally	• Auscultate lung fields q8h and prn • Encourage to practice deep breathing and controlled coughing exercises 5 times per h while awake • Instruct patient on use of spirometry q2h while awake • Turn patient frequently • Control pain • Plan rest periods
		RATIONALE: *These measures improve the breathing pattern and ventilation.*
4 High Risk for Fluid Volume Deficit *r.t. hemorrhage*	• Shows normal VS, BP	• Assess VS q30 min for 1 h, qh for 2 h, q4h for 24 h
	• H&H, electrolytes WNL	• Monitor lab values and report to physician prn
	• Shows no signs of bleeding	• Assess wound site/dressing q30-60 min until stable, then q4-8h • Administer blood products as ordered • Initiate emergency hemorrhage procedures per standards of care
		RATIONALE: *Detect and prevent excessive blood loss and minimize complications.*

NURSING DIAGNOSES	OUTCOME CRITERIA	INTERVENTIONS
5 Knowledge Deficit *r.t. incisional care, post-op care at home*	• Demonstrates/verbalizes proper technique for dressing/incisional care	• Review with patient conditions necessitating notification of physician or nurse • Instruct patient/family re: incisional care
	• Verbalizes correct limits on activity, medication schedule, dietary requirements, and follow-up care	• Instruct patient on medicine schedule and side effects • Instruct patient on dietary restrictions or interaction with medications • Provide written instructions on D/C • Instruct re: activity limitations • Review importance of medical follow-up visits • Evaluate need for home healthcare referral • Review community resources available for assistance
		RATIONALE: *Providing pertinent instructions will promote self-care and compliance with the postoperative treatment regimen.*

GENERAL

> **OTHER LESS COMMON NURSING DIAGNOSES:** *Urinary Retention; Impaired Gas Exchange; High Risk for Injury; Ineffective Airway Clearance; Constipation; Altered Nutrition: Less than body requirements; Altered Tissue Perfusion; High Risk for Infection*

ESSENTIAL DISCHARGE CRITERIA

- Is physiologically stable with VS WNL
- Is afebrile
- Has clear lungs bilaterally

- Shows wound free from signs of infection
- Controls pain with use of oral analgesics
- Accurately describes recommended home care, medications, activities, and diet

PRESSURE ULCERS

NURSING DIAGNOSES	OUTCOME CRITERIA	INTERVENTIONS
1 Impaired Skin Integrity *r.t. pressure, friction, shear, maceration*	• Demonstrates progressive healing of wound that is consistent with underlying medical conditions	• Assess risk factors that contribute to formation of pressure ulcer using systematic risk assessment - use Norton scale, Braden scale or other - include other etiologic factors such as diagnoses: DM, CHF, PVD, pulmonary disease - include medications (steroids), age, edema, obesity, history of previous pressure ulcers • Assess mobility/activity; make physical therapy referral
	• Experiences no further skin breakdown	• Inspect skin q shift
	• Shows no evidence of pressure areas	• Identify measures to reduce or relieve pressure - establish a turning schedule; alter position q2h for bedbound and qh or more frequently for chair-fast patient - position patient for comfort and minimal pressure on bony prominences • Avoid massage over bony prominences • Determine need for specialty mattress overlays, replacement mattress, specialty beds, cushions
	• Shows no redness, abrasions	• Identify measures to reduce - friction - shear - maintain HOB below 30° if tolerated - use trapeze; turn sheets to reposition - place blankets or pillows between knees - apply powder/cornstarch lightly on surfaces contacting skin
	• Remains free of skin moisture from urine, stool, perspiration, or wound drainage	• Protect skin from urine, stool, moisture from diaphoresis, or other drainage

NURSING DIAGNOSES	OUTCOME CRITERIA	INTERVENTIONS

	• Shows normal lab values for nitrogen balance	• Assess nutritional needs and hydration
		  - actual weight compared with ideal body weight
		  - lab data such as serum albumin, transferrin, total lymphocyte count, creatinine
		  - assess protein, calorie, and vitamin intake
		• Initiate dietary referral

	• Shows progressive wound healing	• Assess, document progressive wound healing
		  - stage, location, shape, dimensions, depth, edges
		  - presence of undermining, characteristics of necrotic tissue, exudate
		  - skin color surrounding wound
		  - presence of edema in tissue surrounding wound
		  - presence of granulation tissue
		  - epithelialization

	• Shows decreasing wound circumference	• Measure wound and chart size initially and intermittently; photograph wound for patient record and include date
		• Perform prescribed topical therapy appropriate for wound that provides
		  - moist wound healing
		  - insulation and protection
		  - debridement (per orders) of necrotic tissue
		  - removal of excessive or pooled exudate
		• Consult with nurse specialist and physician for treatment of necrotic, infected, or deep stage 3-4 pressure ulcers

GENERAL

NURSING DIAGNOSES	OUTCOME CRITERIA	INTERVENTIONS

RATIONALE: *Pressure reduction devices lower interface pressures as compared with standard hospital mattress or chair. Pressure-relieving devices reduce interface pressures to a level below capillary closing pressures, thus preventing further breakdown of skin and tissue. Current evidence indicates that massage over bony prominences may be harmful. Friction reduction reduces skin shear, decreasing surface cling. Maceration from moisture and/or chemical erosion from urine, stool, or other secretions contribute to skin breakdown. Positive nitrogen balance and tissue hydration are necessary for wound healing. Vitamin C is necessary for tissue healing. Vitamin A, B, zinc, and sulfur are associated with healthy skin. A moist environment enhances cellular repair. Necrotic tissue and excess exudate inhibit wound healing.*

2 High Risk for Infection

r.t. altered integumentary system

OUTCOME CRITERIA	INTERVENTIONS

• Remains free of local and systemic infection
  - afebrile, pulse and BP WNL for patient
  - WBC count and differential remain WNL
	• Assess local s/s of infection, i.e., erythema, induration, purulent drainage, malodorous drainage
	• Assess s/s of systemic infection, i.e., fever, leukocytosis, confusion, increased pulse rate, and hypotension

• Shows negative cultures	• Obtain culture and sensitivity for wounds that show clinical s/s of infection or potential for osteomyelitis
• Patient/family identify risks of poor hand-washing, personal and oral hygiene, contact with contagious diseases, and other factors that increase the risk of infection	• Explain basic transmission of disease, including hand-washing and contact with contagious disease

RATIONALE: *All dermal wounds are contaminated; culture and sensitivity are indicated only for evidence of clinical signs of infection or potential for osteomyelitis. For deep wounds, or wounds with sinus tracts, consider culture for anaerobes.*

NURSING DIAGNOSES	OUTCOME CRITERIA	INTERVENTIONS
3 Knowledge Deficit *r.t. pressure ulcer risk and management program*	• Patient/family discuss pathophysiology of disease process, rationale for treatment	• Explain pathophysiology of ulcers • Instruct regarding the risk factors contributing to pressure ulcers and identify risk factors specific to the patient
	• Patient/family participate in care activities	• Instruct regarding pressure relief/reduction measures and measures to reduce shear, friction, and moisture • Schedule major position changes and minor weight shifts, and stress importance of compliance
	• Patient/family discuss and plan for dietary requirements	• Explain nutritional and fluid support
	• Patient/family demonstrate required care skills	• Explain need for routine skin care at least daily and importance of lubrication • Show how to perform routine skin inspection at least every day; look for signs of impending breakdown and when to call physician or nurse; look for signs of healing • Instruct about local care, dressings, and measures to prevent further trauma
	• Patient/family have list of reportable s/s	• Teach s/s of color changes, temperature, pain, presence of drainage and odor to report to physician
	• Patient/family discuss medications: dosage, effects, side effects	• Teach medication administration

	• Patient/family express commitment to consistent follow-up and medical supervision	• Instruct patient/family regarding the recommended management program; include rationale, use of specific products, potential problems, and plan for follow-up
		• Evaluate patient/family learning
		  - ability to describe risk factors, prevention, and management plan
		  - correct demonstration of care
		  - active participation in the treatment plan

GENERAL

NURSING DIAGNOSES	OUTCOME CRITERIA	INTERVENTIONS
		• Recommend appropriate referral to social service, home health agencies or other agency, and follow-up

RATIONALE: *If patient and caregiver are to be central figures in the management program, it is essential to educate them regarding specific procedures and care, their rationale, and potential problems. It is essential to assess their learning for assurance in continuity of care and discharge planning. Resource and referral needs must be determined, and follow-up is essential.*

OTHER LESS COMMON NURSING DIAGNOSES:
Altered Nutrition: Less than body requirements; Sensory/Perceptual Alterations

---

ESSENTIAL DISCHARGE CRITERIA

• Displays evidence of wound healing consistent with underlying medical conditions

• Is free of symptoms of infection

• Patient/family discuss risk for pressure ulcer and describe the management program accurately

• Patient/family demonstrate correct technique for specific care procedures

NURSING DIAGNOSES	OUTCOME CRITERIA	INTERVENTIONS
1 Impaired Physical Mobility *r.t. imposed restrictions on activity secondary to injury, traction*	• Is free from multi-system problems - constipation - pneumonia - skin breakdown - thrombus - contracture - urinary retention, calculi - altered nitrogen balance	• Initiate standard nursing measures to monitor and maintain multi-system integrity during long periods of immobility
		RATIONALE: *Prolonged immobility negatively impacts all body systems as well as nutrition and nitrogen balance, which compound the original problem.*
2 Pain *r.t. injury, traction, and inability to reposition at will*	• Verbalizes, displays freedom from pain - identifies source of discomfort - reports relief from pain	• Assess location, type, and intensity of pain • Determine whether pain is similar to previous episodes or different in some way • Inspect traction apparatus for possible misalignment, weights against bed or floor, or movement of patient toward foot of bed; readjust as necessary without disrupting continuity of weights
	• Identifies medication or activity that reduces/aggravates discomfort	• Medicate at first indication of pain increasing past 5 (on a scale of 0-10) and evaluate • Report sudden increases in pain or changes in location, type, or intensity
	• Participates in care activities and mobility exercises without undue resistance	• Allow as much movement as possible and tolerable depending on type of traction • Provide active and passive ROM to unaffected joints • Provide back rubs and maintain clean, dry linen
	• Alternates periods of activity and rest	• Offer diversional activities and visitors as tolerated

GENERAL

NURSING DIAGNOSES	OUTCOME CRITERIA	INTERVENTIONS

RATIONALE: *Pain subsides once traction begins to reduce muscle spasms and realigns bone. Sudden increases in pain or change in location, type, or intensity requires careful evaluation for complications.*

---

3 Toileting, Bathing/Hygiene Self-Care Deficit

r.t. impaired physical mobility

	• Makes decisions related to timing of self-care activities	• Assess ability to participate in care
		• Identify pre-injury patterns and capabilities regarding hygiene, dressing, nutrition, and toileting
		• Identify movements and tasks that are appropriate for type of traction
		• Inspect skin areas that patient cannot see
	• Participates in self-care activities within limitations of injury and traction	• Allow for patient participation in decisions regarding hygiene, dressing, feeding, and toileting
		• Encourage patient participation in providing own care within limitations
		• Assist in care that patient is unable to provide for self
		• Alter types of food to include finger foods as tolerated; provide straws, water within reach, if possible, and nutritional snacks as indicated
		• Allow time and privacy for toileting needs; offer bedpan at regular intervals
		• Answer call light promptly

RATIONALE: *Participation and involvement allow the patient to remain in control of personal care.*

NURSING DIAGNOSES	OUTCOME CRITERIA	INTERVENTIONS
4 High Risk for Injury *r.t. peripheral neurovascular dysfunction (mechanical compression secondary to musculoskeletal injury and traction)*	• Experiences early detection, prompt management of complications	• Monitor for pain of unusual or increasing intensity or pain not controlled with narcotics • Report any compromise of CMS to physician immediately and document
	• Maintains CMS WNL for individual	• Assess CMS in affected limb as frequently as indicated by severity of injury • Monitor traction apparatus, splints, skin traction, and body alignment for potential to impair circulation or compress nerves • Encourage active extension of fingers or toes of affected limb to indicate increasing impairment • Provide adequate nourishment and fluids to promote adequate circulation • Use aseptic technique to clean pin sites to prevent infection and neurovascular damage
		RATIONALE: *Accurate monitoring and aggressive management of neurovascular problems will minimize complications and allow for uneventful recovery.*
5 High Risk for Disuse Syndrome *r.t. mechanical immobility*	• Maintains functional movement of joints within individual limitations	• Monitor musculoskeletal integrity and loss of muscle tone • Promote and encourage activity as tolerated and indicated by type of traction • Perform passive ROM • Maintain correct body alignment to parts in traction as well as uninjured areas
	• Describes, complies with interventions to prevent complications	• Teach patient/family about the limitations and the appropriate movements allowed in traction; encourage them to assist in those care activities

GENERAL

NURSING DIAGNOSES	OUTCOME CRITERIA	INTERVENTIONS
		• Allow time for patient/family to express feelings and to propose ideas about maximizing normal function

RATIONALE: *These measures help to prevent further musculoskeletal injury, promote activity, and prevent loss of muscle tone which enhance a return to normal once the bone has healed.*

6 Powerlessness

r.t. forced immobility imposed by treatment regimen secondary to injury and traction

- Identifies and expresses feelings of powerlessness
  - identifies those factors that he/she does/can control
  - asks questions regarding injury and treatment
  - acknowledges a future without forced immobility

- Assess family and other support systems and encourage their participation in care and diversional activities
- Observe for sense of powerlessness: depression, lethargy, statements about "no control, no future, helplessness"
- Assist to identify achievable goals to minimize powerlessness
- Establish therapeutic relationship to allow expression of feelings and mutual efforts to manipulate environment
- Praise accomplishments and increased control over own situation
- Provide diversional activities and equipment/materials (writing materials, supports for reading, prism glasses for TV viewing, items from home within visual field)
- Allow patient to control visual and auditory stimuli; be aware of threat of sensory overload as well as deprivation

RATIONALE: *These measures promote psychosocial integrity by increasing the patient's control of the situation.*

OTHER LESS COMMON NURSING DIAGNOSES: *Situational Low Self-Esteem;*
Altered Role Performance; Diversional Activity Deficit; Impaired Skin Integrity;
Altered Tissue Perfusion; Impaired Gas Exchange

ESSENTIAL DISCHARGE CRITERIA

- Experiences complete union of bone fracture or has had surgical stabilization of fracture

- Manages self-care within imposed mobility restrictions or has adequate support system for assistance

- Achieves acceptable pain control with oral analgesics

- Is free from injury and multi-system problems

- Verbalizes accurate understanding of need for continued medical supervision and home care of injured area

URINARY ELIMINATION, ALTERED

NURSING DIAGNOSES	OUTCOME CRITERIA	INTERVENTIONS
1 Urinary Retention *r.t. obstruction or detrusor muscle dysfunction*	• Urinary retention is relieved - frequency, nocturia absent - overflow incontinence absent - postvoiding residuals are < 20 percent of total bladder volume	• Assess voiding patterns and stream • Determine feeling of incomplete emptying • Determine measures patient uses, if any, to assist voiding • Assist with voiding q3-4h • Encourage patient to remain on toilet for 5 min after voiding and to try again • Teach Credé's maneuver to assist with voiding • Consult with physician concerning drugs to stimulate detrusor contraction or to decrease sphincter resistance
	• Exhibits no s/s of UTI	• Assess for presence of UTI • Teach importance of complete bladder emptying regularly • Determine effectiveness of current antibiotics, if any • Consult with physician concerning long-term antibiotic therapy or surgical intervention

RATIONALE: *Acute urinary retention must be relieved to reduce pain and pressure. Timed voiding and voiding reattempts maximize patient's ability to empty bladder and prevent chronic over distention. Medications can modify inadequate detrusor function or outlet obstruction. Chronic retention and urinary stasis or use of catheters may need to be treated with antibiotics to minimize bacteriuria.*

NURSING DIAGNOSES	OUTCOME CRITERIA	INTERVENTIONS

2 Stress Incontinence
 	
r.t. relaxed pelvic musculature
	• Is free of perceived urinary leakage as uncontrollable problem
	-verbalizes satisfaction with control measures
		• Monitor voiding pattern
		  - have patient monitor I&O, or, if not possible, nurse should record I&O
		  - determine causes of incontinence, associated factors (coughing, sneezing)
		
		• Promote adequate daily intake of fluids; if no inhibiting existing conditions, intake should be 2000-3000 mL/day
		
		• Schedule fluid intake
		
		• Avoid fluid containing caffeine or those that have a diuretic effect
		
		• Encourage patient to empty bladder completely when urge is felt; instruct not to wait
		
		• Encourage patient to discuss feelings of isolation due to fear of incontinent episodes
		
		• Instruct to wear protective pads in underwear
		
		• Instruct female patient to do Kegel exercises; teach to perform exercises by tightening pelvic floor muscles as though to stop from urinating; do this for 4 sec and repeat 10 times qid
		
		• Praise patient for participation and success
		
		• Inform patient of surgical options to correct stress incontinence
		
		• Administer sympathomimetic medications as directed
		
		• Consult with physician regarding need for surgical intervention

RATIONALE: *Monitoring information aids in planning interventions and helps patient to participate in his/her own care. Bladder distention increases the potential for infection and for episodes of incontinence. Kegel exercises increase the tone of pelvic muscles.*

GENERAL

NURSING DIAGNOSES	OUTCOME CRITERIA	INTERVENTIONS

3 Urge Incontinence
 	
r.t. urinary leakage associated with neurologic disease, outlet obstruction, bladder infection, or irritation
	• Is free of urgency; returns to continence	• Assess history of UTIs
		
		• Assess for lower urinary tract symptoms: nocturia, dysuria, hesitancy, altered stream straining, hematuria, pain, frequency, urgency, increased leakage
		
		• Assess for evidence of related factors
		  - neurologic disease
		  - bladder outlet obstruction
		  - irritative bladder disorders

	• Is free of risk factors for bladder infection or irritation
	  - urine free of bacteria
	  - post-void residuals within acceptable limits
		• Obtain clean-catch urine specimen or catherize per orders
		
		• Measure post-void residuals
		
		• Increase fluid intake by 1500-2000 mL
		
		• Avoid citrus juices, dark colas, and coffee
		
		• Administer antibiotics and urinary antiseptics as prescribed

		RATIONALE: *Culture and sensitivity tests help to determine cause of infection. Nursing measures help determine other causes of incontinence and aid in treating infections, bladder irritability, and incomplete emptying.*
4 Functional Incontinence *r.t. perceptual/ cognitive impairment*	• Remains continent 90 percent of the time	• Monitor I&O, time, and amount of voiding; record • Assess for other forms of urinary incontinence (stress, reflex, urge, total, retention) • Assess for bladder distention at least q2-3h
	• Remains free of UTI, skin irritation, odor - verbalizes satisfaction with control measures	• Alter environment to maximize access to toilet/commode • Institute bladder training program according to cognitive status, physical abilities, motivation • Provide privacy • Assist to commode or toilet q2h while awake; over time, gradually extend time

NURSING DIAGNOSES	OUTCOME CRITERIA	INTERVENTIONS

- Awaken once during night to void; provide call light within reach at all times
- Assist patient to normal voiding position if possible
  - male should stand, if possible
  - female should sit on commode or toilet with thighs flexed and back supported
- Pour water over perineum, run water, or use Credé's maneuver to encourage voiding at scheduled times
- Assist patient to bathroom as soon as desire to void is expressed
- Praise success
- Clean perineal area immediately; apply creams as needed, when incontinent episodes occur
- Prevent sensory deprivation
  - provide environmental stimuli
  - orient to time, place, and person
  - set clock to alert patient to times to void

RATIONALE: *Active participation on part of the patient may increase likelihood of successful bladder retraining. It also helps him/her to void at regular intervals and decreases episodes of incontinence at night. Normal voiding positioning promotes elimination. Routine hygiene and skin care prevent irritation of urine and skin breakdown. Sensory stimulation increases client awareness of his/her surroundings and decreases episodes of incontinence.*

5 Reflex Incontinence

r.t. neurologic impairment

- Maintains continence between catheterizations

- Determine stimuli that cause emptying of bladder
- Initiate clean intermittent catheterization schedule, q4-6h as needed while awake
- Administer automatic or spasmolytic drugs as prescribed
- Monitor for side effects of drugs: blurred vision, dry mouth, tachycardia

NURSING DIAGNOSES	OUTCOME CRITERIA	INTERVENTIONS
		• If unsuccessful, consider use of condom catheter for males, other containment devices for females
	• Shows no symptoms of UTI	• Teach patient/family application and care of containment device • Consult physician if patient is incontinent around catheter
		RATIONALE: *Since bladder training is not feasible for this diagnosis, restoration of continence is achieved by using drugs to prevent bladder emptying at unscheduled times and by using catheters to provide regular emptying. Alternatively, sealed collection devices can be used instead of long-term indwelling catheters to control chance of bacteriuria. Incontinence around catheter may indicate an obstructed catheter.*
6 Total Incontinence *r.t. neurologic impairment*	• Has no urinary leakage around pad, diaper, or urinary containment device	• Determine when incontinence occurs, and associated sensations • Assess for UTI, fever, lower urinary tract symptoms • Evaluate effectiveness of urinary containment devices: pads, briefs, condom catheters, or adult diapers • Consult with physician regarding other sources of leakage, i.e., fistula
	• Has intact skin integrity	• Assess perineal skin integrity • Evaluate effectiveness of hygiene and skin care products • Teach patient/family regular skin care routine - wash once daily with soap and water; dry thoroughly - use moisture barrier between washings
		RATIONALE: *Urinary containment devices are necessary because normal sphincter function is totally absent. Routine skin hygiene protects the perineal skin integrity from irritation and moisture.*

> ***OTHER LESS COMMON NURSING DIAGNOSES:*** *Impaired Skin Integrity;*
> *Social Isolation; Self-Esteem Disturbance; Body Image Disturbance*

ESSENTIAL DISCHARGE CRITERIA

- Is relieved of urinary retention
- Urine culture results WNL
- WBC count WNL
- Female client understands how to do Kegel exercises

- Verbalizes satisfaction with urinary elimination pattern
- Patient/family verbalize knowledge of how to correctly administer medications
- Patient/family verbalize and demonstrate knowledge of bladder training program and skin care

GENERAL

MEDICAL NURSING

CONTENTS

MEDICAL

Seizure Disorders
Shock
Subarachnoid Hemorrhage
Tuberculosis
Venous Insufficiency (Leg Ulcers)
Wound Infection

ADULT RESPIRATORY DISTRESS SYNDROME

NURSING DIAGNOSES	OUTCOME CRITERIA	INTERVENTIONS
1 Impaired Gas Exchange *r.t. ventilation-perfusion mismatch*	• Maintains adequate ventilation - RR 12-20 breaths/min - H&H WNL - ABGs WNL - pink nail beds, ear lobes, and mucous membranes - SaO$_2$ WNL	• Monitor RR, depth, and LOC qh until stable • Auscultate lungs for rhonchi, crackles, and wheezes • Assess effectiveness of O$_2$ therapy: skin color and CRT, ABGs, H&H, O$_2$ saturation by pulse oximeter • Administer prescribed O$_2$ therapy • Assist patient to Fowler's position • Pace activities to level of tolerance • Administer packed cells, as ordered
		RATIONALE: *Measures to minimize O$_2$ demand and to optimize respiration and circulation of oxygenated blood improve the ventilation perfusion relationship.*
2 Ineffective Breathing Pattern *r.t. decreased lung compliance*	• Exhibits improving respiratory status - 12-20 breaths/min - no s/s of distress	• Inspect for symmetric, adequate breathing pattern • Assess for s/s of respiratory distress (i.e., dyspnea, tachypnea, nasal flaring, restlessness)
	• Achieves optimal PaO$_2$, PaCO$_2$, and vital capacity values	• Assess for tolerance of breathing work • Monitor vital capacity values • Initiate pulmonary toileting • Reassure patient that measures are being taken to ensure safety • Initiate treatment for pain as indicated, without depressing respirations • Notify physician and prepare for intubation and mechanical ventilation if other measures do not improve indicators of respiratory function
		RATIONALE: *These measures determine the effectiveness of breathing and support an optimal breathing pattern. Mechanical ventilation prevents respiratory collapse and maintains adequate ventilation.*

MEDICAL

NURSING DIAGNOSES	OUTCOME CRITERIA	INTERVENTIONS

3 Ineffective Airway Clearance
 	
r.t. pulmonary and interstitial edema
	• Has patent airway
	  - demonstrates ability to clear secretions
	  - breath sounds clear in all areas
		• Assess the patient for ability to move secretions at least q2h
		
		• Assess hydration status (24 h I&O, weight, skin turgor)
		
		• Teach patient and family effective coughing techniques
		
		• Nasotrachial or tracheostomy suctioning prn
		
		• Maintain 45-90° HOB elevation, good body alignment, using pillows and supportive aids to maximize breathing
		
		• Assist with turning q2h

		RATIONALE: *The airway must be cleared of secretions through adequate hydration, effective coughing, and gravity.*
4 Altered Nutrition: Less than body requirements *r.t. anorexia or inability to eat secondary to fatigue*	• Maintains adequate nutritional status - maintains/regains lost body weight	• Monitor for s/s of malnutrition: poor skin turgor, muscle atrophy, decreased subcutaneous fat, weight loss, lethargy, altered mental status, decreased lymphocyte count, abnormal urea levels in 24 h urine sample
	• Passes normal stools	• Auscultate bowel sounds • Note any abnormal eating patterns
	• Takes, swallows, retains at least 80 percent of required nutrients	• Accurately record intake, count calories, weigh daily • Ensure intake of required fluids and nutrients • Provide frequent small meals • Permit special food requests as much as possible • Consider dietary consult regarding food preferences, supplements • Remove evidence of sputum or anything that will hinder patient's appetite • Administer supplemental or enteral IV feedings as ordered

NURSING DIAGNOSES	OUTCOME CRITERIA	INTERVENTIONS

- Aspirate feeding tube before each feeding; do not feed patient if amount of aspirate is more than 50 mL; place patient in semi-Fowler's position; administer tube feedings at a slow drip rate (check for bowel sounds before each feeding)

RATIONALE: *The monitoring of weight, bowel sounds, and oral and parenteral feedings measure the effectiveness of nutritional intake and digestion.*

---

5 Anxiety

r.t. change in health status

- Experiences reduced anxiety - relaxed body posture and facial expressions

- Assess level of anxiety
- Check that O_2 delivery device is functioning properly
- Explain anticipated diagnostic procedures
- Explain alarm systems on monitors and ventilators
- Reassure patient that nurse will be close at hand
- Perform treatments in an unhurried manner; remain calm
- Administer analgesics as ordered
- Encourage verbalization of anxiety
- Provide pen and pad to patient if he/she is unable to speak because of respiratory status
- Allow family/significant other to visit and participate in the care
- Consult with psychiatric liaison, clergy, social service, etc., as indicated

RATIONALE: *These measures prevent detrimental effects of increasing anxiety.*

MEDICAL

NURSING DIAGNOSES	OUTCOME CRITERIA	INTERVENTIONS
6 Knowledge Deficit *r.t. unfamiliarity with the disease process and treatments*	• Patient/family verbalize an understanding of the disease process, procedures, and treatments prior to discharge - pathophysiology - activity/rest - monitoring of status	• Assess patient's/family's level of understanding, ability to comprehend, and any physical limitations regarding discharge regimen • Explain the disease process and correct any misconceptions • Discuss the need for the monitoring equipment and frequent assessments
	• Patient/family demonstrate all required care techniques	• Demonstrate special therapeutic measures and safety precautions • Describe discharge regimen - medications: purpose, dose, side effects, schedule - diet therapy - breathing exercises: diaphragmatic, pursed-lip breathing - correct use of nebulizers and inhalers • Request patient/family to "return demonstrate" therapeutic measures • Encourage any verbalization and/or questions regarding therapeutic procedures
	• Patient/family describe reportable s/s and state why they are significant	• Identify s/s that would require medical attention, especially respiratory infections such as cold, sore throat, fever, cough
	• Patient/family identify specific factors at home that should and can be changed	• Discuss preventative environmental factors - do not smoke - avoid excessively dry air and extremely cold weather - avoid sudden changes in temperature - avoid activities that cause excessive dyspnea - keep environment clean and free from dust - keep filter clean on air conditioner - stress importance of congenial family attitude and avoidance of upsetting situations

NURSING DIAGNOSES	OUTCOME CRITERIA	INTERVENTIONS

RATIONALE: *These measures help to relieve anxiety and increase patient compliance with regimen. This reduces the risk of hospital readmission and makes the patient feel in control of his/her health.*

OTHER LESS COMMON NURSING DIAGNOSES: *Sleep Pattern Disturbance; Powerlessness; Impaired Verbal Communication; High Risk for Infection; Fatigue; High Risk for Aspiration; High Risk for Fluid Volume Deficit*

ESSENTIAL DISCHARGE CRITERIA

- Is free of symptoms of respiratory distress
- Lab values WNL
- Mobilizes secretions

- Has no s/s of infection
- Maintains adequate nutritional status
- Patient/family verbalize/demonstrate required discharge regimen

MEDICAL

ALCOHOLISM, ACUTE PHASE

NURSING DIAGNOSES	OUTCOME CRITERIA	INTERVENTIONS
1 Ineffective Breathing Pattern *r.t. impairment of respiratory center from alcohol consumption*	• Exhibits improving respiratory status - takes at least 12-20 deep, regular respirations/min	• Assess RR, rhythm, and depth q2-4h **RATIONALE:** *These measures detect respiratory depressant effects of drugs and alcohol.*
2 High Risk for Injury *r.t. disorientation and impaired judgment*	• Shows normalizing, stable VS; is afebrile	• Monitor VS q4h for 72 h; q4h for 5 days post-operative; q4h for 10 days while using sedative/hypnotics: tremulousness, tachycardia, hypertension, irritability, restlessness, diaphoresis, N/V
	• Exhibits no signs of hypoxia; LOC status is intact, normalizing	• Consider ICU/SCU placement if - increase in above symptoms - confusion, disorientation, hallucinations - hyperthermia • If altered LOC occurs - monitor TPR, BP q2h while awake for at least 24 h - notify physician for pulse > 100, < 60; temperature > 100.5; BP > 150/90
	• Sustains no seizure-related injury - no falls or near falls - correctly placed restraints - improving LOC	• Seizure management protocol • Institute restraint procedure only as a last resort, with CMS checks at least q2h for soft restraints • Orient to place and time q2-4h, or as indicated • Monitor for oversedation before medicating: notify physician if pulse is < 50 and/or patient is unable to respond to verbal commands • Administer medication to control withdrawal symptoms per physician order: chlordiazepoxide, diazepam, oxazepam, lorazepam (oxazepam or lorazepam preferred for patients over 65 or with liver disease) • When withdrawal symptoms are under control, recommend tapering medication 20 percent per day after the first 24-48 h

NURSING DIAGNOSES	OUTCOME CRITERIA	INTERVENTIONS
		• Assess response to medication (pulse, BP, sedation) - after 1 h if postoperative - after 30 min if IM - after 15 min if IV; if dose was ineffective, notify physician
		RATIONALE: *Protection and medication prevent falls and progression of confusion and delirium tremens.*
3 High Risk for Fluid Volume Deficit *r.t. decreased access to hydrating fluids and diuretic effect of alcohol*	• Maintains stable body weight	• Weigh at same time each day
	• Shows no signs of dehydration - normal fluid and electrolyte balance - good skin turgor, moist mucous membranes	• Monitor I&O, electrolytes • Give IV fluids as ordered • Offer PO fluids as tolerated
		RATIONALE: *Weight is the most accurate indicator of fluid balance. Extra fluids will minimize risk for deficit.*
4 Altered Nutrition: Less than body requirements *r.t. anorexia and alcohol dependency*	• Achieves adequate nutritional status - increased oral intake of balanced diet of carbohydrates, fat, and proteins - takes, retains 80 percent of meals	• Assess type and amount of PO dietary intake • Encourage snacks and well-balanced meals • Consult with dietitian about special diet
	• Shows normal Hb, serum cholesterol, electrolytes	• Monitor CBC, serum cholesterol, electrolytes • Give multivitamins including vitamin B and thiamine as ordered
	• Describes rationale for balanced diet	• Explain reasons for eating a balanced diet and improving nutritional status
		RATIONALE: *Balanced fluids and nutrition prevent Wernicke-Korsakoff and other alcohol-related complications.*

MEDICAL

NURSING DIAGNOSES	OUTCOME CRITERIA	INTERVENTIONS
5 Ineffective Individual Coping *r.t. inability to manage stressors without alcohol*	• Identifies ways to cope with stress	• Assess present coping status • Assist to identify effective and ineffective coping mechanisms • Assist to identify ways to reduce stressors and improve stress response
	• Experiences supportive presence or counseling from family, friend, staff	• Encourage the calming presence of a family member or friend • Initiate appropriate health professional referral
		RATIONALE: *Effective coping requires positive responses to stress and effective coping behaviors.*

OTHER LESS COMMON NURSING DIAGNOSES: *Spiritual Distress; Hopelessness*

ESSENTIAL DISCHARGE CRITERIA

- Is free of symptoms from alcohol withdrawal
- Is free of critically high or low lab values
- Takes, retains required nutrition

- Is free from injury
- Verbalizes plans to begin alcohol dependency treatment program

ALZHEIMER'S DISEASE

NURSING DIAGNOSES	OUTCOME CRITERIA	INTERVENTIONS

1 High Risk for Injury

r.t. wandering, behavioral changes, memory loss, seizure activity

- Remains free of injury

- Check identification bracelet
- Check patient visually frequently
- Place patient close to nurse's station, away from stairs/exits
- Assist with/encourage ambulation frequently
- Remove sharp/dangerous objects from reach
- Calmly direct patient to more positive behaviors as needed
- Institute seizure precautions as indicated per institutional policy/procedure
- Administer hypnotics, neuroleptics, and/or antiseizure medications as needed
- Monitor results; report side effects to physician
- Apply restraints correctly and only as a last alternative

RATIONALE: *Manipulating the environment minimizes risk of injury to self and others. Frequent ambulation tends to decrease restlessness, while restraint application may increase restlessness and agitation. Seizure precautions and medications may be needed late in the disease process. Neuroleptics and hypnotics can effectively treat pugnacity, agitation, and hyperactivity.*

2 Altered Thought Processes

r.t. disease process, memory loss

- Performs ADL independently

- Assess customary routine and environment
- Maintain a structured, consistent environment (furniture, glasses, hair brush)

- Recognizes self and family

- Explain changes in routine, environment
- Provide clock, simple calendar
- Encourage participation of family members in plan of care

MEDICAL

NURSING DIAGNOSES	OUTCOME CRITERIA	INTERVENTIONS
		• Help with use of assistive devices as needed
	• Maintains bowel/bladder continence	• Assist to bathroom q2h while awake, less frequently at night (schedule diuretics to peak during awake hours as needed)
		• Communicate in slow, short phrases, minimizing distractions
		• Administer ergoloid mesylates, cholinergics, esterase inhibitors, and/or antidepressants as indicated
		• Monitor effects; report adverse effects to physician
		RATIONALE: *A consistent, dependable environment tends to minimize symptomatic manifestations. Frequent reorientation is needed because of short-term memory loss. Use of assistive devices and scheduled elimination prolongs independence. A variety of drugs may be considered to improve cognition, depending on stage of disease. Antidepressants are used since depression is common with these patients.*
3 Feeding, Bathing/Hygiene, Dressing/ Grooming Self-Care Deficit *r.t. progressive disease process*	• Demonstrates minimal self-care deficits	• Monitor I&O
		• Maintain fluid intake at 2000 mL/day unless contraindicated
		• Assess urine for cloudiness or odor
		• Assist with feeding as indicated or use IV or NG feedings per protocol; elevate head to prevent aspiration
		• Administer oral hygiene q2-4h
		• Assist with daily hygiene care
		• Administer eye care q2-4h if indicated
		• Perform intermittent urinary catheterization per hospital routine
		• Maintain regular bowel function

NURSING DIAGNOSES	OUTCOME CRITERIA	INTERVENTIONS
		RATIONALE: *Regular oral hygiene may be needed to remove secretions and promote comfort. Assistance with elimination may be needed to prevent constipation and alterations in urinary elimination.*

4 Sleep Pattern Disturbance
 	
r.t. sensory alterations
	• Sleeps throughout the night	• Assess for factors that interfere with sleep
		• Establish HS routine
		  - bathing, toileting, oral care
		  - reduce noise and distractions
		  - offer back rub or snack
		• Encourage passive as well as strenuous daytime activity
		• Discourage afternoon naps
		• Discourage fluid, food, caffeine intake, strenuous activity before bedtime
		• Administer hypnotic drugs as needed to induce sleep

		RATIONALE: *Identified causes of sleep disturbance can be eliminated or minimized to achieve adequate quality sleep.*
5 Anticipatory Grieving *r.t. loss of loved one*	• Patient/family verbalize feelings of impending loss	• Encourage patient/family to describe feelings of loss • Explore past effective and ineffective coping behaviors • Assist patient/family in identifying sources of social support • Allow use of denial, but do not reinforce • Do not confront patient/family with distorted perception • Demonstrate acceptance of intense feelings • When appropriate, provide information regarding disease progression, prognosis, and treatment

MEDICAL

NURSING DIAGNOSES	OUTCOME CRITERIA	INTERVENTIONS
		• Allow flexible visiting hours to promote family interaction; acknowledge family needs for rest and health
		• Evaluate need for referral such as social services
		RATIONALE: *Encouraging expression of feelings and family participation will help the patient and family work through the stages of the grieving process.*

OTHER LESS COMMON NURSING DIAGNOSES: *Altered Nutrition: Less than body requirements; Altered Urinary Elimination; High Risk for Impaired Skin Integrity; Ineffective Family Coping; Knowledge Deficit; Sensory/Perceptual Alterations; Impaired Physical Mobility; Anxiety; Powerlessness; Social Isolation*

ESSENTIAL DISCHARGE CRITERIA

• Demonstrates minimal self-care deficits

• Remains free of traumatic injury

• Demonstrates optimal level of orientation

• Achieves adequate, quality sleep

• Patient/family begin to work through grieving process

ANEMIA, PERNICIOUS

NURSING DIAGNOSES	OUTCOME CRITERIA	INTERVENTIONS
1 Activity Intolerance *r.t. fatigue, weakness and malaise*	• Performs ADL without use of supplemental O_2 and with stable VS	• Schedule rest periods after activity and meals • Increase activity level gradually **RATIONALE:** *Pacing of activity reduces tissue O_2 demand.*
2 High Risk for Injury *r.t. sensory and motor loss, alteration in mental status*	• Remains free of injury	• Assess for confusion, changes in mentation, and irritability q2-4h or as indicated • Provide assistance for walking, daily activities, and transferring • Provide bed rest with side rails up to prevent fatigue and falls • Instruct patient to call for assistance when needed • Clear room of excess items • Keep feet covered and warm **RATIONALE:** *Eliminate safety hazards associated with high risk of injury for the debilitated patient.*
3 Altered Nutrition: Less than body requirements *r.t. changes in gastrointestinal mucosa*	• Passes normal stools	• Monitor for diarrhea or constipation; treat as indicated
	• Takes, retains at least 80 percent of meals	• Monitor I&O every shift • Encourage oral intake of vitamins, iron, and protein • Consult nutritionist to provide a balanced diet • Offer small, frequent feedings
	• Mouth is clean and free of irritation	• Provide oral care before and after meals and at mealtime **RATIONALE:** *Altered mucous membranes interfere with the ingestion and absorption of nutrients, fluids, and electrolytes.*

MEDICAL

NURSING DIAGNOSES	OUTCOME CRITERIA	INTERVENTIONS
4 Constipation *r.t. gastrointestinal mucosal atrophy*	• Bowel elimination is normal pattern for patient	• Monitor bowel elimination • Offer a glass of warm water 30 min before breakfast • Encourage intake of 8-10 glasses of fluids each day • Assist in establishing a regular time for elimination • Assist to normal semisquatting position for elimination
		RATIONALE: *Constipation requires nursing intervention to assist the patient in maintaining homeostasis.*
5 Knowledge Deficit *r.t. unfamiliarity with chronicity of disease and treatment protocol*	• Patient/family discuss pathophysiology of disease process, rationale for treatment	• Discuss precautions in the use of heat therapy • Emphasize skin and oral care • Instruct that vitamin B_{12} injections and frequent medical evaluations must be continued for life • Refer to home health for maintenance therapy
		RATIONALE: *Increased knowledge can prevent other complications by stressing the need for continuous parenteral vitamin therapy regimen.*

OTHER LESS COMMON NURSING DIAGNOSES: Sleep Pattern Disturbance; Fluid Volume Deficit; Impaired Gas Exchange; High Risk for Impaired Skin Integrity; Diarrhea

ESSENTIAL DISCHARGE CRITERIA

- Is able to perform ADL to the usual degree without using supplemental O_2
- Remains free of injury

- Exhibits adequate nutritional status and GI function
- Verbalizes plans to return to lab for follow-up blood work and to schedule follow-up visit with physician

ANEMIA, SICKLE CELL (ACUTE CRISIS)

NURSING DIAGNOSES	OUTCOME CRITERIA	INTERVENTIONS
1 Pain *r.t. sickle cell occlusion of microcirculation*	• Verbalizes/displays reasonable comfort	• Identify severity and location of pain: joints, extremities, chest, abdomen, headache • Teach use of 0-10 descriptive pain scale
	• Reports comfort following analgesia	• Administer narcotic analgesics as ordered • Provide teaching to patient and family to decrease fear of "addiction"
	• Identifies medication or activity that reduces or aggravates discomfort - identifies source of comfort	• Position and support painful areas • Provide other pain relief measures: heat application, relaxation techniques, breathing exercises, distraction • Ensure adequate rest • Administer O_2 prn as ordered
	• Takes, retains required fluids	• Monitor I&O • Encourage oral intake of fluids; administer IV fluids (3 L/d) as ordered
		RATIONALE: *Tissues and organs are susceptible to occlusion, hypoxia, and resulting pain. Narcotics are necessary to control moderate and severe pain. Nonpharmacologic measures minimize and focus attention away from pain. Hemodilution reverses sickle cell agglutination.*
2 High Risk for Infection *r.t. disease process, inadequate defenses*	• If free of s/s of systemic or local infection - VS WNL - WBC count, ABGs, H&H WNL - ECG WNL	• Monitor VS q4h; notify physician as indicated • Assess for s/s of infection every shift in the lungs, long bones, urinary tract, and skin • Monitor WBC count, ABGs, H&H, ECG • Encourage early ambulation and pulmonary hygiene • Promote adequate nutrition and fluid intake

MEDICAL

NURSING DIAGNOSES	OUTCOME CRITERIA	INTERVENTIONS
	• Experiences no adverse effects of antibiotics	• Administer antibiotics as ordered; report any side effects
		RATIONALE: *The stress of compromised nutritional state and infection can precipitate or complicate a crisis.*
3 Knowledge Deficit *r.t. unfamiliarity with crisis prevention information*	• Avoids situations that can precipitate a crisis	• Discuss factors that are known to precipitate a crisis: infection, dehydration, exposure to cold, physical and emotional stress, hypoxia (smoking, high altitudes) • Describe the nature of the disease and treatment strategies with patient/family • Offer opportunities for questions and expressions of fear and anger
		RATIONALE: *Avoidance of these situations can lengthen crisis-free intervals. Improved understanding of the illness enhances compliance with treatment regimen.*

OTHER LESS COMMON NURSING DIAGNOSES: *Altered Tissue Perfusion (cardiopulmonary, renal, gastrointestinal, and/or peripheral); High Risk for Injury; Impaired Skin Integrity*

ESSENTIAL DISCHARGE CRITERIA

• Verbalizes comfort

• Shows no evidence of infection

• Avoids/identifies situations that precipitate crisis

ARTHRITIS

NURSING DIAGNOSES	OUTCOME CRITERIA	INTERVENTIONS
1 Pain *r.t. joint/muscle inflammation, degeneration, deformity*	• Verbalizes/displays freedom from pain	• Assess pain (severity and joints involved) q2-4h
	• Reports comfort following analgesia	• Administer narcotic analgesics and NSAIDs as ordered to meet patient's individual needs for pain management
	• Identifies medication or activity that reduces or aggravates discomfort	• Help patient identify pain relief measures that have helped in the past; encourage ventilation of thoughts • Provide moist heat and massage to affected joints • Teach relaxation techniques
	• Alternates periods of activity and rest	• Rest and splint joints when warm and swollen
		RATIONALE: *These measures provide comfort and reduce pain, stiffness, and inflammation. This disease is a long-term, chronically painful condition and requires optimal pain management for maximum mobility and self-care.*
2 Impaired Physical Mobility *r.t. musculoskeletal deformity, pain, decreased muscle strength*	• Uses measures to regain and maintain satisfactory range of joint motion	• Assess range of joint motion, deformity, and signs of inflammation • Apply warm, moist heat prior to ROM exercises • Provide active and passive ROM; inflamed joints should only be moved to the point of pain • Instruct in isometric exercises for use during acute phases • Turn q2h and provide for periods of activity and rest • Assess need for OT/PT
	• Demonstrates use of adaptive devices to increase mobility	• Instruct use of assistive devices (foot board, slings, supports, raised toilet seats)

MEDICAL

NURSING DIAGNOSES	OUTCOME CRITERIA	INTERVENTIONS
		• Encourage patient to assist with ADL as much as possible, allowing ample time for activity • Encourage verbalization regarding limitations in mobility
		RATIONALE: *These measures promote joint mobility, relieve pain, prevent stiffness and contractures, and identify factors that interfere with mobility.*
3 Activity Intolerance *r.t. systemic inflammation, anemia, impaired mobility*	• Tolerates activity or adjusts to decreased energy level	• Assess energy level and response to activity
	• Shows H&H WNL	• Assess for occult blood loss (stool, urine, emesis) and monitor H&H
	• Identifies factors that reduce activity tolerance	• Provide for progressive increase in activity as tolerated • Provide for periods of activity (during times of decreased pain and inflammation) and rest (when joints are inflamed) • Help to identify ways to conserve energy and decrease stress on joints • Provide and encourage a nutritionally balanced diet
		RATIONALE: *Graduated activity maintains strength and reduces fatigue. Provision of essential nutrients support body function and minimize fatigue.*
4 Body Image Disturbance *r.t. change in body structure/function*	• Describes a more positive self-concept and acceptance of self	• Assess concerns about condition and role performance • Encourage active performance and effective coping strategies in usual roles and treatment plan • Encourage patient to ventilate feelings about disease and body changes • Encourage significant others to maintain open communication with patient

NURSING DIAGNOSES	OUTCOME CRITERIA	INTERVENTIONS
		• Offer support and encouragement; stress strengths unique to patient
		• Encourage patient to participate in local support groups and rehabilitation services
		RATIONALE: *These measures promote a positive, accepting, and realistic body image.*
5 Bathing/Hygiene, Toileting Self-Care Deficit *r.t. decreased strength/endurance, ROM, and pain*	• Is able to perform ADL with use of assistive devices, and other resources as needed	• Assess ability to perform ADL
		• Assist patient to identify self-care deficits and factors that interfere with ability to perform ADL
		• Provide modified utensils and other equipment as needed to perform ADL
		• Encourage patient to do as much as possible on their own; praise progress
		RATIONALE: *Self-care promotes independence, self-esteem, and maintains mobility.*

6 Impaired Home Maintenance Management
 	
r.t. knowledge deficit regarding the disease, PT, medicines, alterations in lifestyle
	• Demonstrates understanding of home care management and follow-up care
	  - medications
	  - diet
	  - PT
	  - home safety
	  - support networks
	  - equipment, assistive services
	  - commitment to consistent follow-up care regimen
		• Assess knowledge of disease, medications, need for continued PT, and lifestyle modifications; provide teaching as needed

		• Assess home environment in relation to safety, resources, and support systems
		• Assist patient/family to identify and acquire home care needs including equipment, social services, and home healthcare
		• Encourage to continue with healthcare regimen including medications, PT, and diet
		RATIONALE: *Competence of patient and family promotes a feasible discharge date and helps assure a safe and therapeutic home environment.*

MEDICAL

OTHER LESS COMMON NURSING DIAGNOSES: Sleep Pattern Disturbance; Fatigue; High Risk for Infection; Altered Sexuality Patterns; Altered Role Performance; Ineffective Individual Coping

ESSENTIAL DISCHARGE CRITERIA

- Experiences satisfactory pain relief
- Perform ADL at the most optimal level, independently or with resources
- Verbalizes understanding of medications, diet, and PT needs
- Verbalizes acceptance of self

NURSING DIAGNOSES	OUTCOME CRITERIA	INTERVENTIONS
1 Ineffective Airway Clearance *r.t. excess mucus production, bronchoconstriction, mucosal edema*	• Exhibits airway clearance 　- maintains patent airway 　- demonstrates effective cough for mucous expectoration 　- therapeutic theophylline level of 10-20 µg/mL	• Monitor airway clearance 　- monitor for therapeutic theophylline level 　- assess for contributing/causative factors, e.g., allergens, cold weather 　- auscultate anteroposterior lung sounds for full ventilation and vesicular breath sounds in all lung fields 　- assess amount, color, consistency, and odor of sputum production 　- administer, maintain theophylline at therapeutic levels
	• Shows no sternal retractions, nasal flaring	• Assess for sternal and intercostal retractions, nasal flaring upon inspiration, and chest heaving
	• Shows VS WNL	• Assess VS q1-4h
	• Exhibits no alteration in baseline LOC	• Monitor for changes in mental status from baseline
	• Mobilizes, expectorates lung secretions	• Assist patient with nebulizer or IPPB treatment as ordered • Encourage 2-3 L of fluid intake daily if not contraindicated • Assist to Fowler's position or to a leaning-forward position over a bedside table • Provide chest physiotherapy and postural drainage if not contraindicated • Prepare for emergent intubation and resuscitation if respiratory status worsens
	• Demonstrates competence 　- inhaler 　- coughing techniques	• Teach correct use of inhaler, coughing techniques
	• Identifies precipitating factors	• Assist to identify precipitating factors

RATIONALE: *Measures to prevent, identify, and treat inadequate airway clearance will maintain a patent airway. Optimal theophylline levels produce an optimal outcome while minimizing toxic effects.*

MEDICAL

NURSING DIAGNOSES	OUTCOME CRITERIA	INTERVENTIONS

2 Ineffective Breathing Pattern
 	
r.t. fear and decreased lung expansion
	• Maintains adequate O_2 exchange
	  - SaO_2 WNL
	  - 12-20 deep, regular respirations/min
		• Assess ABGs
		• Monitor continuous pulse oximetry
		• Assess rate, depth, and regularity of respirations
		• Assess response to breathing difficulties

	• Identifies, describes fears	• Listen carefully to explore sources and nature of fears • Instruct patient on controlled breathing techniques; provide emotional support
		RATIONALE: *Assessment measures help evaluate the effectiveness of breathing. Controlled breathing techniques improve oxygenation while decreasing the work of breathing.*
3 Activity Intolerance *r.t. inadequate O_2 supply to meet tissue demands*	• Demonstrates methods that reduce activity intolerance	• Assess current and baseline activity tolerance
	• Meets ADL needs without SOB	• Assess for nonrespiratory contributors to activity intolerance • Assess VS before, during, and 3 min after activity • Encourage patient to make decisions about alternating activity with rest • Provide O_2 therapy as prescribed by the physician • Instruct patient to provide support for arms when performing tasks requiring arm strength • Instruct regarding hazards of smoking; refer to smoking cessation program if appropriate • Teach use of incentive spirometer • Provide appropriate assistive devices; consult OT if necessary • Consult PT for specific reconditioning exercises as approved by physician

NURSING DIAGNOSES	OUTCOME CRITERIA	INTERVENTIONS

- Instruct about importance of optimal nutrition; consult dietitian as indicated

RATIONALE: *Assessment techniques help determine the nature and effectiveness of O₂ supply/demand relationship. Patient teaching and other interventions to support breathing and oxygenation will promote optimal recovery.*

OTHER LESS COMMON NURSING DIAGNOSES: *Impaired Gas Exchange; Ineffective Management of Therapeutic Regimen; Self-Care Deficit; High Risk for Infection; Impaired Home Maintenance Management; Knowledge Deficit; Altered Nutrition: Less than body requirements; Sleep Pattern Disturbance; Anxiety; Impaired Verbal Communication*

ESSENTIAL DISCHARGE CRITERIA

- Maintains patent airway
- Shows respiratory pattern WNL
- Shows ABGs WNL

- Patient/family verbalize understanding of causes of asthma exacerbations
- Demonstrates competence to meet basic ADL at home

MEDICAL

CANCER, ADVANCED

NURSING DIAGNOSES	OUTCOME CRITERIA	INTERVENTIONS

1 Altered Nutrition: Less than body requirements
 	
r.t. loss of appetite or dysphagia, side effects of treatment, obstruction by tumor
	• Achieves, maintains adequate nutritional status
	  - normal serum electrolytes
	  - normal GI functioning
		• Assess for s/s of dehydration, GI function; report abnormal lab values

	• Maintains weight	• Weigh daily and record
	• Swallows, retains feedings	• Assess patient's ability to eat and swallow
	• Takes, retains 80 percent of meals	• Maintain daily dietary intake record • Modify environment to reduce stress • Observe for fit of dentures; provide appropriate foods for ease of chewing
	• Has no vomiting	• Medicate prior to meals to reduce nausea and vomiting • Provide oral anesthetics prior to meals
	• Patient/family discuss/participate in diet planning	• Incorporate family and significant others into nutritional care • Encourage family to prepare foods that cater to patient's likes and dislikes concerning high calorie diet
		RATIONALE: *These measures are designed to monitor nutritional status, promote eating and digestion, prevent vomiting, and involve the patient and family in meal planning.*

2 Altered Role Performance
 	
r.t. change in physical abilities, change in patterns of responsibility
	• Identifies realistic perception of abilities
	  - accepts limitations
	  - discusses ways to change lifestyle to foster goal accomplishment
		• Encourage patient to make a list of individual strengths that will assist with role change
		• Encourage to make a list of goals and responsibilities
		• Assist to explore new ways to accomplish goals with existing limitations
		• Provide realistic patient/family education regarding patient's condition that assists them in adjusting to change in patient's role
		• Refer to counseling as needed

NURSING DIAGNOSES	OUTCOME CRITERIA	INTERVENTIONS
		• Refer to community support agencies as needed
		RATIONALE: *Empathy and a supportive environment assist the patient in making role changes. Family and community resources help with the mastery of a new role.*
3 Pain (chronic) *r.t. disease process (metastasis)*	• Verbalizes, displays freedom from pain	• Assess pain level using scale noting location, duration, intensity • Medicate routinely based on patient's desired comfort level
	• Verbalizes comfort following administration of analgesia	• Monitor the effectiveness of medications used to alleviate pain
	• Exhibits normal bowel sounds	• Set up bowel program to avoid constipation
	• Identifies medication or activity that reduces/aggravates discomfort	• Maintain written records of pain medications and obtained relief • Teach patient/family about appropriate use of pain/bowel medications • Instruct patient/family to keep records of pain medications and obtained relief • Modify environment to reduce anxiety and stress • Teach patient/family alternative methods for controlling pain (distraction techniques)
	• Alternates periods of activity and rest	• Plan daily routines around pain medication
		RATIONALE: *Pain assessment helps determine the effectiveness of interventions. Patient and family involvement in determining and using factors that help alleviate pain enhances comfort and the quality of life.*

MEDICAL

NURSING DIAGNOSES	OUTCOME CRITERIA	INTERVENTIONS
4 Altered Oral Mucous Membrane *r.t. treatment, decreased flora, infection*	• Oral mucosa are intact and without lesions	• Monitor membranes for lesions; immediately report presence of lesions
	• Demonstrates procedures to care for oral cavity	• Teach to brush teeth and thoroughly rinse after each meal and at bedtime • Use soft toothbrush for brushing teeth • Do not use mouthwash with alcohol • Keep lips well lubricated • Avoid spicy, citrus, or hot foods
	• Maintains adequate fluid and nutritional intake	• Keep membranes moist • Encourage to drink adequate fluids (100 mL qh)
		RATIONALE: *Fluid and food intake decreases when it causes discomfort. Changing the taste, temperature, and texture of foods improves intake.*

5 Impaired Physical Mobility
 	
r.t. weakness, neuromuscular skeletal impairment, pain
	• Participates in physical activities
	  - has physical strength and ability to care for self independently
	  - demonstrates ability to use assistive equipment
		• Monitor tissue status and document
		• Medicate for pain/discomfort prior to physical activity
		• Rotate positions to maintain adequate circulation to tissues
		• Assist with passive ROM exercises and active ROM exercises on a routine daily basis
		• Obtain appropriate assistive devices
		• Teach patient/family/significant other appropriate use of assistive devices and specific exercises
		• Refer to PT as needed

		RATIONALE: *These interventions promote the mobility, circulation, and functioning of joints and limbs. Involving the patient/family in the safe use of assistive devices promotes maximum independence.*

NURSING DIAGNOSES	OUTCOME CRITERIA	INTERVENTIONS
6 Ineffective Individual Coping *r.t. personal vulnerability, terminal illness*	• Verbalizes fears and asks for help when needed	• Encourage patient to verbalize fears
	• Demonstrates ability to solve problems	• Assist to learn methods for solving problems
	• Communicates needs to family/others	• Encourage and instruct patient about open communication • Provide mental and physical diversion such as reading, music • Keep patient/family informed of realistic prognostic factors • Openly discuss care with patient/family
	• Is free of self-destructive behaviors	• Refer for counseling when needed • Provide spiritual and religious support as appropriate for the patient/family

RATIONALE: *These interventions provide information and cognitive techniques to improve problem-solving and coping.*

OTHER LESS COMMON NURSING DIAGNOSES: *Altered Tissue Perfusion; High Risk for Injury; Altered Urinary Elimination; Impaired Verbal Communication; Fear; High Risk for Infection; Knowledge Deficit*

ESSENTIAL DISCHARGE CRITERIA

- Maintains optimal nutrition
- Verbalizes acceptable level of comfort
- Ambulates frequently, using assistive devices as needed

- Accepts limitations and demonstrates effective coping strategies
- Verbalizes knowledge of disease process, therapeutic regimen, and reportable s/s

MEDICAL

CEREBROVASCULAR ACCIDENT

NURSING DIAGNOSES	OUTCOME CRITERIA	INTERVENTIONS
1 Altered Tissue Perfusion (cerebral) *r.t. inadequate blood supply, increased intercranial pressure, decreased cerebral oxygenation*	• Exhibits stable VS	• Monitor VS q1-4h
	• Displays unchanged or improved neurologic status - LOC - mentation, verbal responses - pupil/eye movement - grip - headache - dizziness - seizure activity	• Assess neurologic signs q1-4h; notify physician of changes immediately • Monitor pertinent lab values • Administer and monitor effect of medications (antihypertensive, antiseizure, diuretics, steroids, blood thinners) • Elevate HOB • Institute seizure precautions • Restrain only if absolutely necessary (Note: restraints may contribute to agitation, which will further increase intercranial pressure) • Maintain patent airway • Maintain quiet environment
		RATIONALE: *Monitor neurologic signs and VS frequently to note complications as soon as they occur. Alterations in cerebral blood flow compromise the brain, CSF, and blood volume. Inadequate blood supply and decreased O$_2$ to brain result in necrosis or infarction.*
2 Ineffective Airway Clearance *r.t. obstructed airway, immobility, neurologic deficits*	• Maintains regular RR, rhythm - lungs are clear	• Auscultate lungs and monitor RR and pattern qh • Assess ability to maintain an open airway • Assess secretions, obtain sputum C&S • Encourage coughing and deep breathing q2h
	• Shows ABGs WNL	• Monitor ABGs
	• Shows no s/s of hypoxia/respiratory distress	• Monitor for hypoxia/hypercapnia • Monitor I&O

NURSING DIAGNOSES	OUTCOME CRITERIA	INTERVENTIONS

MEDICAL

| | | • Maintain patent airway
  - side position
  - suction
  - utilize airway adjuncts
  - apply O$_2$ as ordered

• Administer medications (expectorants, bronchodilators, antibiotics) and monitor effects

• Notify physician of changes |

RATIONALE: *A patient with neurologic deficits may not be able to maintain a patent airway. Airway obstruction may be caused by diminished gag/cough reflex, the tongue, mucous aspiration, or decreased mobilization.*

---

3 High Risk for Impaired Skin Integrity

r.t. immobility, neurologic deficits

• Skin is clean, dry, and intact
  - shows no skin breakdown
  - participates with staff/family in repositioning and ambulating
	• Assess integument q2h
	
	• Inspect for incontinence; offer bedpan/assist frequently
	
	• Change position q2h
	
	• Provide skin care (keep clean, dry) q2h and prn, including mouth care
	
	• Utilize pressure prevention devices
	
	• Provide nutritionally balanced diet
	
	• Consult therapists: enteral stomal, physical, and occupational (coordinate)

RATIONALE: *Maintaining clean, dry skin is important because the CVA patient may not sense pain or pressure which may lead to skin breakdown.*

---

4 Altered Nutrition: Less than body requirements

r.t. neurologic deficits, inability to ingest food

• Maintains or regains weight	• Weigh qod
• Shows normal electrolytes	• Monitor I&O, F&E
• Swallows, retains feedings	• Monitor calorie count

CEREBROVASCULAR ACCIDENT

NURSING DIAGNOSES	OUTCOME CRITERIA	INTERVENTIONS
		• Assess gag reflex, swallowing, presence of facial paralysis, sensory/motor function, upper limbs perceptual deficits to determine eating ability; assess bowel sounds • Provide IVF, NGT feedings, or TPN as directed • Initiate emergency measures for choking, as indicated
	• Takes, retains at least 80 percent of meals	• Provide mouth care • Assist with meals as needed and taper to increase patient participation • Advance diet as tolerated, taking into account food preferences • Consult with dietitian to incorporate patient's food preferences
		RATIONALE: *CVA may affect sensory and motor functions related to swallowing, chewing, and coordination of extremities, which can result in nutritional difficulties. Immobility and depression may result in loss of appetite.*
5 Altered Urinary Elimination *r.t. sensory/motor impairment, flaccid bladder, confusion, difficulty communicating*	• Remains free of UTI - VS WNL - urine clear, no foul odor	• Assess VS q1-4h • Assess for urinary cloudiness, foul odor
	• Communicates need to void	• Monitor for incontinence • Palpate bladder • Assess awareness of need to void and ability to communicate same • Offer bedpan frequently • Establish schedule to void • Stimulate urge by positioning and privacy • Insert Foley catheter, if retaining urine; obtain specimen, assess urine character and amount • Increase fluid intake

NURSING DIAGNOSES	OUTCOME CRITERIA	INTERVENTIONS
		RATIONALE: *CVA can cause damage to sensory/motor innervation of bladder. Other factors that can add to elimination problems are inability to communicate need to eliminate, difficulty in ambulating to bathroom, inability to obtain fluids and nutrition without help.*
6 Impaired Verbal Communication *r.t. aphasia, dysarthria, altered thought processes*	• Uses an effective method of communication (verbal/nonverbal)	• Assess ability to communicate • Assess nonverbal behavior • Maintain eye contact • Speak clearly and slowly • Utilize alternative measures (pictures, gestures, writing, bells, etc.) • Converse in simple terms to encourage "yes/no" response • Offer consistent schedule, routines, and repetitions • Involve staff and significant others to enhance communication • Obtain speech therapy consult
		RATIONALE: *CVA can affect ability to communicate resulting in inability to express and/or understand messages. Persons may not be able to express themselves verbally or in writing due to changes in mentation.*

7 Feeding, Bathing/Hygiene, Toileting Self-Care Deficit
 	
r.t. multiple neurologic deficits
	• Achieves optimal level of self-care
	  - appears well-groomed without neglecting affected areas
	  - participates in ADL
		• Encourage participation in ADL to extent of ability
		• Have patient carry out all self-care activities on unaffected side (combing hair, brushing teeth, eating)
		• Provide assistance, as necessary
		• Praise all efforts and attempts
		• Encourage ventilation of feelings

MEDICAL

NURSING DIAGNOSES	OUTCOME CRITERIA	INTERVENTIONS
		RATIONALE: *Neurologic deficits produced by CVA contribute to self-care deficit. Encouraging participation in ADL fosters independence and lessens frustration and depression.*
8 Altered Family Processes *r.t. situation crisis/transition*	• Patient/family demonstrates understanding of treatment regimen	• Encourage involvement of patient/family in care (ADL/ROM)
	• Patient/family demonstrates ability to maintain functional roles	• Explain emotional disorders that may ensue
	• Patient/family express feelings about disability and define realistic goals	• Encourage ventilation of feelings
	• Patient/family identify coping mechanisms and support groups	• Utilize support groups and identify appropriate coping mechanisms • Assist patient/family in making plans for the future (home care, respite care)
		RATIONALE: *Psychological response to CVA may be manifested as frustration, depression, feelings of hopelessness, powerlessness, or grief. Emotional responses to illness must be explored so that appropriate coping mechanisms can be instituted.*
9 Knowledge Deficit *r.t. disease process, treatment, prognosis*	• Patient/family discusses pathophysiology, rationale for treatment	• Explain all treatments/procedures
	• Patient/family expresses concerns, questions	• Encourage questions/provide answers • Utilize patient education materials
	• Patient/family participate in care activities	• Explore resources (community, family) • Manage discharge planning, including appropriate referrals on admission

RATIONALE: *CVA has an unexpected course which makes the need for information to both patient and family imperative. Effective teaching strategies must take into account problems in communication.*

OTHER LESS COMMON NURSING DIAGNOSES: *Impaired Physical Mobility; Impaired Swallowing; Pain; Altered Thought Processes; Spiritual Distress; Hopelessness*

ESSENTIAL DISCHARGE CRITERIA

- Shows stable VS and improved neurologic status
- Has intact skin
- Maintains functional musculoskeletal system
- Maintains weight/nutritional status WNL
- Exhibits restored bladder function
- Uses effective method of communication
- Participates in ADL for self-care

- Patient/family verbalize/demonstrate knowledge and care skills
  - disease process
  - need for follow-up care/compliance
  - medication regime
  - proper feeding, ambulation, and transfer technique
  - coping mechanisms/support groups

MEDICAL

CHEMICAL DEPENDENCY

NURSING DIAGNOSES	OUTCOME CRITERIA	INTERVENTIONS

1 High Risk for Fluid Volume Deficit
 	
r.t. vomiting, diarrhea, inability to tolerate oral fluids
	• Exhibits adequate fluid volume
	  - balanced I&O
	  - urinary output WNL
	  - urinary sp. gr. WNL
	  - VS WNL
	  - no nausea, vomiting
	  - moist mucous membranes
	  - presence of bowel sounds
	  - no abdominal distention
		• Monitor I&O q8h
		• Monitor urinary sp. gr. every void or as indicated
		• Assess VS q4h or as indicated
		• Inspect mucous membranes, skin turgor q4h
		• Assess for nausea, anorexia q4-8h
		• Assess bowel sounds q2-4h or as indicated
		• Provide preferred fluids
		• Explain reason for high fluid intake
		• Discuss with patient/family need for fluids and graduation to solids as tolerated
		• Administer parenteral fluids as ordered
		• Administer prescribed medications designed to control or substitute for illicit drug or medication
		• Identify areas of probable noncompliance for special dietary counseling or referrals

		RATIONALE: *Early detection and prompt management of fluid deficit are essential to prevent dehydration which interferes with treatment of primary medical diagnosis.*

2 Altered Nutrition: Less than body requirements
 	
r.t. anorexia, diarrhea, hyperactivity; lethargy associated with effects of illicit drugs or medications
	• Is able to take required calories
	  - receives, retains oral, parenteral feedings (specify calories required for patient)
	  - no vomiting
	  - no significant change in LOC
	  - no undue hyperactivity
		• Monitor effects of dietary intake q8h
		  - monitor I&O q8h: caloric intake, nausea, or vomiting
		  - assess LOC for significant irritability or lethargy q4-8h
		• Provide nutritious supplements during and between meals
		• Provide frequent small snacks, meals
		• Include patient in dietary management

NURSING DIAGNOSES	OUTCOME CRITERIA	INTERVENTIONS
	• Patient, family discuss typical dietary habits; identify problems; plan for improved methods of nutritional intake	• Assist patient, family to discuss typical dietary habits, to identify problem areas, and to plan for dietary improvements that are feasible to maintain
	• Patient, family identify community resources to foster compliance with required nutritional regimen	• Discuss and provide list of nutrition counseling, support groups, free nutrition/feeding centers in community
		RATIONALE: *A high caloric and highly nutritive diet is required to counteract the gastrointestinal side effects associated with drug use.*
3 Sensory/ Perceptual Alterations (visual, auditory, kinesthetic) *r.t. effects of illicit drugs or medications*	• Maintains stable LOC - no hypertension or tachycardia - no significant mood swings - no extreme lethargy - no extreme hyperirritability - no pupillary or visual changes	• Monitor VS q4h • Assess LOC baseline, then at 4-8 h intervals • Inspect pupils for response to light
	• Experiences no violent outbursts	• Assess mood for depression, hyperactivity, loss of self-control • Administer prescribed medications to produce calming, stabilizing emotional status
	• Experiences no falls	• Monitor LOC q4-8h • Keep padded side rails up or bed in lowest position • Assist to bathroom and other ambulation
		RATIONALE: *Protection from accidental self-harm is essential when the drug produces altered perceptions and imbalance and when it creates emotional volatility.*

MEDICAL

NURSING DIAGNOSES	OUTCOME CRITERIA	INTERVENTIONS

4 Anxiety

r.t. loss of control, memory loss, fear of withdrawal

- Participates in discussion of plans for "maintaining" while in hospital
  - understands primary reason for hospitalization
  - understands that keeping the chemical dependency in stable state is necessary during hospitalization

- Monitor for covert illicit drug consumption

- Discuss rationale for treatment of primary diagnosis in conjunction with the secondary problem of chemical dependence

- Reassure that the goal is to avoid withdrawal symptoms during hospitalization for a primary acute illness problem

- Discuss community resources for follow-up in breaking the chemical dependency

RATIONALE: *A chemically dependent person who is hospitalized for another primary medical diagnosis needs to understand and to cooperate with dual therapeutic regimens.*

> ***OTHER LESS COMMON NURSING DIAGNOSES:*** *Sleep Pattern Disturbance; Fatigue; High Risk for Violence: Self-directed or directed at others; Noncompliance; Powerlessness*

ESSENTIAL DISCHARGE CRITERIA

- Is physiologically stable for primary admitting problem
- Is hydrated on oral fluids
- Is alert, oriented

- Affirms need to comply with prescribed dietary plan
- Patient, family affirm need to seek help with chemical dependence; possess list of potential resources

CHOLECYSTITIS, CHOLELITHIASIS

NURSING DIAGNOSES	OUTCOME CRITERIA	INTERVENTIONS
1 Pain *r.t. inflammation and obstruction of biliary system*	• Verbalizes/displays freedom from pain - reports relief following analgesia	• Assess/monitor location, severity, frequency, duration, and causative and alleviating factors related to the pain q4h • Administer analgesics and monitor response • Avoid use of morphine • Instruct to report pain promptly
	• Identifies medication or activity that reduces or aggravates discomfort	• Anticipate need for analgesics or alternate nonpharmacologic methods of pain relief
	• Alternates periods of activity and rest	• Manipulate the environment to eliminate sources of stress and discomfort
		RATIONALE: *Morphine sulfate constricts the common duct sphincter. Giving pain medication prior to experiencing moderate to severe pain greatly increases effectiveness.*
2 Altered Nutrition: Less than body requirements *r.t. nausea, vomiting, NPO status, flatulence, anorexia*	• Maintains body weight	• Weigh daily until weight stabilizes
	• Has no vomiting	• Monitor I&O • Maintain NGT drainage to depress stomach and relieve nausea and vomiting
	• Shows lab values WNL - electrolytes - amylase - CBC - BUN - bilirubin - serum albumin	• Monitor lab values • Administer IV fluids as ordered
		RATIONALE: *The elimination of gastric juices decreases the secretion of bile. Interventions replace fluid and electrolyte loss as a result of vomiting and NGT drainage.*

MEDICAL

NURSING DIAGNOSES	OUTCOME CRITERIA	INTERVENTIONS
3 Fluid Volume Deficit *r.t. diminished intake (NPO status); nausea, vomiting, nasogastric suction*	• Maintains balanced I&O	• Monitor I&O q8h
	• Shows VS, BP WNL	• Monitor VS, BP q4h
	• Displays good skin turgor, moist mucous membranes	• Assess skin turgor/mucous membranes each shift
	• Shows electrolytes WNL	• Monitor electrolytes daily • Assess nausea, vomiting, and abdominal distention q8h
		RATIONALE: *NPO status predisposes to dehydration. Frequent assessments are necessary to monitor fluid volume status.*
4 Anxiety *r.t. diagnostic procedures, recurrence of symptoms, pain, hospitalization, possible surgery*	• Verbalizes decrease in anxiety level	• Encourage verbalization of feelings and listen attentively
	• Appears relaxed with only mild signs of anxiety, restlessness, fear	• Teach patient relaxation techniques • Manipulate the environment to reduce stressors/stimuli • Keep patient informed and involved in plan of care • Provide accurate information on disease, tests, etc. • Provide reassurance and comfort
		RATIONALE: *Intensity of anxiety varies depending on the perceived severity of the threat and the success or failure of the patient's coping mechanisms.*
5 Sleep Pattern Disturbance *r.t. pain, fear, unfamiliar surroundings (hospitalization), pruritus, jaundice*	• Verbalizes that he/she feels rested	• Plan nursing interventions to reduce/eliminate interruptions in sleep pattern
	• Demonstrates no sleeplessness or related behaviors: irritability, restlessness, lethargy, interrupted sleep patterns	• Provide for a quiet environment with minimal stimuli/comfortable temperature

NURSING DIAGNOSES	OUTCOME CRITERIA	INTERVENTIONS
	• Identifies factors that prevent/induce sleep	• Allow patient to verbalize concerns/fears that may be preventing sleep • Provide normal sleep aids, i.e., correct number of pillows, bath, massage, reading materials • Administer hypnotics/sedatives as ordered
		RATIONALE: *Quality of and ability to sleep are indicators of physiological, psychological, and spiritual health.*
6 Knowledge Deficit *r.t. disease process, medical/surgical management, alterations in lifestyle*	• Patient/family list reportable s/s	• Assess patient's knowledge level and allow learner to identify important aspects
	• Patient/family participate in care activities	• Establish learning goals in collaboration with patient/family
	• Patient/family discuss patho-physiology of disease; plan for required relaxation, activity, diet	• Provide information about disease, contributing factors, s/s, plan for management including lifestyle changes, i.e., diet, weight control • Allow time for interpretation of material learned
		RATIONALE: *Learning depends on physical/emotional readiness. The patient needs to be free of pain and extreme anxiety. Retention of information is increased by utilizing various methods of instruction to stimulate various senses.*

MEDICAL

> **OTHER LESS COMMON NURSING DIAGNOSES:** *Ineffective Breathing Pattern; High Risk for Injury; High Risk for Infection*

ESSENTIAL DISCHARGE CRITERIA

- Is afebrile, with stable VS
- Tolerates low fat diet
- Reports that pain is absent or minimal

- Is free of sleeplessness and fatigue
- Verbalizes knowledge of disease, diet, and treatment plan including medications and follow-up

CHRONIC OBSTRUCTIVE PULMONARY DISEASE

NURSING DIAGNOSES	OUTCOME CRITERIA	INTERVENTIONS

1 Ineffective Breathing Pattern
 	
r.t. tracheobronchial obstruction and fatigue
	• Exhibits improving respiratory status
	  - ABGs, vital capacity parameters are optimal for condition
	  - at least 12-20 deep, regular respirations per min
		• Assess RR, rhythm, depth, and quality q2-4h
		• Monitor ABGs
		• Report s/s of respiratory acidosis and/or worsening condition
		• Provide mechanical ventilation care as indicated
		• Identify factors that contribute to breathing difficulty

	• Cooperates with care activities that reduce dyspnea, fatigue	• Assess for tiring relative to the work of breathing • Place in semi to high Fowler's • Instruct/assist with diaphragmatic and pursed lip breathing • Instruct coughing, deep breathing, and use of incentive spirometer q2h • Maintain pulmonary toilet
	• Returns to baseline for amount and color of secretions	• Suction as necessary to remove secretions
		RATIONALE: *Frequent assessment and intervention improve breathing, facilitate ventilation, clear lung secretions, and prevent further deterioration in respiratory function.*
2 Fluid Volume Deficit *r.t. decreased fluid intake*	• Shows normal VS, BP, serum electrolytes	• Monitor VS, BP q2-4h • Monitor skin turgor, electrolytes, I&O, daily weight q8h • Report s/s of decreasing fluid volume
	• Has no frank or occult blood in emesis, stools	• Assess for gastrointestinal bleeding secondary to physiologic stress

	• Shows no s/s of dehydration
	  - takes oral fluids
	  - paces activities
		• Encourage fluids of at least 2500 mL/day unless contraindicated
		• Provide frequent rest periods

MEDICAL

NURSING DIAGNOSES	OUTCOME CRITERIA	INTERVENTIONS
		RATIONALE: *Adequate hydration prevents complications which could lead to hypovolemic shock. Increased fluids help to loosen secretions, enabling expectoration of mucus.*
3 Altered Nutrition: Less than body requirements *r.t. fatigue, SOB, anorexia*	• Maintains adequate nutritional status - maintains, regains weight • Takes, retains 80 percent of meals	• Assess for s/s of malnutrition: weight loss, anorexia • Provide high protein diet with frequent feedings that are easy to chew and swallow; avoid gas-producing food and carbonated beverages • Provide frequent oral care **RATIONALE:** *Frequent feedings lessen fatigue. Air-filled stomach makes breathing harder.*
4 High Risk for Infection *r.t. debilitated state, inability to expectorate adequately, drug-induced immunosuppression*	• Exhibits normal temperature • Shows negative cultures	• Monitor temperature q4h • Collect sputum for culture and sensitivity • Monitor visitors for colds, etc. • Teach to avoid crowds and ill people **RATIONALE:** *Protection from exposure to acute upper respiratory infection is important in preventing complications.*
5 Knowledge Deficit *r.t. unfamiliarity with disease state, treatment regimen*	• Patient/family discuss accurate knowledge of pathophysiology, rationale for treatment	• Reinforce explanation of disease, medications, and equipment

NURSING DIAGNOSES	OUTCOME CRITERIA	INTERVENTIONS
	• Patient/family list medications, dosages, effects, side effects - demonstrates correct use of inhaler • Patient/family have list of reportable s/s	• Discuss drugs, side effects, follow-up care, and symptoms to report to healthcare provider • Discuss use and misuse of inhalers
	• Avoids activities that aggravate condition	• Discuss aggravating factors: excessive dryness, temperature changes, pollens, tobacco smoke
		RATIONALE: *Knowledge decreases anxiety and leads to better cooperation with treatment.*

MEDICAL

OTHER LESS COMMON NURSING DIAGNOSES: *Anxiety; Ineffective Airway Clearance; Impaired Gas Exchange; Fatigue; Impaired Physical Mobility*

ESSENTIAL DISCHARGE CRITERIA

- Exhibits good air exchange
- Shows improved ABGs
- Is free of infection
- Maintains stable weight

- Patient/family verbalize understanding of medication therapy and importance of taking medication as prescribed
- Has list of s/s to report to healthcare provider

CIRRHOSIS OF THE LIVER

NURSING DIAGNOSES	OUTCOME CRITERIA	INTERVENTIONS

1 Altered Nutrition: Less than body requirements
 	
r.t. insufficient protein intake, impaired absorption of fat-soluble vitamins and nutrients, anorexia
	• Maintains adequate nutritional status
	  - normal albumin levels
	  - normal serum, BUN, glucose, creatinine
		• Assess protein and glucose lab values
		  - serum albumin levels
		  - serum BUN, glucose, and creatinine
		• Assess need for liquid supplements or high calorie snacks between meals

	• Takes, retains at least 80 percent of meals, snacks	• Measure dietary intake by calorie count • Offer small, frequent feedings • Administer tube feedings if unable to maintain adequate oral intake (unless patient has esophageal varices) • Limit protein if encephalopathy is present • Maintain Na restriction to prevent progression of ascites
	• Affirms need to maintain required nutrition	• Instruct and emphasize importance of good nutrition
	• Patient/family verbalize accurate knowledge of diet; affirm commitment to comply	• Discuss with patient/family need to avoid alcohol as a source of dietary intake • Consult nutritionist for follow-up
		RATIONALE: *Protein catabolism requires dietary supplements of protein and calories.*
2 Altered Thought Processes *r.t. increased circulating ammonia levels, electrolyte imbalances*	• Is oriented to time, person, place	• Assess for development of asterixis or apraxia • Determine baseline LOC, orientation; assess for changes q4-8h and prn
	• Shows ammonia levels within acceptable limits	• Monitor ammonia levels • Anticipate use of neomycin sulfate orally, enterally, or rectally

102

NURSING DIAGNOSES	OUTCOME CRITERIA	INTERVENTIONS
	• Remains free of injury related to altered mentation	• Apply soft restraints only as necessary to protect patient
		• Place tongue blade and airway at bedside; provide padded bed rails
		• Monitor for increased muscle tone in extremities
		• Minimize sensory stimuli; reorient to surroundings q2h and prn
		• Explain all procedures, medications, and treatments
		• Avoid sedatives and hypnotics; if necessary, use lorazepam, oxazepam, or promethazine
	• Family/caregiver asks questions, expresses concerns	• Provide opportunity for family to ask questions and obtain information; offer support
		RATIONALE: *Medications are partially metabolized in the liver and may depress LOC, respirations, or BP. Protein catabolism creates increased serum ammonia which also affects LOC. Frequent monitoring of LOC and preventative protection by caregivers are essential.*
3 Ineffective Breathing Pattern *r.t. encephalopathy, diaphragmatic elevation*	• Exhibits improved respiratory status - normal VS, SaO_2	• Assess VS, SaO_2, mental status q2-4h and prn
	• Takes 12-20 deep, regular respirations/min	• Assess respiratory character, pattern, rate q2-4h and prn
	• Shows improving skin color	• Assess skin color q4h and prn
		• Perform TCDB and incentive spirometry q1-2h and prn
		• Elevate HOB 30°
		• Administer supplemental O_2
	• Returns to baseline for color, amount of secretions	• Suction as needed to assist in removal of secretions

MEDICAL

NURSING DIAGNOSES	OUTCOME CRITERIA	INTERVENTIONS
		RATIONALE: *General debilitation puts patient at risk for respiratory infections. Good pulmonary toilet is essential because ascites puts pressure on the diaphragm, reducing lung capacity.*
4 Fluid Volume Deficit *r.t. hemorrhage from esophageal and gastric varices and/or coagulopathies*	• Shows normal VS, BP	• Monitor circulating volume - assess VS, BP, CVP (if available) q2-4h and prn
	• Shows no bleeding	• Monitor PT, PTT, platelet levels and H&H • Monitor for s/s of GI hemorrhage - decreased BP - tachycardia - bright red or coffee-ground emesis, melena - hematochezia - positive stool or emesis guaiac • Inspect for presence of ecchymosis, petechiae, and/or spontaneous bleeding from mucous membranes • Keep NGT on constant or low intermittent suction • Irrigate NGT prn as needed to maintain patency • Lavage NGT until clear if NG fluid appears bloody as directed
	• Exhibits normal blood values for bleeding, clotting factors - stable/normal H&H with supplemental products - coagulation values WNL	• Use small gauge needles (20-22 gauge) for venipuncture except for blood administration; apply prolonged, gentle pressure after injections
	• Achieves balanced I&O	• Monitor I&O q8h • Anticipate use of vasopressin IV and nitroglycerin

NURSING DIAGNOSES	OUTCOME CRITERIA	INTERVENTIONS

RATIONALE: *Constant and frequent monitoring of fluid volume variables prompts early detection and management of negative trends. Vasopressin reduces blood flow to the abdominal organs, reducing portal pressure and portal blood flow. Nitroglycerin products help counteract the increased afterload induced by vasopressin.*

OTHER LESS COMMON NURSING DIAGNOSES: *High Risk for Injury; Impaired Skin Integrity; Activity Intolerance; Ineffective Individual Coping; Self-Esteem Disturbance; Impaired Physical Mobility; Pain; Anxiety; Knowledge Deficit*

ESSENTIAL DISCHARGE CRITERIA

- Shows H&H, clotting factors, fluids and electrolytes within acceptable parameters
- Is oriented to person, place, time
- Maintains stable weight
- Takes, retains adequate nutrition with positive nitrogen balance
- Exhibits effective respiratory pattern without distress

MEDICAL

COLITIS, ULCERATIVE

NURSING DIAGNOSES	OUTCOME CRITERIA	INTERVENTIONS
1 Fluid Volume Deficit *r.t. diarrhea, bleeding, sequestering of fluid in the bowel (toxic megacolon), nausea and vomiting*	• Displays good skin turgor, moist mucous membranes	• Assess skin turgor, mucous membranes
	• Achieves balanced I&O	• Measure and record all fluid intake and measurable output including diarrhea
	• Shows normal serum electrolytes	• Assess serum laboratory values and observe for the development of imbalances • Administer the prescribed volumes of fluids and electrolytes
		RATIONALE: *Inadequate intravascular volume disrupts recovery. Electrolyte imbalances may accompany fluid loss. Profuse diarrhea leads to loss of fluids and electrolytes.*
2 Diarrhea *r.t. intestinal inflammatory process*	• Manifests decrease in the number and volume of stools per day; stools are of normal consistency	• Assess pattern of bowel elimination: frequency, consistency, color, amount, presence of blood, mucus, pus • Observe for fever, tachycardia, lethargy, leukocytosis • Maintain a clean, dry, and odor-free environment
	• Perineal skin is clear, clean, intact	• Provide gentle but thorough perineal care • Administer medications (corticosteroids, antidiarrheals) • Observe for side effects of steroids if given on a long-term basis

	• Displays positive coping behaviors
	  - paces activities
	  - participates in care
	  - discusses concerns
	  - seeks support from family, staff as needed
		• Provide for periods of rest
		
		• Reinforce patient's positive strategies for dealing with stress; teach positive coping strategies if necessary

NURSING DIAGNOSES	OUTCOME CRITERIA	INTERVENTIONS
		RATIONALE: *Assessment of bowel elimination assists in evaluation of therapy. Good perineal care prevents irritation. Physical rest and control of stress provide some relief from diarrhea by decreasing intestinal motility. Pharmacotherapy is aimed at either decreasing inflammation or directly suppressing the immune system. Medications include anti-inflammatory, antibacterial, antimetabolic, antibiotic, anti-infective, and antidiarrheal agents.*
3 Altered Nutrition: Less than body requirements *r.t. diarrhea, pain, inflammatory process, maldigestion, malabsorption, anorexia, nausea and vomiting*	• Maintains, regains weight	• Monitor weight daily
	• Takes, retains at least 80 percent of meals	• Monitor patient's acceptance and tolerance of food type and amount taken orally • Consult dietitian and reinforce teaching of diet
	• Patient/family participate in diet planning	• Involve appropriate family members/friends in nutritional plan and teaching

	• Shows normal lab values
	  - WBC count
	  - H&H, blood glucose
	  - electrolytes
	  - serum albumin
		• Assess WBC count, H&H, blood glucose, electrolytes, serum albumin

	• Shows no negative effects of TPN
	  - local infection
	  - elevated temperature
		• If on TPN
		  - assess IV site
		  - maintain sterility of the line
		  - change dressing at least 3 times weekly
		  - assess for complications of IV therapy

	• Has no vomiting
	• Passes normal stools
		• If on enteral nutrition
		  - care for NGT
		  - assess abdominal distention, diarrhea, nausea and vomiting, tube placement

MEDICAL

NURSING DIAGNOSES	OUTCOME CRITERIA	INTERVENTIONS

		• If on oral diet
		  - encourage food high in calories, protein, vitamins, and carbohydrates
		  - instruct about possible danger of raw fruits, vegetables, condiments, whole grain cereals, gas-forming and fried foods, alcohol, and iced drinks
		  - encourage small, frequent feedings/meals
		• Maintain good oral hygiene

RATIONALE: *The intake of protein, carbohydrates, fats, vitamins, and other nutrients are necessary to maintain resistance to infection, promote tissue repair, and enhance the effectiveness of steroids. During an acute exacerbation of the disease, energy requirements are increased because of the inflammatory process, fever and the catabolic effects of steroid therapy. TPN, if needed, allows the inflamed bowel to rest and the depleted body to restore itself.*

4 Impaired Skin Integrity

r.t. diarrhea, malnutrition, dehydration

	OUTCOME CRITERIA	INTERVENTIONS
	• Maintains integrity of skin	• Ensure skin in the anal regions is kept clean and dry • Gently wash with plain water and pat dry; avoid soap • Use a protective barrier on skin; do not use toilet paper (use squirt bottle instead of wiping) • Provide treatments for perianal fissures as ordered • Use pressure reduction surfaces as appropriate
	• Takes, retains required fluids, foods	• Maintain hydration • Increase protein and carbohydrate intake to maintain a positive nitrogen balance

RATIONALE: *The skin needs to be protected from damage due to enzymatic intestinal drainage. If the patient is dehydrated and malnourished, the skin is at further risk.*

NURSING DIAGNOSES	OUTCOME CRITERIA	INTERVENTIONS
5 Ineffective Individual Coping *r.t. chronicity of disorder*	• Verbalizes feelings related to emotional state	• Explain all diagnostic tests and procedures, what the patient will experience and feel, and what preparations are involved • Provide support during and after the procedures
	• Identifies personal coping patterns and strengths	• Allow time and provide opportunities for ventilation of fears, anger, frustrations, and questions • Involve family members/friends whenever possible
	• Makes decisions and follows through with appropriate actions to deal with issues related to health status	• Consult other professionals (such as social workers) to deal with issues of finances, employment, and coping with a chronic illness • Refer to support groups and organizations as appropriate
		RATIONALE: *Patients who are involved in their own care are informed and have resources that enhance control and reinforce effective coping skills. Involvement of family/friends provides support and helps the patient cope.*
6 Knowledge Deficit *r.t. lack of information or recall*	• Patient/family discuss pathophysiology of disease process, rationale for treatment • Patient/family verbalize knowledge of complications • Patient/family list reportable s/s	• Educate patient/family about ulcerative colitis - the recurrence and significance of symptoms and early signs of complications (such as toxic megacolon)
	• Patient/family discuss/verbalize knowledge of medications	• Review medications (including purpose, effects, and side effects of prescribed drugs and the rationale for compliance)
	• Patient/family discuss relaxation, activity, diet	• Provide surveillance for - diet - need for rest, optimal nutrition, and stress management (including the utilization of a variety of coping skills)

MEDICAL

NURSING DIAGNOSES	OUTCOME CRITERIA	INTERVENTIONS
	• Patient/family verbalize knowledge of follow-up appointments	• Discuss follow-up needs - support groups and organizations - the need for regular monitoring of disease and therapy

RATIONALE: *Knowledge about the illness and the results of diagnostic tests and therapy may help to decrease anxiety and enable realistic goal-setting. Knowledge about the recurrence and significance of certain symptoms is necessary so that the patient will seek help early to avoid serious complications.*

OTHER LESS COMMON NURSING DIAGNOSES: *Sleep Pattern Disturbance; Impaired Social Interaction; Body Image Disturbance; Altered Family Processes; Pain; Activity Intolerance; Altered Sexuality Patterns*

ESSENTIAL DISCHARGE CRITERIA

- Lab values WNL
- Experiences decrease in the number and volume of stools per day so that dehydration is no longer a risk
- Has positive nitrogen balance
- Identifies situations that create stress and anxiety and how to cope/obtain help

- Maintains skin integrity
- Patient/family verbalize accurate knowledge of physiology of disease, potential complications
- Patient/family list/discuss medications/regimen, dietary management
- Possesses written follow-up appointments

CONGESTIVE HEART FAILURE

NURSING DIAGNOSES	OUTCOME CRITERIA	INTERVENTIONS

1 Decreased Cardiac Output
 	
r.t. decreased pumping ability of the heart
	• Shows improved cardiac output
	  - systolic BP = or > 95 mmHg
	  - HR < 100 BPM; strong bounding pulse
	  - urinary output + 50 mL/h
		• Assess for changes in BP, HR, heart sounds, peripheral pulses, and signs of decreased tissue perfusion, such as cool skin, diaphoresis q4h
		
		• Report any decrease in BP systolic < 85 mmHg or 20 mmHg decreased from baseline
		
		• Report any HR > 100 BPM
		  - minimize activity; require complete bed rest and explain rationale
		
		• Monitor ECG for dysrhythmia
		
		• Monitor serum digitalis levels periodically

		RATIONALE: *Incidence of digitalis toxicity is high due to narrow margin between therapeutic and toxic ranges. Digitalis increases heart pump efficiency, which improves tissue perfusion and decreases pulmonary congestion.*
2 Fluid Volume Excess *r.t. compromised regulatory mechanism*	• Achieves, maintains balanced I&O	• Monitor I&O, serum electrolytes, and calculate 24 h fluid balance
	• Shows stable body weight	• Monitor daily weights
	• Shows decreased dyspnea, cyanosis; reduced neck vein engorgement; reduced, absent edema	• Assess for changes in breath sounds, RR and depth, neck vein distention and peripheral edema
	• Shows normal VS, acceptable BP	• Monitor PCWP (in the presence of a PA catheter)
	• Displays no edema	• Note increased amount of sputum, dyspnea, tachypnea, orthopnea, cough, and increased fatigue • Observe for anasarca • Elevate feet when sitting
	• Shows serum Na, K WNL	• Limit fluid intake and salt intake; teach rationale for these limitations • Administer drugs that will alleviate fluid excess/congestion: diuretics, inotropic and unloading agents

NURSING DIAGNOSES	OUTCOME CRITERIA	INTERVENTIONS

- Maintain semi-high Fowler's position
- Administer O_2 as ordered
- Monitor SaO_2
- Refer to home health for home O_2, as indicated

RATIONALE: *Increased fluid in lungs restricts oxygenation producing these symptoms, which may indicate left heart failure. Venous congestion in the systemic circulation indicates right-side heart failure. Several factors can result in tissue edema. These include increased vascular fluid resulting from decreased cardiac output, increased hydrostatic pressure, and decreased colloidal holding pressure.*

3 Impaired Gas Exchange

r.t. increased pulmonary capillary pressure and alveolar-capillary membrane changes

- Shows $SaO_2 > 90$ percent (when lying flat for measurement only)

- Displays improved respiratory function
  - absent or decreased SOB, dyspnea
  - respirations unlabored
  - RR WNL
  - decreased crackles on auscultation
  - clearing chest x-rays

- Monitor ABGs and/or SaO_2 regularly

- Monitor respiratory function q2h: SOB, dyspnea, orthopnea, tachypnea, use of accessory muscles, loud gurgling respirations, cough, restlessness, confusion
- Assess breath sounds: degree of crackles
- Assess characteristic of pulmonary secretions: pink, frothy secretions
- Place in high Fowler's position
- Suction q2-4h (if necessary)
- Provide O_2 support, e.g., nasal cannula, O_2 mask, or mechanical ventilation
- Monitor chest x-rays
- Administer medications that will relieve pulmonary congestion
- Prepare for intubation and assisted ventilation, if required
- Consult with respiratory therapist as indicated

NURSING DIAGNOSES	OUTCOME CRITERIA	INTERVENTIONS

RATIONALE: *These measures improve tissue oxygenation and minimize respiratory distress.*

---

4 Activity Intolerance

r.t. decreased cardiac output, insufficient O_2 for ADL

- Exhibits minimal cardiovascular distress with simple ADL (i.e., eating, personal hygiene), procedures, or treatments

- Assess patient's cardiovascular response to activities: tachycardia, increasing SOB or dyspnea, hypotension or hypertension, dysrhythmias
- Explain and discuss with patient those activities that potentiate cardiovascular distress
- Check VS before and after an activity
- Advance activity from commode privileges to ambulation with minimal assistance
- Provide rest between activities
- Encourage verbalization regarding limitations
- Refer to a cardiac rehabilitation for a progressive ambulation and activity program

RATIONALE: *Pacing of activities in collaboration with patient increases his/her psychological morale and provides concrete examples of appropriate and inappropriate activities.*

---

5 Impaired Skin Integrity

r.t. prolonged bed rest, peripheral edema, decreased cardiac output

- Maintains skin free of ulcerations

- Assess skin condition q2-4h
- Reposition q2h
- Keep skin dry at all times
- Provide a pressure-relieving device, i.e., high float mattress, airflow mattress, heel protectors

RATIONALE: *Relieving pressure areas improves tissue perfusion, ensuring skin integrity.*

MEDICAL

NURSING DIAGNOSES	OUTCOME CRITERIA	INTERVENTIONS
6 Knowledge Deficit *r.t. lack of exposure to disease process and/or treatment plans*	• Patient/family discuss pathophysiology of disease process, rationale for treatment	• Review symptoms associated with the disease process: SOB, rapid weight gain, edema, and easy fatigability
	• Patient/family discuss medications: dosage, effects, side effects	• Explain actions and side effects of medications, i.e., furosemide, digoxin, capoten, dobutamine
	• Patient/family discuss rest, activity, diet	• Explain importance of decreased Na intake in the diet; if necessary, refer to a dietitian for detailed instructions
	• Patient/family participate in care activities; discuss rationale, risk factors	• Explain patient and family role in controlling risk factors to prevent acute episodes of CHF
	• Patient/family express concerns, ask questions, seek clarification	• Provide verbal and written instructions • Encourage patient and family to ask questions

RATIONALE: *A patient's participation in the plan of care and in the planning of his/her lifestyle changes increase the effectiveness of the required treatment regimen.*

> ***OTHER LESS COMMON NURSING DIAGNOSES:*** *Anxiety;*
> *Altered Tissue Perfusion (cardiopulmonary); Diversional Activity Deficit;*
> *Altered Nutrition: Less than body requirements; Spiritual Distress; Pain*

ESSENTIAL DISCHARGE CRITERIA

• Exhibits decreased s/s of respiratory distress/dysfunction: absence of SOB at rest or on minimal exertion; absence or decreased crackles; unlabored breathing

• Tolerates simple ADL (eating, bathing, toileting, etc.) without cardiovascular compromise

• Skin is free from ulcerations

• Verbalizes understanding of regimen for disease process and participates actively in the plan of care

• Verbalizes understanding of s/s to report to physician

DEEP VENOUS THROMBOSIS

NURSING DIAGNOSES	OUTCOME CRITERIA	INTERVENTIONS

1 Altered Tissue Perfusion (peripheral)
 	
r.t. venous interruption of flow
	• Is free of s/s of DVT
	  - distal pulses on affected extremity WNL for patient
	  - warm extremity
	  - absence of pain
		• Assess status of venous circulation
		  - diminished or absent peripheral pulses
		  - unusual warmth and redness or coolness and cyanosis
		  - leg pain
		  - sudden severe chest pain
		  - dyspnea
		  - tachypnea
		
		• Monitor for increase in circumference of calf or thigh

	• Shows anticoagulation studies within therapeutic range	• Monitor for s/s of anticoagulant therapy complications (bleeding gums, petechiae, epistasis) • Administer, monitor results of anticoagulant therapy qd
	• Complies with required treatment and preventative measures	• Elevate affected extremity above heart level • Encourage PO intake and adequate hydration • Discourage smoking • Administer analgesic and warm, moist heat for leg pain as ordered • Restrict activity as ordered (usually bed rest 4-7 d) • Assess circulatory flow in affected extremity with Doppler at least q2-4h • Consult physician regarding use of alternating-pressure stockings

RATIONALE: *DVT causes insufficient or absent blood flow to affected limb. This results in life-threatening and painful complications. Specific monitoring techniques detect complications and prevent potentially life-threatening problems.*

MEDICAL

NURSING DIAGNOSES	OUTCOME CRITERIA	INTERVENTIONS

2 Knowledge Deficit

r.t. unfamiliarity with medical regimen

- Describes disease process: factors contributing to symptoms; procedure(s) for disease control

- Explain that lifestyle changes and new learning takes time to integrate
  - provide printed material regarding anticoagulant therapy and risk factor reduction
  - explain whom to contact with questions

RATIONALE: *DVT, particularly in the lower extremities, is the main predisposing factor for pulmonary emboli.*

OTHER LESS COMMON NURSING DIAGNOSES: *Pain; Impaired Skin Integrity; Anxiety*

ESSENTIAL DISCHARGE CRITERIA

- Shows VS WNL

- Shows adequate anticoagulation levels as indicated by PT, PTT, or clotting time

- Shows no signs of DVT

- Verbalizes correct knowledge of anticoagulant therapy management

- Verbalizes realistic plans to reduce risk factors for recurrence of DVT

DIABETES MELLITUS

NURSING DIAGNOSES	OUTCOME CRITERIA	INTERVENTIONS
1 Altered Nutrition: More than body requirements *r.t. excess dietary intake or ineffective utilization of nutrients*	• Achieves, maintains normal blood glucose and glycosylated Hb levels	• Monitor blood glucose and Hb
	• Achieves, maintains IBW	• Weigh daily • Instruct regarding patient-specific diet • Identify barriers to attainment of IBW • Identify interventions to overcome barriers to IBW • Initiate patient-specific exercise programs
		RATIONALE: *Attainment of IBW alters need for insulin and improves utilization of available insulin.*
2 Altered Nutrition: Less than body requirements *r.t. inadequate dietary intake or ineffective utilization of body nutrients*	• Demonstrates normal blood glucose and glycosylated Hb levels	• Monitor blood glucose and Hb
	• Achieves, maintains IBW	• Instruct regarding ideal patient-specific diet • Administer oral hypoglycemic agent or insulin
		RATIONALE: *Weight loss is reflective of poor glycemic control.*
3 High Risk for Fluid Volume Deficit *r.t. diuretic effects of hyperglycemia*	• Urinary sp. gr. WNL • Serum electrolytes WNL	• Maintain adequate hydration of at least 2000 mL/d in adult by oral or IV route, unless contraindicated

	• Shows no evidence of glycosuria
	  - no orthostatic BP, pulse changes
	  - skin turgor intact
		• Support dietary compliance
		• Administer oral hypoglycemic agent or insulin as directed

		RATIONALE: *Attainment of normal glycemic levels removes diuretic stimulation.*

MEDICAL

117

NURSING DIAGNOSES	OUTCOME CRITERIA	INTERVENTIONS
4 Sensory/ Perceptual Alterations (visual) *r.t. diabetic retinopathy*	• Is free of anatomic and physiologic ocular changes associated with DM	• Administer correct dose of oral hypoglycemic agent or insulin
	• Maintains normal vision with or without assistive devices	• Instruct in the importance of obtaining visual exams at recommended intervals
		RATIONALE: *Maintenance of normal glycemic control delays or attenuates sequelae of DM. Regular periodic visual screening detects early changes and prompts timely treatment.*
5 High Risk for Injury *r.t. sensory/perceptual alterations in tactile sensation associated with neurologic and vascular changes*	• Maintains intact sensory response to tactile stimulation, temperature, and pressure	• Instruct regarding awareness of this possible sequelae
	• Experiences no injury, tissue damage	• Instruct in importance of daily feet examination • Identify and eliminate potential environmental hazards for injury
		RATIONALE: *Awareness of injury-producing situations may eliminate possible injury.*
6 High Risk for Infection *r.t. hyperglycemia*	• Is free from s/s of infection - no breaks in skin - no skin rashes associated with elevated blood glucose	• Inspect skin q8h • Provide regular bathing • Apply emollients to dry skin • Instruct regarding s/s of infection
		RATIONALE: *Normal glycemic control lowers risk for infections and improves healing. Intact skin lowers risk of infection.*

NURSING DIAGNOSES	OUTCOME CRITERIA	INTERVENTIONS
7 Altered Sexuality Pattern *r.t. effects of chronic illness*	• Reports satisfaction with sexual activity	• Administer correct dose of oral hypoglycemic agent or insulin • Propose altered sexual activities based on limitations of disease • Eliminate possibility of infection, i.e., UTI or vaginitis • Provide support in ventilation of feelings
		RATIONALE: *Maintenance of normal glycemic control may delay or attenuate sequelae of DM, such as impotence. Providing alternatives improves quality of life.*
8 Knowledge Deficit *r.t. unfamiliarity with information resources*	• Is free of s/s of hypoglycemia	• Maintain regular, consistent dietary intake • Alter insulin dosage or dietary intake prior to exercise • Maintain proper dose, time, and site rotation for insulin administration
	• Patient/family demonstrate correct technique for insulin injection	• Teach correct techniques related to insulin injections
	• Describes, follows recommendations for management of hypoglycemic episodes	• Instruct regarding prevention and management of hypoglycemic episodes • Instruct where to obtain information resources, supplies • Consult with educator knowledgeable of diabetes
		RATIONALE: *Maintenance of regular dietary intake and accommodations for exercise prevent hypoglycemia. If hypoglycemic symptoms occur, timely response prevents further problems.*

MEDICAL

NURSING DIAGNOSES	OUTCOME CRITERIA	INTERVENTIONS
9 Body Image Disturbance *r.t. chronic disease*	• Maintains a positive body image	• Provide support in ventilation of feelings
	• Demonstrates prescribed self-care recommendations	• Instruct in self-care measures regarding diet, hygiene, exercise, foot care, medication administration, blood glucose monitoring
	• Verbalizes confidence in ability to manage the disease	• Discuss importance of periodic health screening measures • Provide information regarding support groups, home health, and/or American Diabetes Association

RATIONALE: *Providing instruction and support in self-management of chronic disease increases the patient's competence.*

> **OTHER LESS COMMON NURSING DIAGNOSES:** *Impaired Skin Integrity; Anxiety; Altered Urine Elimination; Activity Intolerance; Ineffective Family Coping: Compromised; Noncompliance; Self-Care Deficit*

ESSENTIAL DISCHARGE CRITERIA

• Maintains normal body weight

• Shows blood glucose, serum electrolytes WNL

• Is free of injury related to impaired sensory responses

• Demonstrates self-administration of insulin, using correct techniques

• Verbalizes knowledge of diet plan

• Describes s/s of hypoglycemia and its management

• Describes s/s of reportable complications

• Has follow-up appointment with care provider

DISSEMINATED INTRAVASCULAR COAGULATION

NURSING DIAGNOSES	OUTCOME CRITERIA	INTERVENTIONS
1 Fluid Volume Deficit *r.t. bleeding*	• Shows VS WNL	• Assess VS qh and prn during bleeding episode
	• Maintains sufficient circulatory volume - normal LOC - normal BP - moist mucous membranes - stable, normal weight - normal serum electrolytes, H&H - normal urinary volume	• Assess LOC qh • Assess lungs, heart, jugular veins for fluid balance • Assess mucous membranes for hydration • Monitor daily weights, I&O, H&H
	• Shows no evidence of bleeding - no increase in abdominal girth - no petechiae, ecchymosis - no frank or occult blood in excretions - no bleeding from skin cuts, abrasions	• Auscultate abdomen • Assess skin for petechiae and ecchymotic areas • Determine presence of blood in stool, emesis, urine, and sputum • Determine presence of abdominal pain • Monitor serum electrolytes and UA • Enforce complete bed rest during bleeding episodes • Avoid using injections or razors • Provide gentle care to skin, mucosa, nails, injection sites • Administer heparin as ordered • Notify physician, administer blood components, and IV fluids as indicated
		RATIONALE: *These assessments determine degree of blood loss and need for further replacement and help prevent further complications, i.e., renal failure. Safety measures prevent further bleeding.*
2 Impaired Gas Exchange *r.t. arterial hypotension*	• Maintains adequate O_2 exchange - clear breath sounds	• Assess skin color and temperature • Auscultate breath sounds • Position in Semi-Fowler's with legs elevated • Alternate rest with activity when bed rest is no longer necessary

MEDICAL

NURSING DIAGNOSES	OUTCOME CRITERIA	INTERVENTIONS
		• Administer O₂ prn as ordered
	• Shows balanced ventilation perfusion ratios	• Monitor lab results
		RATIONALE: *These measures monitor the adequacy of breathing and tissue oxygenation and detect needs for further balancing O₂ supply and demand. Positioning and pacing promote chest expansion and cardiac output.*
3 Altered Tissue Perfusion (cardio-pulmonary) *r.t. interrupted blood flow*	• Shows VS WNL • Has pulses present	• Monitor apical and peripheral pulses qh
	• Shows ABGs, H&H WNL	• Administer antiarrhythmics, cardiotonics, and vasoactive drugs as ordered
		RATIONALE: *These measures determine pumping action of heart and correct dysrhythmias, slow HR, and improve cardiac output.*
4 Fear *r.t. bleeding*	• Is oriented, alert, and calm	• Encourage verbalization of fears • Correct distorted perceptions; orient to the environment; explain procedures
		RATIONALE: *Verbalization helps the patient identify real sources of fear. This helps to reduce fear of the unfamiliar and to strengthen effective coping strategies.*

> **OTHER LESS COMMON NURSING DIAGNOSES:**
> *Altered Urinary Elimination; Sensory/Perceptual Alterations; Anxiety; Pain*

ESSENTIAL DISCHARGE CRITERIA

- Shows H&H, ABGs, serum electrolytes, VS, I&O WNL
- Is calm, alert, and oriented
- Patient/family verbalize knowledge of follow-up plan

MEDICAL

GASTROINTESTINAL BLEEDING

NURSING DIAGNOSES	OUTCOME CRITERIA	INTERVENTIONS

1 Altered Tissue Perfusion (renal, cerebral, cardiopulmonary, gastrointestinal, peripheral)

r.t. blood loss

- Exhibits adequate tissue perfusion
  - stabilized VS; no dysrhythmias
  - adequate urine output
  - warm skin
  - palpable peripheral pulses
  - baseline cognitive function
  - bowel sounds
  - H&H WNL
  - ABGs WNL

- Maintain strict I&O
- Monitor VS q15 min during acute phase, then q30 for 1 h and qh for 4 h; include orthostatic VS
- Monitor skin for coolness, pallor, diaphoresis, delayed CRT and weak, thready pulse
- Assess for s/s of hypoxia, e.g., decreased LOC
- Assess for s/s of myocardial ischemia and dysrhythmias
- Monitor H&H and platelets
- Assess for adequacy of drug treatment
- Administer IV fluids including blood products
- Monitor effectiveness of O$_2$ therapy/pulse oxymetry

RATIONALE: *Stable VS, adequate urinary output, warm/dry skin, absence of abdominal pain, normal pulse oxymetry, and baseline cognitive function are good indicators of tissue perfusion, which must be maintained to prevent irreversible system failure.*

---

2 Fluid Volume Deficit

r.t. blood loss

- Shows normal circulating volume
  - BP WNL
  - CRT < 3 sec
  - balanced fluids and electrolytes
  - stable body weight
  - no evidence of bleeding

- Montor BP, I&O
- Assess CRT
- Observe for bleeding; note characteristics of emesis; heme test emesis or NG output
- Monitor stool characteristics; heme test all stools
- Observe other possible sites of bleeding, e.g., drains, tubes; liver (palpate)
- Weigh daily
- Assess abdomen for increased pain, tenderness, and distention
- Insert NGT, if indicated
- Auscultate for hyperactive bowel sounds q8h

NURSING DIAGNOSES	OUTCOME CRITERIA	INTERVENTIONS
		• Prepare for surgery if indicated
		RATIONALE: *Continued blood and fluid loss from any source without replacement can lead to hypovolemic shock, hypoperfusion, and, if untreated, death.*
3 Anxiety *r.t. bleeding threat to health status*	• Verbalizes feelings	• Inform of procedures and treatments • Provide a calm, restful environment
	• Appears relaxed with decreased signs of anxiety and restlessness	• Note behavior clues, e.g., restlessness, anxiety, irritability, combativeness
	• Exhibits no physiologic s/s of anxiety	• Monitor physiologic responses, e.g., tachypnea, palpitations, vertigo, headache, tingling sensations (distinguish from s/s of shock) • Medicate for anxiety, if indicated • Protect from injury, if indicated • Demonstrate relaxation techniques, if appropriate
		RATIONALE: *These interventions help reduce anxiety and support patient's coping skills, thus decreasing psychological stress response.*
4 Knowledge Deficit *r.t. unfamiliarity with GI bleeding and treatment*	• Patient/family verbalizes knowledge about the illness, s/s, treatments, surgical interventions	• Assess patient/family understanding of the illness and readiness to learn • Explain disease process, any treatments or procedures, or surgical interventions
	• Lists and describes medications: dosages, effects, side effects	• Review medications and follow-up care

MEDICAL

NURSING DIAGNOSES	OUTCOME CRITERIA	INTERVENTIONS

	• Recognizes s/s of complications and why they should be reported	• Teach s/s to report to PCP
		  - coffee ground emesis
		  - red blood in the stools
		  - black tarry stools
		  - increased weakness, dizziness, restlessness
		  - cool, clammy skin
		  - increased discomfort, tenderness, or distention

	• Selects correct foods from list and correctly explains why	• Instruct patient regarding proper diet
	• Identifies probable correlations between bleeding and lifestyle; proposes feasible changes	• Encourage patient/family verbalization of the relationship between the bleeding, illness, and any lifestyle behaviors

RATIONALE: *Increased knowledge reduces anxiety and improves compliance and outcome.*

OTHER LESS COMMON NURSING DIAGNOSES: *Decreased Cardiac Output; Altered Nutrition: Less than body requirements; High Risk for Aspiration; Altered Oral Mucous Membrane; Activity Intolerance; Pain*

ESSENTIAL DISCHARGE CRITERIA

- Manifests no evidence of bleeding
- Shows H&H, electrolytes, platelets, BUN WNL
- VS WNL

- Understands s/s of recurrent GI bleeding and what to do

NURSING DIAGNOSES	OUTCOME CRITERIA	INTERVENTIONS
1 Impaired Gas Exchange *r.t. altered alveolar membrane changes*	• Maintains adequate O_2 exchange	• Auscultate breath sounds • Assess RR, depth, regularity, ease • Assess for cough • Monitor pulmonary function studies
	• ABGs WNL	• Monitor ABGs
	• Exhibits no symptoms of respiratory distress	• Provide chest physiotherapy, postural drainage q2-4h or as indicated • Instruct about breathing exercises, relaxation techniques, and energy conservation measures • Assist to high or semi-Fowler's position
	• Shows negative cultures	• Obtain sputum cultures as indicated • Encourage 3-4 L of fluid daily, unless contraindicated • Encourage smoking cessation, if applicable • In collaboration with physician, determine need for ventilatory assistance
		RATIONALE: *Sputum specimens are needed to determine appropriate antibiotic therapy. Chest physiotherapy and hydration open airways and mobilize secretions. Breathing exercises and relaxation techniques decrease respiratory effort and control O_2 demand.*
2 Altered Nutrition: Less than body requirements *r.t. diarrhea, anorexia*	• Exhibits/maintains adequate nutritional status • Maintains or regains weight	• Assess nutritional status: weight, caloric intake, I&O
	• Shows normal H&H, serum electrolytes	• Monitor H&H • Determine need for dietary changes, enteral feedings, TPN; provide vitamin supplements for deficiencies • Correct stomatitis

NURSING DIAGNOSES	OUTCOME CRITERIA	INTERVENTIONS
	• Takes, retains 80 percent or more of meals	• Administer antiemetics as ordered, 30-60 min before eating
		• Provide small, frequent, high calorie, high protein feedings
		• Have favorite foods brought from home
		• Avoid foods that stimulate intestinal motility or extreme temperatures
		• Consult with dietitian
		• Refer to Social Services, AIDS Task Force as indicated
		RATIONALE: *Assessment of nutritional status and lab values help determine lost nutrients that need replacement. Mouth care, antiemetics, and assistance with dietary selections enhance the intake and retention of essential nutrients.*
3 Diarrhea *r.t. enteric pathogens or chemotherapy*	• Resumes usual bowel habits	• Assess elimination pattern: amount and frequency of stools, associated abdominal pain (cramping), presence of blood, fat, undigested food
		• Monitor 24 h I&O
	• Shows VS WNL	• Monitor VS q4h
	• Maintains perianal skin integrity	• Provide perianal skin care after each stool with nonabrasive soap, water, and soft cloths or sponges
		• Provide sitz baths as indicated for comfort
		• Obtain stool cultures
		• Administer prescribed antibiotics and/or antidiarrheal agents (anticholinergics or opiates)

NURSING DIAGNOSES	OUTCOME CRITERIA	INTERVENTIONS

RATIONALE: *I&O and weight is monitored to determine degree of fluid deficit and weight loss. VS are monitored for evidence of hypovolemia. Perianal care helps prevent skin breakdown. Antidiarrheal agents decrease intestinal motility and spasms, enhancing absorption of needed nutrients.*

4 Impaired Skin Integrity

r.t. cutaneous effects of HIV infection

- Maintains skin integrity

- Assess skin integrity: lesions, texture, temperature, color, poor healing
- Provide regular oral care, avoiding acidic fluids
- Provide topical viscous anesthetic
- Encourage bland foods of medium temperatures
- If Kaposi's lesions are present, note change in size, color in response to chemotherapy
- Reposition at least q2h
- Encourage mobility within functional limits
- Treat pressure ulcers

RATIONALE: *Methods to improve skin integrity and prevent further breakdown will promote comfort and prevent further infections and complications.*

5 Altered Thought Processes

r.t. HIV encephalopathy

- Thought processes are optimal or improved

- Assess for alterations in mental status
  - interpretation of environment
  - changes in attention
  - routine patterns, emotions
  - LOC
  - orientation

- Is oriented to time, place, person

- Reorient as needed; identify self
- Give one direction at a time; keep conversation reality centered
- Provide clock, simple calendar

MEDICAL

NURSING DIAGNOSES	OUTCOME CRITERIA	INTERVENTIONS
		• Offer positive reinforcement for small accomplishments
		• Assist family in dealing with changes
	• Identifies medication or activity that reduces or aggravates discomfort	• Administer analgesics routinely to prevent pain
		• Ensure calm, restful, undisturbed environment, balanced with diversional stimuli as tolerated
		• Use relaxation techniques
	• Sustains no injury	• Implement measures to decrease risk of injury
		RATIONALE: *Alterations in thought processes may be due to infection, discomfort, side effects of treatment, coping mechanisms, anger, or depression. Interventions are designed to help the patient and family cope with changes, improving or maintaining functional abilities while providing a safe environment.*
6 High Risk for Activity Intolerance *r.t. infection, malnutrition, side effects of therapy*	• Has increased activity tolerance	• Assess degree of activity intolerance
	• Participates in ADL	• Assist with ADL as needed
		• Monitor tolerance to visitors, phone calls
		• Teach energy conservation measures, such as sitting while washing; evaluate response
		• Keep frequently used personal items within reach
		• In collaboration with physician, treat underlying causes of activity intolerance (pain, infection, malnutrition, sleeplessness)
		• Balance exercise with rest as tolerated
		• Consult with PT or OT
		RATIONALE: *Interventions are designed to conserve energy and reduce factors that decrease tolerance to activity.*

NURSING DIAGNOSES	OUTCOME CRITERIA	INTERVENTIONS
7 High Risk for Infection *r.t. disease process, debilitation, and invasive procedures*	• Remains free of new systemic or local infections • Manifests no odors or drainage	• Assess skin, mucous membranes, IV sites for evidence of infection
	• Exhibits normal VS - is afebrile	• Monitor for chills, night sweats, cough, difficulty breathing, white patches in mouth, swollen lymph glands, N/V, urinary urgency/ frequency, visual changes • Monitor VS, temperature q4h
	• Shows normal WBC count	• Monitor WBC count • Use strict asepsis in all invasive procedures • Initiate neutropenic precautions as needed per protocol
	• Experiences no nosocomial infections	• Restrict contact with infected persons • Maintain strict hand-washing before and after patient care • Provide clean environment
		RATIONALE: *Assessment and monitoring will detect early signs of new infection. Limiting exposure to pathogens that could be introduced by invasive procedures or infected persons will prevent nosocomial infections and further complications.*
8 Knowledge Deficit (prevention of infection transmission) *r.t. unfamiliarity with information*	• Verbalizes understanding of how to prevent transmission of HIV	• Teach importance of personal hygiene • Strongly urge patient and sexual partner to avoid exposure to body fluids • Strongly discourage IV drug abuse
		RATIONALE: *An understanding of how HIV is transmitted to other individuals increases the probability that the patient will not spread the disease to his/her contacts.*

MEDICAL

> **OTHER LESS COMMON NURSING DIAGNOSES:** *Pain; Social Isolation; Anxiety; Spiritual Distress; Body Image Disturbance; High Risk for Injury; Altered Protection; Ineffective Airway Clearance; Fluid Volume Deficit*

ESSENTIAL DISCHARGE CRITERIA

- Maintains optimal respiratory status
- Maintains adequate nutritional status
- Resumes usual bowel habits
- Has intact skin integrity

- Has optimal thought processes
- Displays improved tolerance to ADL
- Experiences no nosocomial infections
- Verbalizes understanding of how HIV is transmitted

INTESTINAL INFLAMMATION

NURSING DIAGNOSES	OUTCOME CRITERIA	INTERVENTIONS
1 Fluid Volume Deficit *r.t. inadequate intake/excessive loss of fluids (secondary to vomiting and diarrhea)*	• Achieves, maintains balanced I&O	• Monitor I&O q8h
	• Shows VS, BP WNL	• Monitor VS q4h
	• Shows serum electrolytes WNL	• Assess serum electrolytes as indicated
	• Has urinary sp. gr. WNL	• Measure urinary sp. gr. q shift
	• Has decreasing diarrhea	• Document the number and consistency of stools on chart • Assess need for IV fluids; may need to be NPO until GI upset decreases
	• Is alert, oriented	• Observe mental status changes and lethargy that may indicate fluid/electrolyte disturbances
	• Maintains stable body weight	• Weigh daily
	• Shows decreasing signs of dehydration - moist mucous membranes, good skin turgor	• Perform assessment of skin turgor, sunken eyes q4-8h
	• Takes oral fluids and foods q shift	• Offer PO fluids q1-2h (at least 30 mL) per orders; initially may need to start with ice chips • Provide fluids of choice; encourage fluids suitable for replacing electrolytes (flat 7-Up, sodas, nondairy drinks, tea, or gelatin) • As soon as fluids are tolerated, include fluids high in Na and K, such as bouillon, fruit juices • Avoid high fat or high residue foods/fluids • Include cultural and religious preferences when planning teaching

RATIONALE: *Vomiting and diarrhea may cause loss of essential electrolytes, especially H, Cl & K, and may produce alkalosis. Close monitoring and fluid and electrolyte replacement are essential.*

MEDICAL

NURSING DIAGNOSES	OUTCOME CRITERIA	INTERVENTIONS
2 **Altered Nutrition: Less than body requirements** *r.t. inadequate intake and impaired GI absorption*	• Maintains normal GI function - has no vomiting - decreasing steatorrhea	• Observe characteristics of vomitus and document • Keep NPO until acute symptoms subside • Offer clear liquids such as ice chips and 7-Up before other foods • Assess bowel sounds q shift
	• Takes, retains 80 percent of meals	• Provide frequent oral hygiene • Provide small, frequent meals of bland food • Encourage high calorie foods/fluids that can be easily digested and tolerated (may want to avoid high liquid intakes immediately prior to food and may take liquid after food instead) • Provide pleasant surroundings for eating
	• Patient/family identify ways to improve access to food	• Assess ability to access food (affordability, meal preparation, demands on energy level, etc.), when returns to the home situation • Consult with dietitian regarding need for supplements
		RATIONALE: *Identifying and avoiding foods that cause irritation enhance absorption of important nutrients.*
3 **Knowledge Deficit** *r.t. disease process and treatment*	• Identifies s/s to report to PCP • States underlying causes of gastroenteritis	• Teach s/s of dehydration to report
	• Has list of medications: dosage, effects, side effects	• Discuss OTC medications and their common side effects
	• Affirms need for high fluid intake	• Discuss importance of taking in 2500-3000 mL of fluids until diarrhea resolves

NURSING DIAGNOSES	OUTCOME CRITERIA	INTERVENTIONS
	• States correct method for food preparation at home and what methods to avoid	• Teach patient the following food preparation methods - cook food thoroughly - refrigerate foods requiring refrigeration (4-9°C, 35-45°F) - sanitize cutting instruments before preparing raw foods (chicken, raw meat, vegetables) - avoid unpasteurized milk and unchlorinated H_2O
	• Identifies food and product irritants that aggravate gastroenteritis	• Teach patient to avoid alcohol, caffeine or caffeinated beverages, spicy foods, highly seasoned or irritating foods and nicotine
		RATIONALE: *Improper food preparation is often the cause of gastroenteritis. Caffeine is a CNS stimulant and increases pepsin secretion. Nicotine reduces pancreatic bicarb secretion thus inhibiting the neutralization of acid. Nicotine also increases muscle activity of bowels which produces nausea and vomiting.*

MEDICAL

OTHER LESS COMMON NURSING DIAGNOSES: *Pain; High Risk for Impaired Skin Integrity*

ESSENTIAL DISCHARGE CRITERIA

• Maintains adequate hydration

• Maintains adequate caloric intake to meet nutritional needs

• Identifies causative factors and/or avoids irritating foods/substances

INTESTINAL OBSTRUCTION

NURSING DIAGNOSES	OUTCOME CRITERIA	INTERVENTIONS
1 Pain *r.t. physical obstruction, distension and/or strangulation of the intestines*	• Reports, displays freedom from pain	• Assess level of pain using analogue pain scale q2h
	• Identifies medication or activity that reduces or aggravates discomfort - identifies source of comfort	• Assess for rebound tenderness, guarding, and increasing pain • Administer/monitor prescribed analgesics • Provide supportive care during procedures, i.e., nasoenteral intubation • Position for comfort: from side to side; ambulate as tolerated
		RATIONALE: *Monitoring detects signs of peritonitis and perforation. Alleviating pain related to mechanical or neurogenic blockage of bowel helps minimize complications. Promoting ambulation minimizes intestinal side effects of narcotic analgesics.*
2 Fluid Volume Deficit *r.t. decreased fluid intake, vomiting, diarrhea and gastric suctioning*	• Maintains adequate fluid volume - normal VS, BP - balanced I&O - normal serum electrolytes - good skin turgor, moist mucous membranes	• Monitor VS q4h • Measure and record all I&O • Monitor pertinent lab values (electrolytes, urinary sp. gr., Hb) • Assess skin, mucous membranes q4h • Administer IV fluids as prescribed to replace/maintain fluid balance • Offer frequent mouth care • Irrigate NGT with N/S q4h • Notify physician of change in status
		RATIONALE: *Monitoring of lab values determines hydration status, acid/base balance, and potential for hypovolemic shock. Irrigating with N/S prevents electrolyte loss.*

NURSING DIAGNOSES	OUTCOME CRITERIA	INTERVENTIONS
3 Anxiety *r.t. life-threatening symptoms of bowel obstruction and hospitalization*	• Demonstrates reduced anxiety - patient/family express concerns, identify coping strengths	• Assess patient/family concerns • Assess previous life stressors and effective/ineffective coping mechanisms • Ascertain specific anxieties and provide specific therapeutic responses (patient education regarding diagnosis, treatment, and prognosis) • Encourage to describe anxieties

RATIONALE: *Exploring anxiety and effective coping mechanisms with the patient and family help reduce anxiety.*

OTHER LESS COMMON NURSING DIAGNOSES:
Altered Oral Mucous Membrane; Knowledge Deficit

MEDICAL

ESSENTIAL DISCHARGE CRITERIA

• VS, BP hydration status WNL

• Verbalizes comfort

• Demonstrates reduced anxiety

LEUKEMIA, ACUTE PHASE

NURSING DIAGNOSES	OUTCOME CRITERIA	INTERVENTIONS

1 High Risk for Infection
 	
r.t. decreased resistance secondary to abnormal WBCs
	• Remains free of infection and sepsis
	  - blood leukocyte count WNL
	  - normal VS
	  - afebrile
	  - no urinary RBCs, WBCs, or casts
		• Assess for s/s of any infection q shift
		• Monitor WBC count and differential daily
		• Check blood studies for evidence of specific pathogens
		• Take and record VS q4h; notify physician as ordered
		• Monitor urinary studies
		• Instruct about importance of self-hygiene, including oral care qid
		• Place patient in reverse isolation
		• Post sign to remind staff and visitors to wash hands frequently and not enter room if ill

	• Experiences no adverse effects of antibiotics	• Give antibiotics and neutrophil-stimulating medications as ordered
		RATIONALE: *Protection prevents exposure and improves resistance to pathogens.*
2 Altered Tissue Perfusion (cardio-pulmonary) *r.t. blood loss and chemotherapy*	• Demonstrates minimal fatigue during ADL	• Assess for dizziness, tachycardia, headache, dyspnea with activity and modify as needed
	• Shows improving H&H	• Monitor daily H&H
	• Tolerates progressive activity increases	• Assist in organizing activities to minimize unnecessary exertion; plan for rest periods • Administer PRBCs as ordered, O_2 as needed for SOB • Encourage gradual increase in activities, including exercise, per physician's orders
		RATIONALE: *A balanced combination of rest and activity maintains muscle strength and function.*

NURSING DIAGNOSES	OUTCOME CRITERIA	INTERVENTIONS
3 Altered Tissue Perfusion (peripheral) *r.t. decreased platelets and bleeding*	• Risk of bleeding is minimized - no evidence of injury or bleeding from trauma	• Assess for s/s of bleeding q shift: petechiae, hematomas, epistaxis, blurred vision, headache, blood in urine or stool
	• BP WNL	• Monitor BP q4h
	• Shows normalizing lab values - platelets - H&H	• Monitor platelet count, H&H daily
	• Experiences minimal or no bleeding from invasive procedures	• Prevent possible trauma by minimizing invasive procedures and by instructing on ADL restrictions (e.g., no razors, strenuous activities) • Post sign to inform others of bleeding precautions • Administer platelets as ordered
		RATIONALE: *It is necessary to assess adequacy of clotting elements and to prevent bleeding.*
4 Altered Nutrition: Less than body requirements *r.t. anorexia and increased metabolic rate*	• Maintains/regains weight	• Monitor weight at least qod
	• Takes, retains 80 percent of meals	• Monitor amount of meals taken • Provide diet with emphasis on protein, vitamins, and calories
	• Has no vomiting	• Assist with meal selection to make foods available that prevent aversions, nausea, oral pain • Give antiemetics as needed • Consult with dietitian, if special meals are required
	• Patient/family identify prescribed foods	• Encourage family to bring in small portions as allowed by prescribed diet
		RATIONALE: *Prevention of nausea and vomiting and the tailoring of meals promote optimal nutrition, weight maintenance, and antibody enhancement.*

MEDICAL

NURSING DIAGNOSES	OUTCOME CRITERIA	INTERVENTIONS
5 Knowledge Deficit *r.t. unfamiliarity with condition, nutritional requirements, and drug therapy*	• Demonstrates adequate understanding of disease and treatment plan - nutrition - reportable s/s - medications - infection prevention - pain control - activity - family concerns, questions	• Assess patient's/family's knowledge base regarding treatment plan • Allay patient's and family's fears • Provide additional teaching as needed - fluid balance and nutrition - reportable s/s (infection, bleeding) - medications, antibiotics - preventing infection and injury - pain relief strategies
	• Patient/family participate in care activities	• Establish patient's and family's roles in the treatment plan
	• Patient/family express commitment to consistent follow-up	• Assist patient/family to direct questions to health team members, physician, MSW, community health agencies

RATIONALE: *A knowledgeable and competent patient/family are likely to successfully manage long-term care needs.*

OTHER LESS COMMON NURSING DIAGNOSES: *Altered Urinary Elimination; Diarrhea; Pain; Anxiety; Spiritual Distress; Body Image Disturbance; Social Isolation; Altered Sexuality Patterns; Altered Oral Mucous Membrane*

ESSENTIAL DISCHARGE CRITERIA

- Is free of any life-threatening infection, bleeding, or injury
- Is free of critically low CBC and platelet values
- Body weight and VS WNL
- Performs ADL with minimal discomfort or fatigue

MENINGITIS, BACTERIAL OR VIRAL

NURSING DIAGNOSES	OUTCOME CRITERIA	INTERVENTIONS
1 High Risk for Infection *r.t. presence of pathogens in CSF and respiratory secretions*	• Has normal breath sounds	• Assess lungs for adventitious breath sounds q4h • Assess depth and quality of respirations q4h
	• Is afebrile	• Monitor temperature q4h • Administer antimicrobial agents as ordered; assess for side effects • Explain the purpose of respiratory isolation to patient and significant other • Observe respiratory isolation precautions for 24 h from the initiation of antimicrobial therapy
		RATIONALE: *These measures minimize complications and prevent the transmission of the disease.*
2 Altered Tissue Perfusion (cerebral) *r.t. inflammation/ edema of the brain and meninges*	• Demonstrates no evidence of increased ICP - decreased LOC - increased BP with widened pulse pressure - unequal pupillary response	• Monitor LOC q4h • Assess respiratory pattern and rhythm q4h • Assess for presence of unequal pupillary response q4h • Assess HR and rhythm q4h
	• Demonstrates adequate cerebral perfusion - no evidence of apnea (after hyperventilation) or Cheyne-Stokes respirations - no evidence of bradycardia or arrhythmias	• Report abnormalities in neurologic status to physician • Elevate head slightly • Instruct not to strain or bear down when defecating • Assist in activities that require effort such as coughing and vomiting
	• Demonstrates negative Kernig's and Brudzinski's sign	• Note presence of Kernig's and Brudzinski's sign
	• Displays no nuchal rigidity	• Assess presence of nuchal rigidity
		RATIONALE: *Frequent monitoring prompts early detection and management of increased ICP.*

MEDICAL

NURSING DIAGNOSES	OUTCOME CRITERIA	INTERVENTIONS
3 Hyperthermia *r.t. infectious process*	• Maintains temperature WNR	• Monitor q2h for temperature of 102°F or above, otherwise q4h
	• Maintains balanced I&O	• Monitor fluid I&O • Administer antipyretics as ordered • Administer cooling measures - bath with tepid water or alcohol; hypothermia blanket as ordered
		RATIONALE: *Cooling measures and antipyretics reduce fever and hypermetabolic state and ensure comfort and compensate for fluid loss associated with elevated temperature.*
4 Pain (acute) *r.t. inflammation of meninges and brain*	• Reports reasonable comfort	• Assess location, intensity, quality, and duration of pain associated with headache, fever, general aching
	• Reports comfort following analgesia	• Administer prescribed analgesics; evaluate effects of pain medications given
	• Identifies activities that reduce or aggravate discomfort	• Provide comfort measures such as ice bag on head or cold wash cloth on forehead • Maintain quiet environment • Keep room dark if photophobia is present • Maintain position of comfort with head slightly extended • Assist with bath, hygiene, and feeding as needed • Provide passive ROM exercises or supervise implementation of active ROM
		RATIONALE: *Comfort measures and analgesia relieve head and muscle aches/pain.*

NURSING DIAGNOSES	OUTCOME CRITERIA	INTERVENTIONS
5 High Risk for Injury *r.t. seizure activity, generalized weakness, vertigo, ataxia, altered LOC*	• Remains free of injury	• Ensure that side rails are up • Keep side rails padded • Keep soft roll or plastic airway and suction equipment ready at bedside • Maintain bed rest during acute phase • Maintain quiet environment • Provide restraints as ordered • Provide close supervision when getting out of bed • Apply restraints correctly if absolutely necessary
	• Exhibits stable, improving LOC	• Administer tranquilizers and antiseizure drugs as indicated
		RATIONALE: *Interventions minimize onset of seizure activity and other symptoms and prevent occurrence of injury.*
6 Anxiety *r.t. communicability of disease condition; lack of knowledge regarding illness; hospitalization*	• Verbalizes knowledge of the situation	• Instruct regarding the disease process, diagnostic procedures, and treatments
	• Verbalizes measures to control/prevent the spread of the infectious agents	• Instruct regarding the extent of isolation precautions
	• Exhibits relaxed appearance	• Include family and significant other when providing instructions • Encourage family and significant other to participate in caring for patient • Provide opportunities to verbalize needs and concerns
		RATIONALE: *Knowledge, predictability, and support alleviate anxiety.*

MEDICAL

> ***OTHER LESS COMMON NURSING DIAGNOSES:*** *Ineffective Breathing Pattern;*
> *Ineffective Airway Clearance; Impaired Physical Mobility; Bathing/Hygiene Self-Care Deficit;*
> *High Risk for Fluid Volume Deficit; Fluid Volume Excess*

ESSENTIAL DISCHARGE CRITERIA

- Is afebrile
- Is free of pain
- Is free of injury related to altered LOC

- Is able to manage ADL; if unable, home health assistance is obtained
- Parent/family are aware of needs and resources

MULTIPLE MYELOMA

NURSING DIAGNOSES	OUTCOME CRITERIA	INTERVENTIONS
1 Pain *r.t. bone destruction from disease and possible fractures*	• Reports acceptable comfort level	• Assess for evidence of fracture • Teach use of 0-10 descriptive pain scale
	• Identifies medication or activity that reduces or aggravates discomfort	• Encourage verbalization of measures such as narcotic analgesics, positioning, and alignment that prevents or decreases pain • Provide teaching to patient and family to decrease fear of "addiction" • Provide other preventative and relief measures such as heat, firm mattress, braces, distraction, positioning, appropriate body mechanics
		RATIONALE: *Narcotics are necessary to control moderate and severe pain or to reduce or eliminate pain associated with muscle spasms. Prevention and treatment of pain should include the patient's prior pain experience.*
2 High Risk for Infection *r.t. decreased resistance secondary to low WBC count*	• Is free of s/s of systemic infection - VS WNL	• Assess for s/s of infection - take and record VS q4h; notify physician as indicated
	• Lab values WNL or negative for pathogens	• Monitor WBC count and differential daily • Check blood studies for evidence of specific pathogens
	• Maintains urine free of cloudiness	• Inspect urine q8h
	• Has clear breath sounds bilaterally	• Instruct about importance of self-hygiene including oral care qid and pulmonary function (coughing and deep breathing)
	• Remains free of nosocomial infection	• Place in reverse isolation • Post sign to remind staff and visitors to wash hands frequently and not enter room if ill

MEDICAL

NURSING DIAGNOSES	OUTCOME CRITERIA	INTERVENTIONS
	• Is free of adverse effects of antibiotics	• Give antibiotics as ordered
		RATIONALE: *These measures prevent additional exposure to pathogens and detect bacteremia and sepsis.*
3 Altered Tissue Perfusion (peripheral) *r.t. bleeding*	• No evidence of injury or bleeding from trauma	• Assess for s/s of bleeding q shift: petechiae, hematomas, epistaxis, blurred vision, headache, blood in urine or stool
	• Shows H&H WNL	• Monitor platelet count, H&H daily
	• Risk of bleeding is minimized	• Prevent possible trauma by minimizing invasive procedures and by instructing on ADL restrictions (e.g., no razors, strenuous activities) • Post sign to inform others of bleeding precautions • Administer platelets and blood as ordered
		RATIONALE: *Monitoring assesses the adequacy of clotting elements and protection helps to prevent bleeding.*
4 Activity Intolerance *r.t. impaired O2 transport secondary to diminished RBC count*	• Demonstrates normal VS, perfusion, and minimal fatigue during ADL	• Assess for dizziness, tachycardia, headache, dyspnea with activity and modify as needed • Assist in organizing activities to minimize unnecessary exertions; plan for rest periods • Administer O2 as needed for SOB • Encourage gradual increase in activities, including exercise, as tolerated
		RATIONALE: *Progressive activity maintains muscle strength and function while providing adequate rest.*

NURSING DIAGNOSES	OUTCOME CRITERIA	INTERVENTIONS
5 Altered Urinary Elimination *r.t. renal obstruction from disease and increased uric acid*	• Shows balanced I&O	• Monitor I&O; report discrepancies
	• Shows creatinine, BUN, uric acid WNL	• Administer hydration (3 L/d) and medications (e.g., allopurinol) as ordered • Monitor renal function lab values as ordered • Encourage diet low in Ca and phosphorus • Give acidic juices, avoiding bicarbonates and carbonated beverages

RATIONALE: *Hydration and monitoring of renal function promote prevention of irreversible renal failure. Slightly acid urine helps to prevent the formation of calculi.*

MEDICAL

OTHER LESS COMMON NURSING DIAGNOSES: *Impaired Physical Mobility; Fluid Volume Excess; Altered Nutrition: Less than body requirements*

ESSENTIAL DISCHARGE CRITERIA

• Reports/displays sustained comfort

• Is free of infection, bleeding, or injury

• Maintains balanced daily I&O

• Ambulates freely with minimal fatigue

MULTIPLE SCLEROSIS

NURSING DIAGNOSES	OUTCOME CRITERIA	INTERVENTIONS
1 Ineffective Airway Clearance *r.t. fatigue*	• Exhibits improving pulmonary function - normal RR, depth, ease - mobilizes secretions	• Assess lung sounds q2-4h depending on condition • Assess respirations and degree of respiratory effort and cough reflex • Position for maximum respiratory expansion and control of respiratory secretions • Avoid neck flexion if immobile
	• Is free of respiratory complications	• Plan for rest periods • Assist and teach to cough and deep breathe q2-4h and as needed • Keep NPO as indicated • Suction oral pharynx as needed • Prepare to assist with ventilation if indicated
		RATIONALE: *Suctioning clears obstructions and prevents risk of aspiration. Inadequate chest excursion contributes to stasis of lungs and predisposes to infections and other respiratory complications.*
2 Altered Urinary Elimination *r.t. neuromuscular impairment*	• Is continent	• Assess degree of functional disability • Initiate bladder program as indicated and ordered - assess function and voiding pattern (frequency, urgency, incontinence) - assist as needed with scheduling voiding and fluid intake - measure I&O - catheterize intermittently as indicated
	• Empties bladder using method most appropriate (i.e., self-catheter)	• Teach Credé's maneuver and/or self-catheterization as indicated
	• Describes realistic plans to manage bladder program	• Teach diet to keep urine acidic - regular voiding times - fluid management (2000-3000 mL/d, intake q2h, restrict fluids at night) - prevention and s/s of urinary infection

NURSING DIAGNOSES	OUTCOME CRITERIA	INTERVENTIONS
		RATIONALE: *Mechanical or manual assistance may be necessary to overcome effects of demyelinization on elimination.*
3 Impaired Verbal Communication *r.t. dysarthria from neuromuscular impairment*	• Expresses self with minimum impairment	• Identify method to communicate basic needs • Explore with patient/family alternative methods of communication as needed • Encourage slow, deliberate speech • Provide upright, supported position • Provide adequate rest periods • Encourage person as well as family to verbalize feelings as long as able • Consult with speech pathologist
		RATIONALE: *Ability to communicate alleviates despair, frustration, and fear.*
4 Impaired Physical Mobility *r.t. neuromuscular weakness*	• Improves, maintains level of mobility	• Provide maximum possible mobilization
	• Demonstrates measures to increase mobility	• Teach to perform active/passive ROM at least qid • Encourage use of affected limbs as much as possible • Encourage time out of bed (chair or ambulating) to maximum of ability
	• Demonstrates use of adaptive devices to increase mobility	• Observe and teach use of adaptive devices (walkers, canes, wheelchairs, etc.)

MEDICAL

NURSING DIAGNOSES	OUTCOME CRITERIA	INTERVENTIONS

	• Uses safety measures to minimize potential for injury	• Teach safety precautions
		  - protect areas with decreased sensation from temperature extremes
		  - discuss how to recover from falls with decreased perception of legs
		  - instruct to check placement when changing positions or going through doorways
		  - instruct to shift position and lift buttocks in chair or bed q15 min
		  - instruct in wheelchair safety if appropriate
		
		• Instruct patient to walk with feet wide apart, to widen base of support and increase walking stability

RATIONALE: *Musculoskeletal activities improve circulation and muscle tone, prevent contractures, enhance sense of achievement, and decrease sense of powerlessness.*

OTHER LESS COMMON NURSING DIAGNOSES: *Altered Nutrition: Less than body requirements; Anxiety; Feeding, Bathing/Hygiene, Toileting Self-Care Deficits*

ESSENTIAL DISCHARGE CRITERIA

- Displays increased mobility
- Displays effective coughing and breathing patterns

- Is able to communicate
- Empties bladder using appropriate method

MYOCARDIAL INFARCTION (POST CCU)

NURSING DIAGNOSES	OUTCOME CRITERIA	INTERVENTIONS

1 Activity Intolerance
 	
r.t. insufficient oxygenation for ADL secondary to myocardial ischemia
	• Tolerates ADL by discharge
	  - no complaints of pain
	  - no SOB
	  - no tachycardia
		• Monitor effectiveness of medications (nitrates, beta blockers, Ca channel blockers); teach patient to use nitroglycerin SL properly
		
		• Assess for chest pain, SOB, dizziness, tachycardia, ST-T changes or dysrhythmias
		
		• Encourage gradual progression from bed rest to activity; monitor tolerance at each step of progression
		
		• Allow, encourage rest periods between activities

	• Participates in care activities; asks questions; seeks clarification of rationale for care	• Teach how and when to take pulse and check pulse parameters (before, during, and 3 min after activity) • Teach to conserve energy (pace self, sit rather than stand when possible) • Teach to avoid vagal maneuvers (heavy lifting, straining on stool) • Explain need to avoid exercise for 2 h after meals • Begin cardiac exercise program per protocol • Reinforce need to contact physician if problems, questions, or concerns
		RATIONALE: *Healing is gradual after MI as collateral circulation develops. Decreased cardiac output results in altered tolerance to activity. Nitroglycerin reduces preload and lowers myocardial O_2 demand. Beta blockers lower HR and contractility, thus reducing myocardial O_2 demand. Ca blockers cause coronary and peripheral arterial dilation.*

MEDICAL

NURSING DIAGNOSES	OUTCOME CRITERIA	INTERVENTIONS

2 Decreased Cardiac Output
 	
r.t. loss of myocardial contractility
	• Improved or maintained cardiac output
	  - normal VS, BP
	  - serum electrolytes, cardiac enzymes WNL or improving
	  - no tachycardia, irregular pulse, or third heart sound
	  - urine output WNL
	  - no jugular vein distention
	  - no cyanosis or pallor, diaphoresis
	  - CRT < 3 sec
	  - strong, palpable peripheral pulses
	  - no changes in mentation
	  - no edema or rales
		• Monitor for s/s of decreased cardiac output q1-4h
		• Monitor response to medications
		• Monitor cardiac rhythm; record rhythm strip q4h; notify physician of dysrhythmias and blocks
		• Prevent fluid overload (use caution with IV fluids; monitor I&O)

		RATIONALE: *Decreased cardiac output results in impaired tissue oxygenation. Poor ventricular function causes incomplete ejection of blood from the heart, with pulmonary or systemic congestion as a result. Dysrhythmias can occur as a result of decreased oxygenation.*

3 Anxiety
 	
r.t. actual or perceived threat to biological integrity
	• Demonstrates decreased anxiety
	  - actively participates in care activities
	  - verbalizes decreasing anxiety
	  - has relaxed facial expression and body posture
		• Assess level of anxiety
		  - observe reactions to care activities
		  - spend time using therapeutic communication to allow patient to express feelings
		• Teach how to prevent and manage anginal episodes
		• Give thorough, simple explanations and encourage questions
		• Teach relaxation techniques (progressive relaxation, guided imagery, controlled breathing)

	• Family participates in discussing, planning, providing care and support	• Explore coping mechanisms (support group) • Encourage family participation
		RATIONALE: *Anxiety can be relieved by using relaxation techniques and effective coping skills in response to stress.*

NURSING DIAGNOSES	OUTCOME CRITERIA	INTERVENTIONS
4 Altered Sexuality Patterns *r.t. fear of pain and altered self-concept*	• Identifies ways to facilitate return to prehospitalization sexuality patterns	• Explain that return to sexual activity is usually safe 5-8 weeks post infarction (when patient is able to climb 2 flights of stairs without chest pain) • Encourage patient to see physician before resuming strenuous activity • Teach to avoid sexual activity after large meals or after drinking alcohol • Teach that research has shown risk is low for a cardiac event occuring during non-strenuous sexual activity • Refer to sexual therapist if appropriate
		RATIONALE: *Patients often have concerns regarding sexuality after MI, but are reluctant to discuss these. By bringing up the topic, the nurse conveys the message that it is okay to discuss these concerns.*

5 Ineffective Management of Therapeutic Regimen
 	
r.t. complexity of regimen and lifestyle change implications
	• Describes essential facts
	  - CAD process
	  - causative and contributing factors
	  - regimen for symptom control
	  - reduction of risk factors
		• Assess learning needs and readiness to learn
		
		• Teach required knowledge
		  - normal heart anatomy and function
		  - MI/CAD effects on cardiovascular function
		  - risk factors and how to reduce them (smoking cessation, diet modification, weight and cholesterol control, BP control, stress reduction, exercise
		  - management of angina
		  - when to call/come to hospital (chest pain unrelieved by three nitroglycerin tablets in 15 min and rest, change in character or location of pain, severe fatigue, syncope, dyspnea, palpitations)

	• Verbalizes intent to follow health behaviors necessary or desirable for recovery and for decreased risk of recurrence	• Encourage questions; provide visual aids (handouts, videos, heart models) • Include spouse, caregiver in teaching

MEDICAL

NURSING DIAGNOSES	OUTCOME CRITERIA	INTERVENTIONS
	• Verbalizes knowledge of medication regimen (name of each medication, purpose, dosage, route, frequency, side effects, precautions, and special considerations or actions)	• Teach regimen for each medication

RATIONALE: *The patient needs to know the factors involved in MI and how to reduce these to decrease the risk of a repeat MI. Medications are more effective if taken properly. The patient is more apt to comply with medication regimen if it is well understood.*

OTHER LESS COMMON NURSING DIAGNOSES: Ineffective Breathing Pattern; Pain; Sleep Pattern Disturbance

ESSENTIAL DISCHARGE CRITERIA

- Is free of significant dysrhythmias or heart blocks
- Demonstrates adequate cardiac output (VS WNL, normal color and mental status, urine output WNL, absence of s/s of fluid overload)
- Experiences reduced anxiety
- Tolerates ADLs without pain, SOB, tachycardia
- Describes MI and healing process

- Identifies own risk factors and measures to reduce them
- Describes medication regimen
- Identifies s/s to report to physician and when to report to hospital
- Verbalizes sexual concerns

PANCREATITIS

NURSING DIAGNOSES	OUTCOME CRITERIA	INTERVENTIONS
1 Altered Nutrition: Less than body requirements *r.t. loss of nutrients from vomiting, inadequate fluid intake, fever and diaphoresis*	• Maintains/regains weight	• Weigh daily

	• Has decreasing GI symptoms
	  - diarrhea
	  - steatorrhea
	  - vomiting
		• Monitor output, especially stools for diarrhea, steatorrhea, and nasogastric output

	• Has adequate energy to perform ADL
	  - takes, retains 80 percent of meals
	  - normal blood glucose levels
		• Control nausea by providing small frequent feedings high in carbohydrates, protein; low in fat; bland; no stimulants (caffeine); no alcohol (least stimulating to the pancreas)
		
		• Administer insulin as indicated
		
		• Monitor blood glucose levels
		
		• Obtain dietary consult if indicated

		RATIONALE: *Adequate intake must be maintained without stimulating pancreatic secretions. Weight loss, malabsorption of fats, and hyperglycemia are problems related to pancreatic inflammation.*
2 Fluid Volume Deficit *r.t. nausea, vomiting, NG suction, decreased intake*	• Maintains balanced I&O	• Monitor I&O and electrolytes
	• Maintains stable body weight	• Weigh every day
	• Shows normal VS, BP	• Monitor VS q4h

	• Exhibits no s/s of dehydration
	  - moist mucous membranes
	  - normal skin turgor
		• Assess for signs of cardiac failure
		
		• Plan initial goal of 2000-2500 mL per day
		
		• Administer IV fluids as ordered
		
		• Electrolytes WNL

		RATIONALE: *Weight is the most accurate indicator of fluid balance. Shock is a possibility because of vasoactive peptides released from the inflamed pancreas. Extra fluids minimize risk of deficit.*

MEDICAL

NURSING DIAGNOSES	OUTCOME CRITERIA	INTERVENTIONS
3 Pain *r.t. inflammation, edema, distention of pancreas, peritoneal irritation, obstruction of the biliary tract*	• Verbalizes/displays reasonable comfort - no rigidity of abdomen	• Assess pain experience: determine intensity, location, and other accompanying symptoms • Teach to avoid foods that cause abdominal pain; emphasize that alcohol must be avoided completely
	• Reports comfort following analgesia	• Administer analgesics (preferably meperidine) as ordered to prevent pain; ascertain how long medication provides relief
	• Identifies medication or activity that reduces or aggravates discomfort	• Encourage frequent position changes • Provide calm, quiet environment
		RATIONALE: *Meperidine is preferred because it causes less spasm of smooth muscles than opiates. Pain may increase pancreatic enzymes and delay recovery.*
4 Ineffective Breathing Pattern *r.t. pulmonary complications*	• Exhibits improving respiratory status • Takes at least 12-20 deep, regular respirations/min	• Assess RR, depth and rhythm, breath sounds, sputum, cough, elevated diaphragm, fluid accumulation
	• Maintains SaO$_2$ WNL	• Monitor ABGs • Place patient in semi-Fowler's position to promote deep respirations, unless contraindicated
		RATIONALE: *Respiratory assessment provides early detection of ARDS. Taking deep breaths, coughing, and positioning clears airways and reduces atelectasis.*
5 Knowledge Deficit *r.t. new treatment regimen of dietary and alcohol restrictions, preventative measures, and follow-up care*	• Discusses relaxation, activity, diet	• Reinforce diet; emphasize eliminating pancreatic stimulants, especially alcohol; refer to detoxification program as indicated
	• Patient/family discuss medications and insulin therapy: dosages, schedules, effects, side effects	• Instruct patient/family regarding medications and insulin therapy as indicated

156

NURSING DIAGNOSES	OUTCOME CRITERIA	INTERVENTIONS
	• Patient/family have list of s/s of complications to report to physician	• Instruct about possible complications of disease, reportable s/s; provide written materials
		• Refer family to use support systems whether at home or in community

RATIONALE: *Knowledge of the illness and essential treatments may decrease repeat hospitalizations.*

OTHER LESS COMMON NURSING DIAGNOSES: *High Risk for Activity Intolerance; Impaired Home Maintenance Management; High Risk for Injury*

ESSENTIAL DISCHARGE CRITERIA

- Respiratory function WNL
- Reports relief of pain and discomfort

- Demonstrates improved fluid and nutritional status
- Verbalizes understanding of diet and avoidance of alcohol

MEDICAL

PARKINSON'S DISEASE

NURSING DIAGNOSES	OUTCOME CRITERIA	INTERVENTIONS

1 Impaired Swallowing

r.t. neuromuscular impairment

- Displays minimal difficulty with swallowing

- Assess presence of gag reflex
- Assess ability to chew/swallow
- Assess nutritional status
  - calorie count
  - 3 d intake record
- Incline HOB up 90° with meals and 30 min after
- Avoid thin liquids
- Provide bite-sized pieces
- Provide adequate time for meal consumption
- Teach how to reduce swallowing difficulty
  - avoid speaking while eating
  - move tongue to back of mouth with swallowing
  - keep chin down with swallowing
  - make conscious effort to swallow accumulated saliva
- Prepare to suction as needed
- Consult with speech/swallowing specialist

RATIONALE: *Elevated HOB aids swallowing and digestion. Thick liquids and solids are better tolerated in a patient with dysphagia. Putting chin down and proper tongue movement promote swallowing. Suctioning removes obstruction and provides patent airway.*

2 High Risk for Injury (external)

r.t. impaired postural reflexes, bradykinesia, akinesia, rigidity, tremor, and propulsive or retropulsive gait

- Remains free of injury

- Assess ability to ambulate independently
- Assess for orthostatic hypotension
- Assess BP and pulse before and after activity
- Assess environment for safety hazards and remove throw rugs, electrical cords, clutter
- Assess patient with frequent falls for levodopa toxicity
- Instruct patient to make position changes slowly

NURSING DIAGNOSES	OUTCOME CRITERIA	INTERVENTIONS
		• Encourage upright posture with ambulation and wide-based gait
		• Encourage use of nonskid slippers, eyeglasses if worn

RATIONALE: *Elders are prone to orthostatic hypotension due to impaired baroreceptor function; Parkinson's disease exacerbates this (position changes will minimize). Monitoring VS can determine activity tolerance. Falls can be a warning sign of levodopa toxicity.*

NURSING DIAGNOSES	OUTCOME CRITERIA	INTERVENTIONS
3 Impaired Physical Mobility *r.t. bradykinesia, rigidity, tremor, and impaired postural reflexes*	• Maintains full ROM	• Assess gait, balance
	• Demonstrates mobility at maximum potential	• Assess effectiveness of medication on mobility
		• Assess present activity level and encourage exercise - minimum 3x/week - 30 min sessions - ambulation, leg/arm lifts
	• Is free of new contractures	• Assist with ROM and stretching exercises every day
		• Provide instructions with ambulation - rock side to side - swing arms - "step" over imaginary line
		• Space activity with rest
		• Provide raised toilet seat
		• Consult with OT/PT for devices which facilitate ADL and self-care

RATIONALE: *Exercise prevents deconditioning of muscles and promotes maintenance of ROM. Exercise techniques can improve ambulation and decrease tremors.*

MEDICAL

NURSING DIAGNOSES	OUTCOME CRITERIA	INTERVENTIONS

4 Impaired Verbal Communication *r.t. dysarthria*	• Is able to communicate his/her needs effectively	• Assess patient's ability to speak clearly and understand simple messages
		• Assess for sensory deficits (auditory, visual)
		• Approach in an unhurried manner
		• Encourage all speech efforts
		• Teach speech techniques
		  - speak slowly
		  - use short sentences or phrases
		  - take deep breaths between words
		  - carefully enunciate, emphasizing consonants
		  - speak aloud in front of mirror
		  - exercise facial muscles
		• Ask questions requiring simple or yes/no answers when speech is difficult
		• Explore alternate means of communication (letter board, typewriter, magic slate)
		• Consult with physician to refer for speech therapy evaluation

		RATIONALE: *Sensory deficits compound communication difficulties. Speaking aloud in front of a mirror allows patient to see lip/tongue movement; facial exercise helps maintain flexibility of facial musculature.*
5 Bathing, Grooming, and Toileting Self-Care Deficits *r.t. bradykinesia, rigidity, and tremors*	• Participates in self-care	• Assess patient's self-care abilities and deficits; document in chart • Provide environment conducive to safety • Provide adequate time for ADL completion • Assist with self-care activities, allowing patient to do as much as possible for him- or herself • Consult with OT regarding appliances to assist with ADL
		RATIONALE: *Providing adequate time and encouragement promotes a patient's independence. Many OT appliances are available which can encourage self-care.*

NURSING DIAGNOSES	OUTCOME CRITERIA	INTERVENTIONS
6 Constipation *r.t. immobility, anticholinergic drug therapy*	• Has soft bowel evacuation every 1-3 days	• Assess and document bowel sounds and bowel elimination patterns (time, amount, character) • Assess dietary habits • Encourage fluid intake to 2-3 L/day unless contraindicated • Educate about importance of eating foods rich in fiber • Encourage mobility • Consider use of stool softeners/laxatives as intervention of last resort
		RATIONALE: *In fluid volume deficit, the body absorbs more water from the colon. Fiber provides more bulk in the stool. Activity promotes peristalsis. Stool softeners and laxatives, although sometimes necessary, can lead to atonic colon.*

7 Ineffective Individual and Family Coping
r.t. progressive chronic illness, multiple self-care deficits
	• Patient/family discuss disease process, care needs; identify required support services	• Assess patient/family level of knowledge regarding disease process, community resources
		
		• Provide information to patient/family
		  - disease process
		  - local support groups
		  - respite or day care services, if available

	• Identifies appropriate coping mechanisms
	
	• Demonstrates problem-solving skills
		• Assess, foster present effective coping mechanisms and problem-solving skills
		  - provide calm, nonjudgmental environment
		  - assist patient/family in identifying coping strategies that have been successful in the past
		  - encourage social activities
		  - encourage verbalization of fears, anxiety, frustration

MEDICAL

NURSING DIAGNOSES	OUTCOME CRITERIA	INTERVENTIONS

RATIONALE: *Previously successful coping strategies may be applied to this situation. A nonjudgmental environment is conducive to a trusting nurse-family relationship. Support services assist the family with coping difficulties. Social activities prevent isolation and increase self-esteem.*

OTHER LESS COMMON NURSING DIAGNOSES: *Ineffective Airway Clearance; Altered Nutrition: Less than body requirements; Anxiety; Altered Thought Processes; Altered Urinary Elimination*

ESSENTIAL DISCHARGE CRITERIA

- Maintains ideal body weight (considering height and age)
- Is free of constipation
- Meets self-care needs
- Is able to communicate with staff/family effectively
- Mobility status is maintained or improved

- Experiences no complications of immobility
- Is free from injury
- Patient/family identify appropriate resources to meet their needs
- Patient/family demonstrate effective problem-solving skills

NURSING DIAGNOSES	OUTCOME CRITERIA	INTERVENTIONS
1 Ineffective Airway Clearance *r.t. excessive mucous production*	• Exhibits normal RR, depth, and ease	• Assess RR, rhythm, and depth q2-4h
	• Has no adventitious breath sounds upon auscultation	• Auscultate lung sounds q2-4h
	• Mobilizes secretions	• Turn, cough, and deep breathe q2h • Suction prn • Provide chest physiotherapy q8h • Elevate HOB 30-45° • Encourage intake of 2-3 L fluid intake qd • Administer medications as ordered (mucolytics, expectorants, bronchodilators)
		RATIONALE: *These measures promote removal of excess mucus and decrease mucous production.*
2 Impaired Gas Exchange *r.t. inflammation of alveolar-capillary membrane*	• Demonstrates improved oxygenation by ABGs WNL	• Monitor ABGs, ventilation perfusion as ordered
	• Exhibits balanced ventilation perfusion	• Assess mental status q2-4h • Assess HR and rhythm q2-4h • Administer O2 as ordered by physician
	• No cyanosis	• Assess for cyanosis (peripheral and central) q2-4h
	• Exhibits no use of accessory muscles for breathing	• Assess for use of accessory muscles for breathing q2-4h
	• ADL activity tolerance without SOB	• Assess for SOB with activity • Maintain bed rest • Organize care to include rest periods
		RATIONALE: *These measures decrease body O2 demand and monitor balance between supply and demand of O2.*

MEDICAL

NURSING DIAGNOSES	OUTCOME CRITERIA	INTERVENTIONS
3 High Risk for Infection *r.t. invasion of respiratory tract from bacteria or virus*	• Experiences no adverse effects of antibiotics	• Administer medications as ordered (antibiotics, antivirals)
	• Shows negative cultures	• Monitor sputum cultures as ordered
	• Mobilizes secretions	• Instruct patient to expectorate sputum raised with coughing rather than swallowing
	• Experiences no nosocomial infection	• Monitor chest x-rays as ordered • Monitor VS q2-4h • Demonstrate and encourage good hand-washing • Limit exposure to any other infection • Encourage adequate nutrition and rest
		RATIONALE: *These measures decrease and eliminate invading organisms and monitor the effectiveness of treatment.*
4 Altered Nutrition: Less than body requirements *r.t. decreased intake*	• Exhibits/maintains adequate nutritional status • Maintains, regains weight	• Weigh qod
	• Takes, retains 80 percent of meals	• Offer small, frequent meals • Encourage balanced meals (protein, carbohydrates, fats, and vitamins) • Offer easy to ingest and digestible foods • Schedule chest physiotherapy 30 min before meals • Offer mouth care before meals and prn • Eliminate offensive odors and sights before meals • Provide quiet atmosphere and decreased stimulation during meals • Allow adequate time for client to eat • Provide O_2 as ordered per nasal cannula

NURSING DIAGNOSES	OUTCOME CRITERIA	INTERVENTIONS
	• Patient/family demonstrate knowledge of diet	• Determine food preference

RATIONALE: *Improve intake by reducing fatigue, dyspnea, and unpleasant taste in mouth. Provide pleasant, unhurried atmosphere and client preferences to encourage increased intake. O2 demand may increase while eating.*

OTHER LESS COMMON NURSING DIAGNOSES: *Sleep Pattern Disturbance; High Risk for Fluid Volume Deficit; Pain; Ineffective Breathing Pattern; Fatigue; Knowledge Deficit; Hyperthermia*

ESSENTIAL DISCHARGE CRITERIA

• Is free of adventitious breath sounds

• Has no cyanosis or SOB

• Consumes, retains adequate calories

• Verbalizes understanding of and medications or treatments to be continued at home

• Verbalizes understanding of importance and ways to balance activity and rest

• Verbalizes s/s for which physician needs to be notified

MEDICAL

PNEUMOTHORAX

NURSING DIAGNOSES	OUTCOME CRITERIA	INTERVENTIONS

1 Ineffective Breathing Pattern
 	
r.t. air in pleural cavity and decreased lung expansion
	• Exhibits improving respiratory status
	  - takes 12-20 deep, regular respirations/min
	  - returns to baseline for amount, color of secretions
		• Assess RR, rhythm, and depth q2h
		• Auscultate lungs q2-4h
		• Administer O_2 therapy as ordered
		• Suction as needed to remove secretions
		• Assist in balancing rest and activity, O_2 supply and demand
		• Position patient for maximum breathing comfort
		• Plan to assist with chest tube insertion if indicated

		RATIONALE: *These measures determine the effectiveness of breathing pattern and optimize breathing efforts by providing a patent airway, optimal lung expansion, and supplemental O_2.*

2 Impaired Gas Exchange
 	
r.t. air and/or fluid in the pleural space
	• Exhibits effective gas exchange
	  - normal ABGs and serum electrolytes
	  - normal VS
	  - normal ECG
	  - balanced I&O
	  - urinary output WNL
	  - SaO_2 WNL
	  - no increasing restlessness, irritability
		• Monitor chest tube for drainage and/or air leak
		• Monitor VS q2-4h
		• Monitor ABGs, serum electrolytes
		• Monitor ECG as indicated
		• Monitor I&O
		• Assess adequacy of renal output
		• Assess for s/s of hypoxia: increasing restlessness, irritability

	• Achieves, maintains full expansion of affected lung
	  - normal breath sounds
	  - clearing chest x-ray
		• Auscultate breath sounds q2-4h

		RATIONALE: *Air and/or fluid in the pleural space impedes normal gas exchange and tissue oxygenation throughout the body.*

NURSING DIAGNOSES	OUTCOME CRITERIA	INTERVENTIONS
3 High Risk for Infection *r.t. impaired skin integrity at chest tube insertion site and limited mobility*	• Remains free of s/s of local and systemic infection - no odors or drainage around or through tube site	• Monitor for signs of local and systemic infections (elevated temperature, redness, warmth, drainage at insertion site) • Maintain strict asepsis when changing chest tube insertion site dressing
	• Shows normal CBC	• Preview daily lab work for changes in WBC, wound culture results
	• Shows no adverse effects of antibiotics	• Administer antibiotics as ordered
	• Exhibits normal breath sounds	• Assist with frequent position change and/or ambulation • Encourage patient to deep breathe
		RATIONALE: *The chest tube insertion site may be a portal of entry for infectious organisms. Limited mobility may lead to pooling of pulmonary secretions which become a medium for bacterial growth.*

4 Anxiety
 	
r.t. feelings of dyspnea and pain
	• Displays relief from anxiety
	  - relaxed body posture and facial expressions
	  - verbalizes sense of reduced anxiety
		• Remain with patient during procedures; explain all procedures
		• Listen actively to patient/family concerns about treatment
		• Administer analgesics and sedatives as ordered
		• Promote uninterrupted rest
		• Encourage alternatives in relaxation/distraction (music, guided imagery)

		RATIONALE: *Feelings of pain and dyspnea may cause anxiety, which complicates breathing difficulty and recovery.*

MEDICAL

> **OTHER LESS COMMON NURSING DIAGNOSES:**
> *Knowledge Deficit; Pain; Ineffective Airway Clearance; Fear*

ESSENTIAL DISCHARGE CRITERIA

- Achieves adequate lung re-expansion and breathing pattern

- ABGs, serum electrolytes WNL
- Is free from infection

PULMONARY EMBOLISM

NURSING DIAGNOSES	OUTCOME CRITERIA	INTERVENTIONS

1 Impaired Gas Exchange
 	
r.t. ventilation/perfusion imbalance
	• Exhibits effective gas exchange
	  - ABGs, serum electrolytes WNL
	  - balanced I&O
	  - 12-20 respirations/min, nonlabored; with pink earlobes, lips, and nail beds
	  - normal LOC
		• Assess cardiopulmonary status q2-4h
		  - monitor ECG and ABGs
		  - monitor I&O
		  - inspect the rate, rhythm, depth, and effort of breathing
		  - auscultate the chest to assess for full ventilation with vesicular sounds in all lung fields and with normal heart sounds
		  - note s/s of increasing restlessness, irritability, confusion
		
		• Monitor VS q2-4h
		
		• Maintain bed rest during active pulmonary embolism, then proceed with ambulation as soon as possible
		
		• Continuous O_2 by mask or cannula, per order
		
		• Prepare for diagnostic studies: chest x-ray, ECG, blood tests, lung perfusion scans, pulmonary arteriography
		
		• Consult with physician about appropriateness of initiating heparin therapy if not already begun
		
		• Prepare to initiate preoperative care or emergency resuscitative efforts in case of cardiopulmonary instability

		RATIONALE: *Vascular obstruction of pulmonary circulation produces decreased pulmonary oxygenation, resulting in hypoxemia and possible medical emergency.*

2 High Risk for Injury (internal)
 	
r.t. altered clotting factors and anticoagulant therapy
	• Experiences no further complication from anticoagulant therapy
	  - no s/s of bleeding
		• Monitor for signs of bleeding
		  - mucous membranes
		  - urine
		  - stool
		  - sputum

	• Manifests stable, improving LOC	• Assess neurologic status q1-4h and prn

MEDICAL

NURSING DIAGNOSES	OUTCOME CRITERIA	INTERVENTIONS
	• Coagulation studies are within therapeutic range	• Monitor coagulation studies • Provide antiembolytic devices, as ordered, i.e., TEDs, SCDs

	• Experiences no bleeding as side effect of anticoagulant therapy	• Administer anticoagulants as ordered
		• Apply direct pressure to puncture sites (3-5 min) to control bleeding
		• Avoid constipation and straining; use stool softeners or mild laxatives as ordered
		• Instruct patient in safety measures
		  - use electric razor
		  - use soft toothbrush
		  - ambulate with care to avoid trauma
		  - avoid aspirin and aspirin-containing products
		  - avoid sharp objects
		  - wear appropriate foot coverings

		RATIONALE: *These measures prevent or detect bleeding related to decrease in clotting ability of the blood.*

3 Anxiety
r.t. hypoxia and feelings of impending doom
	• Experiences reduced symptoms of anxiety
	  - verbalizes feeling less anxiety
	  - relaxed facial expression
		• Assess level of anxiety; monitor physiologic responses
		• Stay with patient and offer reassurance and support
		• Maintain calm and quiet environment
		• Listen to patient's description of feelings
		• Communicate in a quiet, calm voice using simple words and brief, concise statements
		• Explain all treatments and interventions
		• Assist patient to use coping strategies, i.e., relaxation techniques, imagery, and music

		RATIONALE: *Threats to biologic integrity elicit stress responses which can be minimized by supportive care.*

NURSING DIAGNOSES	OUTCOME CRITERIA	INTERVENTIONS
4 Activity Intolerance *r.t. insufficient oxygenation in relation to demand*	• Performs ADL without respiratory distress - monitors own fatigue level - alternates rest/activity	• Assess response to increase in activity and patterns of fatigue • Teach patient to monitor response to activity and to alter or cease activity when s/s of anoxia (increased pulse rate, dyspnea) or fatigue are present • Teach to alternate periods of activity and rest • Teach methods of conserving energy, i.e., sit instead of stand to perform tasks • Support and encourage activity to level of tolerance
		RATIONALE: *Reducing the rate of cellular metabolism and demand for O$_2$ decreases fatigue.*
5 Ineffective Management of Therapeutic Regimen *r.t. complexity of anticoagulant therapy*	• Patient/family verbalizes understanding of post-hospitalization management of anticoagulant therapy	• Teach patient/family about medications: name, dosage, time of administration, purpose, and side effects; provide appropriate written material • Explain importance of ongoing medical follow-up and monitoring, i.e., regular coagulation studies as ordered • Advise to wear/carry medical alert information regarding treatment with anticoagulants
	• Patient/family describes s/s requiring medical evaluation	• Teach to check stools, urine, and sputum for blood • Remind of need to report sudden, sharp chest pain, SOB, or increased RR
	• Patient/family verbalizes understanding of measures to prevent recurrence	• Instruct about prevention - avoid prolonged sitting or standing - elevate legs when sitting - do not cross legs - use antiembolytic devices if ordered - exercise regularly to tolerance level with planned rest periods - avoid constipation and straining

MEDICAL

NURSING DIAGNOSES	OUTCOME CRITERIA	INTERVENTIONS

RATIONALE: *Providing the patient with adequate information regarding treatment regimen, warning signs, and preventative measures reduces anxiety, enhances compliance, and supports continuity of care after discharge.*

OTHER LESS COMMON NURSING DIAGNOSES:
Ineffective Breathing Pattern; Pain; Knowledge Deficit

ESSENTIAL DISCHARGE CRITERIA

- Maintains optimal level of ABGs, serum electrolytes, and cardiopulmonary assessment
- Reports, displays reduced feelings of anxiety
- Shows no evidence of bleeding

- Performs ADL without respiratory distress
- Patient/family have sufficient information to comply with discharge regimen

RENAL CALCULI

NURSING DIAGNOSES	OUTCOME CRITERIA	INTERVENTIONS
1 Pain *r.t. inflammation, obstruction, and abrasion of the urinary tract*	• Verbalizes/displays reasonable comfort - relaxed body posture, facial expression	• Assess location, duration, quality, and movement of pain experience
	• Reports comfort following analgesia	• Administer analgesics, antiemetics, narcotics, and/or antispasmodics as ordered (do not delay in giving pain medicine when needed, as pain can be quite severe)
	• Identifies medication or activity that reduces/aggravates discomfort	• Promote a quiet, restful environment • Encourage fluids, especially water, if not contraindicated • Strain urine to obtain stone sample for laboratory analysis
		RATIONALE: *Consistent analgesia and comfort measures produce sustained relief from the acute pain of renal calculi. Straining urine for stones aids in identifying causes of pain.*

2 Anxiety
r.t. unfamiliar procedures, i.e., ESWL, IVP, and other radiographic and laboratory procedures
	• Displays, expresses reduced anxiety
	  - asks questions, seeks clarification
	  - affirms sense of reduced anxiety
	  - relaxed body posture, facial expressions
		• Teach patient and/or family member regarding pre-, intra-, and postprocedural events, as appropriate, before the procedure occurs
		• Encourage and answer questions regarding the procedures
		• Provide an environment that promotes learning (free of distractions; calm, unhurried manner)
		• Use simple, brief explanations
		• Remain with the patient when appropriate or possible
		• Provide continuity of care as much as possible
		• Include family as much as possible
		• Administer antianxiety medications as ordered

MEDICAL

NURSING DIAGNOSES	OUTCOME CRITERIA	INTERVENTIONS
		• Consult or refer to other healthcare personnel as appropriate
		RATIONALE: *Moderate to severe anxiety can decrease an individual's ability to synthesize information and problem-solve.*

NURSING DIAGNOSES	OUTCOME CRITERIA	INTERVENTIONS
3 Ineffective Management of Therapeutic Regimen *r.t. lack of knowledge regarding dietary component*	• Describes specific dietary changes to prevent recurrence of renal calculi	• Assess the patient's knowledge level regarding type of stone and its treatment regimen • Explain factors that contribute to stone formation • Instruct regarding ordered diet therapy: low Na, low Ca, low protein, and/or low oxalate diets • Provide instructions regarding prescribed medication therapy: thiazide diuretics, allopurinol • Provide patient with realistic choices about the various aspects of care
	• Expresses intent to practice required dietary changes	• Individualize teaching plan to fit patient's learning needs; consider factors that may impact readiness to learn - physical: illness state, fatigue, pain - psychosocial: age, current knowledge level, emotional status, cultural background, intelligence, past experiences • Consult dietitian to assess current diet and modifications needed • Facilitate family involvement
		RATIONALE: *These measures provide the necessary resources to make the needed dietary changes. Successful management depends on the person believing that behavior change will be beneficial and that he/she can make the change.*

NURSING DIAGNOSES	OUTCOME CRITERIA	INTERVENTIONS
4 High Risk for Infection *r.t. urinary stasis and/or irritation of tissue by calculi*	• Remains free of s/s of systemic/local infection - normal VS, BP - normal CBC - clear urine - no dysuria, frequency - no complaints of flank pain	• Monitor for s/s of pyelonephritis - chills, fever, increased WBC count (leukocytosis) - bacteria or pus in urine - hematuria - costovertebral angle pain - dysuria - frequency - loin or flank pain
	• Shows negative cultures	• Evaluate cultures and sensitivities • Encourage fluids, unless contraindicated
	• Practices appropriate precautions to prevent recurrences	• Use aseptic technique when emptying or handling urinary drainage devices
	• Experiences no nosocomial infection	• Administer antibiotics, antispasmodics as ordered • Reassess continued need for indwelling catheter

RATIONALE: *Protection prevents infections and associated complications.*

MEDICAL

> **OTHER LESS COMMON NURSING DIAGNOSES:** Noncompliance; Fluid Volume Excess; Altered Urinary Elimination; Knowledge Deficit

ESSENTIAL DISCHARGE CRITERIA

- Is free of pain
- Is free of s/s of infection
- Verbalizes understanding of dietary changes that need to be made

- Verbalizes understanding of prescribed medication regimen
- Describes s/s which should be reported
- Affirms knowledge of required follow-up appointments

RENAL FAILURE, ACUTE

NURSING DIAGNOSES	OUTCOME CRITERIA	INTERVENTIONS

1 Altered Tissue Perfusion (renal)
 	
r.t. damage to nephrons from hypovolemia, ischemia, toxins, stenosis, or obstruction
	• Shows improved tissue perfusion
	  - serum electrolytes, BUN, creatinine, pH WNL
	  - RR, rhythm WNL
		• Monitor serum lab values
		• Assess for Chvostek's and Trousseau's sign
		• Assess RR, rhythm
		• During oliguric phase, provide bed rest, assisting with ADL

	• Is free from adverse effects of medications	• Administer ordered medications with care, decreasing dosage or increasing intervals between doses • Avoid nephrotoxic drugs • Provide protein-sparing diet
		RATIONALE: *Lab values assessment reflects kidney's ability to regulate wastes, fluids, and electrolytes. Bed rest conserves energy and promotes recovery. Nephrotoxic or high-dose drugs damage kidneys that are already compromised. Decreased protein intake modifies build-up of additional nitrogen.*
2 Fluid Volume Excess (oliguric) *r.t. Na and water retention*	• Achieves balanced I&O	• Monitor I&O
	• Shows serum Na, K WNL	• Monitor serum levels, ECG, CVP as available
	• Achieves normalizing stable body weight	• Assess weight daily
	• Shows BP, VS WNL	• Assess VS, breath sounds q4h
	• Shows BUN, creatinine WNL	• Monitor BUN/creatinine ratios
	• Displays no edema	• Monitor edema, JVD
	• Urine output WNL	• Monitor urinary output q1-2h • Administer diuretics as ordered; monitor response
		RATIONALE: *Assessment measures help identify changes in fluid and electrolyte status. Changes in K related to diuretic therapy may be manifested in ECG changes.*

NURSING DIAGNOSES	OUTCOME CRITERIA	INTERVENTIONS
3 High Risk for Fluid Volume Deficit (diuretic) *r.t. active losses and compromised regulatory mechanisms*	• Displays good skin turgor, moist mucous membranes	• Assess CRT, oral mucous membranes, skin turgor
	• Shows no s/s of dehydration - fluids and electrolytes WNL	• Monitor serum electrolytes • Administer vasoconstrictors, fluids, and electrolytes as ordered
		RATIONALE: *Identify electrolytes lost via body fluids. Increase systemic resistance, BP and renal blood flow; replace losses, and ensure adequate circulating volume.*
4 Altered Nutrition: Less than body requirements *r.t. changes in GI tract and restricted diet*	• Exhibits adequate nutritional status	• Strictly monitor food intake • Administer parenteral or enteral feedings as indicated
	• Maintains normal GI function	• Assess bowel function/bowel sounds at least q8h
	• Has no vomiting	• Monitor for nausea, vomiting, anorexia • Give good mouth care before oral feedings
	• Patient/family demonstrate knowledge of dietary restrictions	• Instruct regarding ideal carbohydrate, protein, Na, and vitamin intake • Refer complex problems to dietitian
		RATIONALE: *Food intake is monitored to ensure adequate intake within limits prescribed. N/V decreases intake of needed nutrients. A team approach to renal diet management enhances the achievement of optimal nutritional status.*
5 High Risk for Infection *r.t. suppressed immune response*	• Remains free of local and systemic infection	• Monitor for s/s of infection in secretions, exudates, and fever • Inspect skin q8h
	• Shows normal CBC	• Monitor WBCs

MEDICAL

177

NURSING DIAGNOSES	OUTCOME CRITERIA	INTERVENTIONS
		• Maintain strict asepsis of indwelling catheter and any invasive procedure
		• Promote pulmonary hygiene
		• Use measures to prevent skin breakdown
		• Avoid exposure to persons with infections
		• Encourage regular hand-washing, bathing, and adequate rest and nutrition
	• Experiences no adverse effects of antibiotics	• Administer prescribed antibiotics on a timely basis
		RATIONALE: *Monitoring helps detect early on any infection. Measures to improve immunity and minimize exposure to pathogens help prevent complications for these high-risk patients.*
6 Knowledge Deficit *r.t. lack of exposure to ARF and its treatment*	• Patient/family discuss pathophysiology of disease process, rationale for treatment	• Instruct patient/family regarding the cause of ARF - expected course of recovery
	• Patient/family list reportable s/s, demonstrate required skills	• Have patient/family demonstrate VS, I&O, weight measurements
	• Verbalizes knowledge of follow-up appointments • Discusses relaxation, activity, and diet	• Explain the schedule of medical follow-up - diet and fluid restrictions, which may or may not continue - exercise and rest as indicated/ prescribed
	• Patient/family list medications	• Explain medications: purpose, dose, schedule, and side effects
		RATIONALE: *Providing necessary information will enhance patient/family participation and improve compliance with the treatment regimen.*

> **OTHER LESS COMMON NURSING DIAGNOSES:** *Sensory/Perceptual Alterations; Altered Family Processes; Ineffective Individual Coping; Altered Thought Processes; Self-Care Deficit*

ESSENTIAL DISCHARGE CRITERIA

- Shows serum electrolytes, renal function tests WNL or optimal
- Has stable fluid balance
- Demonstrates optimal nutritional status, stable body weight
- Is free of s/s of infection or skin breakdown
- Patient/family verbalize/demonstrate knowledge of ARF and treatment

MEDICAL

RENAL FAILURE, CHRONIC

NURSING DIAGNOSES	OUTCOME CRITERIA	INTERVENTIONS
1 Altered Tissue Perfusion (renal) *r.t. nephron destruction and inability to maintain renal functions*	• Shows improved renal tissue perfusion	• Assess for Chvostek's and Trousseau's signs • Monitor ECG if available
	• Renal function tests WNL or stable	• Monitor serum electrolytes, BUN, creatinine, H&H
	• Shows stable body weight	• Monitor weight daily
	• Achieves balanced I&O	• Monitor I&O for 24h
	• Shows normal VS	• Monitor VS at least q4-8h

	• Shows acceptable BP, mentation	• Monitor for fluid excess
		  - orthostatic BP
		  - mental status
		  - RR and effort
		  - JVD
		  - CVP, pulmonary artery pressures as available

	• Displays no edema	• Offer limited intake over 24 h
	• Experiences no adverse effects of medications	• Administer medications carefully, decreasing dose, adjusting intervals, if needed, according to response • Administer diuretics; monitor response • Avoid use of magnesium-based antiacids • Administer hemo- or peritoneal dialysis as indicated, per institutional policy/procedure

RATIONALE: *Changes in serum K levels are manifested in ECG changes. Serum levels reflect impairment of kidneys' excretory and nonexcretory functions. Monitoring for adverse effects of drugs helps determine effectiveness as well as side effects of drugs, such as hypokalemia. Offering fluids on a 24 h basis helps prevent nocturnal dehydration.*

NURSING DIAGNOSES	OUTCOME CRITERIA	INTERVENTIONS
2 Altered Nutrition: Less than body requirements *r.t. GI changes and anorexia*	• Exhibits/maintains adequate nutritional status	• Monitor lab data
	• Has no vomiting	• Assess for nausea, vomiting, anorexia
	• Takes, retains 80 percent or more of meals	• Monitor and encourage food intake as prescribed • Provide oral hygiene before meals • Encourage food intake as prescribed • Provide patient's food preferences within dietary restrictions • Administer antiemetics as prescribed • Refer complex nutritional aspects to dietitian
		RATIONALE: *N/V decreases adequate intake of needed nutrients. Monitor intake to determine compliance with prescribed diet. Give and monitor antiemetics to improve timing for best results. Using a team approach to dietary management improves patient satisfaction and compliance with treatment regimen.*
3 Knowledge Deficit *r.t. CRF and treatment regimen*	• Patient/family discuss pathophysiology of disease process, rationale for treatment	• Assess readiness to learn, knowledge and understanding of CRF • Explain the nature of CRF
	• Patient/family verbalize knowledge of complications, expected course, and prognosis	• Assist patient to identify ways to incorporate changes and treatment into lifestyle • Discuss renal dialysis and transplantation • Explain avoidance of infection
	• Patient/family list reportable s/s	• Explain s/s to report to physician
	• Patient/family demonstrates self-observation skills	• Demonstrate monitoring VS, BP, I&O, weight
	• Patient/family express commitment to consistent medical follow-ups	• Explain the plan for medical follow-up

MEDICAL

NURSING DIAGNOSES	OUTCOME CRITERIA	INTERVENTIONS
	• Patient/family discuss relaxation, activity, diet	• Explain personal hygiene, rest, exercise, restricted protein, Na, K, and fluid intake
	• Patient/family verbalize knowledge of medications	• Provide written information about medications: purpose, dose, interval, and side effects
		RATIONALE: *Providing the necessary information facilitates patient self-care, family participation and improves compliance with the therapeutic regimen.*
4 High Risk for Infection *r.t. suppressed immune response*	• Remains free of local and systemic infections	• Assess for s/s of infection in drainage
	• Manifests no odors or drainage	• Assess skin for integrity, pruritus, excoriations
	• Exhibits normal VS	• Assess for chills
	• Is afebrile	• Monitor temperature q4h
	• Shows normal CBC	• Monitor WBCs
	• Shows negative cultures	• Monitor cultures
	• Is free of urinary cloudiness or foul odor	• Practice strict hand-washing technique • Avoid exposing patient to people with infections • Ensure aseptic technique for any invasive procedure • Encourage regular personal hygiene, bathing, adequate nutrition, and rest
		RATIONALE: *Assess for infection for early detection and treatment. Use and teach hand-washing and hygiene to decrease exposure to pathogens. Maintaining skin integrity protects the patient from pathogens.*

NURSING DIAGNOSES	OUTCOME CRITERIA	INTERVENTIONS
5 Altered Thought Processes *r.t. uremia and toxic accumulation of chemicals*	• Thought processes are normal and stable: oriented to time, place, person	• Assess neurologic status: orientation, sleep pattern, LOC, seizure activity, neuropathy • Monitor for behavioral changes • Orient frequently to reality
	• Remains free of injury	• Maintain safety precautions (bed rails up, call light in reach) • Institute seizure precautions as indicated • Allow extra time for patient's response, questions • Provide a balance of rest with activity
		RATIONALE: *Neurologic changes reflect uremic effects on CNS. Reorientation minimizes disorientation related to isolation and lack of information. Safety precautions reduce injury. Allowing extra time for patient's response helps compensate for short-term memory losses. Balanced rest/activity enhances normal sleep/rest patterns.*

MEDICAL

> **OTHER LESS COMMON NURSING DIAGNOSES:** *High Risk for Impaired Skin Integrity; Activity Intolerance; Self-Esteem Disturbance; Feeding, Bathing/Hygiene, Toileting Self-Care Deficits; Sexual Dysfunction; Body Image Disturbance; Altered Family Processes*

ESSENTIAL DISCHARGE CRITERIA

- Shows renal function tests WNL or stable
- Maintains normal fluid balance
- Is free of infection and injury

- Is oriented, with stable thought processes
- Demonstrates optimal nutritional status
- Patient/family are knowledgeable about CRF and treatment regimen

RIB FRACTURES (WITHOUT SURGERY)

NURSING DIAGNOSES	OUTCOME CRITERIA	INTERVENTIONS
1 Ineffective Breathing Pattern *r.t. pain and trauma to rib cage*	• Respiratory pattern is effective - ABGs WNL - takes at least 12-20 regular respirations/min	• Inspect thorax for symmetry of respiratory movement • Monitor ABGs • Observe breathing pattern for SOB and use of accessory muscles • Assess emotional response that may cause hyperventilation • Assess for possible complications (pneumothorax, hemothorax) • Assess for pain • Assist to optimal position for breathing (i.e., semi-Fowler's) • Encourage coughing, splinting, deep breathing, and moving • Medicate with analgesics without reducing respirations • Monitor results • Encourage use of incentive spirometry • Teach use of abdominal muscles for breathing **RATIONALE:** *Splinting, positioning and use of abdominal muscles enhance lung expansion and optimal breathing patterns, preventing hypoventilation and possible atelectasis.*
2 Pain *r.t. trauma to rib cage*	• Verbalizes, displays freedom from pain	• Assess pain regularly - use self-rating scale (scale of 0-10) - assess pain in relation to coughing, breathing, moving • Reposition for comfort q2h • Apply ice or chest binder as ordered • Administer analgesics regularly; include bolus "rescue" doses for breakthrough pain; coordinate with lung expansion maneuvers • If pain persists despite analgesics, notify physician, who may consider intercostal nerve block

NURSING DIAGNOSES	OUTCOME CRITERIA	INTERVENTIONS
		RATIONALE: *Alleviating pain promotes deep breathing, coughing, and moving and prevents hypoventilation, atelectasis, pneumonitis, and hypoxemia.*
3 Knowledge Deficit *r.t. lack of exposure to information*	• Discusses nature of chest injury and rationale for treatment	• Explain specific nature of injury, need for coughing, and deep breathing
	• Lists reportable s/s	• Discuss s/s, complications to report to physician: unrelieved pain, difficulty breathing, and associated injuries
	• Lists medications • Verbalizes knowledge of follow-up appointment	• Explain analgesic doses, intervals, and side effects
		RATIONALE: *Providing essential information will facilitate self-care and compliance with postinjury treatment.*

MEDICAL

> **OTHER LESS COMMON NURSING DIAGNOSES:** *Anxiety; Ineffective Airway Clearance*

ESSENTIAL DISCHARGE CRITERIA

• Has effective respiratory pattern

• Takes oral analgesics to alleviate pain

• Verbalizes understanding of follow-up care

SEIZURE DISORDERS

NURSING DIAGNOSES	OUTCOME CRITERIA	INTERVENTIONS

1 High Risk for Injury

r.t. seizure activity

- Sustains no injury from seizure activity
  - exhibits intact neurologic status
  - manifests improving LOC

- Prevent injuries during convulsive activity
  - have side rails up, padded side rails, oral airway or padded tongue blade at bedside, bed in low position, suction and O₂ available
  - institute seizure precautions per unit standards
  - maintain patent airway
  - insert bit block or padded tongue blade only if teeth not clamped
  - do not restrain movements
  - remove objects that could cause injury
  - protect head from injury
  - provide for privacy

- Notify physician immediately if seizure lasts over 10 min or new seizure begins before return of conscious state

- Observe seizure activity; record and report observations
  - note time and any sign of aura or cry
  - note parts of body involved, order of involvement, and character of movements
  - check pupils for deviation, nystagmus, and change in pupil size
  - note tonic and clonic movements
  - note for loss of continence

- Provide safe environment after seizure
  - place on side after seizure to maintain airway
  - provide time to sleep
  - reorient prn
  - evaluate behaviors, weakness, and/or paralysis

RATIONALE: *During a seizure, abnormal movements and/or altered LOC places the patient at risk for injury. Seizure lasting over 10 min may indicate status epilepticus. Recording features of seizure assists in classifying and diagnosing cause of seizures. Inhibited cerebral function during postictal period requires that the patient rest and be reoriented to his environment.*

NURSING DIAGNOSES	OUTCOME CRITERIA	INTERVENTIONS
2 Ineffective Individual Coping *r.t. inability to meet role responsibility and chronic nature of disease*	• Demonstrates coping strategies and realistic perceptions of self	• Assess patient's emotional status • Promote open discussion of feelings and beliefs • Discuss relationship of stress and seizures • Encourage patient and family not to overprotect • Refer to community resources (epileptic organization, counselors)
		RATIONALE: *These interventions provide information and cognitive techniques to improve problem-solving and coping.*
3 Knowledge Deficit *r.t. treatment, diagnostic procedures, and disease*	• Patient/family discuss pathophysiology of disease process, rationale for treatment • Patient/family make realistic statements about expected course of recovery, prognosis	• Teach physiology of seizures, treatment, expected course
	• Patient/family verbalize/discuss knowledge of medications	• Assist patient in determining how to fit drug therapy into own ADL • Teach name, dosage, frequency, toxicity, and side effects as well as to take medication even if seizure-free
	• Patient/family express commitment to consistent medical follow-up	• Stress importance of follow-up to monitor blood levels of anticonvulsant
	• Patient/family discuss relaxation, activity, diet	• Discuss need to avoid alcohol and emotional stress • Discuss need to obtain proper nutrition and rest • Teach to refrain from dangerous activities (usually can drive after seizure-free 1 year)
	• Patient/family discuss safety measures; possess emergency phone numbers	• Teach family how to initiate safety measures • Teach need to wear medical alert bracelet

MEDICAL

NURSING DIAGNOSES	OUTCOME CRITERIA	INTERVENTIONS

RATIONALE: *Failure to take medications exactly as prescribed may precipitate seizures. Dosages of anticonvulsants are difficult to regulate because of high incidence of toxicity and side effects. Alcohol and stress may trigger seizure activity.*

OTHER LESS COMMON NURSING DIAGNOSES: Anxiety; Ineffective Airway Clearance; Ineffective Breathing Pattern; Sensory/Perceptual Alterations; Social Isolation

ESSENTIAL DISCHARGE CRITERIA

- Remains free of traumatic injury
- Demonstrates effective coping strategies

- Verbalizes understanding of disease, treatment regimen, and lifestyle changes

SHOCK

NURSING DIAGNOSES	OUTCOME CRITERIA	INTERVENTIONS

1 Altered Tissue Perfusion (renal, cerebral, cardio-pulmonary, peripheral)
 	
r.t. decreased cardiac output
	• Shows improved tissue perfusion	• Assess for altered tissue perfusion
		  - cool skin temperature
		  - cyanosis
		  - decreased pulses, BP q2h
		  - tachycardia

	• Manifests stable LOC	• Altered mental status
	• Achieves balanced I&O	• Measure I&O q2h or as indicated • Maintain complete bed rest (preferably flat) • Keep patient warm
		RATIONALE: *Assessment helps determine the effectiveness of interventions to improve tissue perfusion. Fluid intake should equal fluid loss. Output volume is needed to determine required fluid intake. Bed rest facilitates circulation while minimizing metabolic needs.*

2 Decreased Cardiac Output
 	
r.t. altered pre-load, after-load, and/or contractility
	• ECG, VS, BP stable, WNL
	• Has urinary output WNL
		• Assess for signs of decreased cardiac output
		  - decreased pulse volume
		  - irregular pulse
		  - fatigue
		  - diaphoresis
		  - hypotension, declining BP
		  - oliguria/anuria

	• BUN, creatinine WNL	• Monitor indices of renal function • Monitor invasive hemodynamic parameters as available, i.e., CVP • Administer drugs that increase heart contractility • Assess cardiovascular response to drug therapy • Plan interventions to minimize O_2 demand
		RATIONALE: *Monitoring invasive and noninvasive parameters helps evaluate clinical status and response to therapy. Planning and pacing care prevent fatigue and minimize O_2 demand.*

NURSING DIAGNOSES	OUTCOME CRITERIA	INTERVENTIONS
3 Fluid Volume Deficit *r.t. blood loss*	• Shows no bleeding, normal CBC	• Monitor loss from GI tract, wounds, drains, other sources of bleeding • Estimate loss from dressings • Monitor CBC
	• Shows no s/s of dehydration • Has stable body weight	• Weigh daily
	• Shows normal fluid and electrolyte balance	• Assess for signs of fluid and electrolyte imbalance: poor skin turgor, weakness, irritability, N/V • Monitor serum electrolytes • Note and report variations • Administer IV fluids, blood, plasma expanders as indicated • Apply pressure dressings, shock trousers as indicated • Closely monitor response to therapy
		RATIONALE: *Fluctuations in fluid deficit variables are excellent indicators of fluid volume balance and identify the effectiveness/ineffectiveness of interventions.*
4 Impaired Gas Exchange *r.t. ventilation/ perfusion imbalance*	• Exhibits adequate O$_2$ exchange - takes at least 12-20 deep, regular respirations/min - lungs clear to auscultations - ABGs, H&H WNL	• Assess respiratory pattern, noting rate, rhythm, use of accessory muscles • Auscultate breath sounds q2h • Assess for signs of increasing pulmonary congestion • Monitor ABGs • Administer O$_2$ as ordered • Prepare for intubation and assisted ventilation as indicated
		RATIONALE: *Monitor/assess respiratory parameters regularly to identify ventilation/perfusion status and need for alternative interventions.*

NURSING DIAGNOSES	OUTCOME CRITERIA	INTERVENTIONS
5 Altered Thought Processes *r.t. decreased cerebral perfusion*	• Demonstrates improved cerebral circulation - alert, oriented to environment	• Assess behavioral and neurologic status response to verbal, tactile stimuli, state of orientation, restlessness, confusion, lethargy, unresponsiveness, seizures • Assess pain as a possible contributor to shock • Assess for spontaneous movement of all extremities, pupillary response, presence of protective reflexes • Report variations to physician

RATIONALE: *Diminished alertness is an early indication of diminishing cerebral perfusion. Early treatment prevents more serious manifestations.*

OTHER LESS COMMON NURSING DIAGNOSES: *Anxiety; Altered Nutrition: Less than body requirements; High Risk for Infection; High Risk for Impaired Skin Integrity*

ESSENTIAL DISCHARGE CRITERIA

• Is alert, oriented, and normotensive

• Has improved cardiac output

• Shows ABGs, serum electrolytes, I&O WNL

SUBARACHNOID HEMORRHAGE

NURSING DIAGNOSES	OUTCOME CRITERIA	INTERVENTIONS

1 Altered Tissue Perfusion (cerebral)
 	
r.t. cerebral trauma, increased ICP
	• Maintains usual/improved LOC, cognition, and sensory motor function	• Obtain, document baseline data
		  - risk factors/underlying pathophysiology status
		  - current treatments, medications, diet
		  - situational and maturational factors
		  - serum chemistries
		
		• Monitor neurologic status for trends, patterns, and changes
		  - use Glasgow Coma scale: eye opening, verbal response, motor response
		  - also assess for visual changes, memory loss, personality changes, headache, dizziness

	• VS stable, WNL	• Monitor VS for signs of increasing ICP
		  - widened pulse pressure
		  - dysrhythmias
		  - respiratory patterns

	• Exhibits PERL	• Inspect pupils for changes
	• Displays intact reflexes	• Monitor and report presence/absence of reflexes
	• Maintains balanced I&O	• Monitor I&O

	• Displays reasonable comfort	• Provide comfort measures
		  - minimize extraneous stimuli
		  - elevate HOB 20-40°, maintaining head-neck alignment
		
		• Assist in implementation of collaborative interventions as indicated
		
		• Administer ordered medications (diuretics, steroids, anticonvulsants, analgesics, antibiotics)
		
		• Coordinate ordered diagnostic procedures

RATIONALE: *Baseline data are needed to identify contributing risk factors that may impede recovery. Identification of changes and trends in LOC, VS determines progression of damage and increased ICP. Rest and quiet environment aid recovery; alignment aids venous drainage.*

NURSING DIAGNOSES	OUTCOME CRITERIA	INTERVENTIONS
2 High Risk for Infection *r.t. instrumentation, invasive diagnostic procedures*	• Remains free of local and systemic infection - afebrile - no localized redness, swelling, drainage around invasive sites	• Monitor VS q4h • Enforce infection control precautions with all invasive procedures - proper hand-washing
	• Participates in learning self-care - recognizes s/s of complications - describes specific realistic plan for follow-up care	• Initiate health teaching as needed with patient and family regarding self-care for preventing infection
		RATIONALE: *These measures prevent nosocomial infection and promote healing.*
3 Knowledge Deficit *r.t. inexperience and unfamiliarity with diagnosis*	• Patient/family participate in care activities	• Involve patient and caregiver in setting care goals (in hospital and for home)
	• Patient/family discuss medications, diet • Patient/family identify specific activities that will be allowed at home	• Patient/family demonstrate knowledge and competence with medications, diet, activity limitations
	• Patient/family recognize reportable s/s: changes in LOC, changes in balance or gait, vomiting, changes in eye movement or size of pupils, headache, seizure activity	• Has specific plan for accessing healthcare professional for immediate attention
		RATIONALE: *Knowledge and competence help patient to maintain accountability for health.*

MEDICAL

> **OTHER LESS COMMON NURSING DIAGNOSES:** High Risk for Aspiration; High Risk for Injury (external); Pain; Bathing/Hygiene, Dressing Self-Care Deficits; Body Image Disturbance; Impaired Physical Mobility; Powerlessness; Impaired Verbal Communication

ESSENTIAL DISCHARGE CRITERIA

- Maintains baseline/normal LOC
- Is afebrile
- Patient/family demonstrate required home care techniques

- Patient/family have list of s/s to report to physician
- Possesses follow-up appointments/referrals for physician and other therapists as indicated

TUBERCULOSIS

1 Ineffective Breathing Pattern

r.t. poor cough effort, necrosis of lung tissue

- Exhibits improving respiratory status
  - at least 12-20 regular respirations/min

  • Assess quality, rate, depth of respirations, use of accessory muscles; record changes

  • Assess q2-4h until stable, then q8h
    - breath sounds
    - VS

- Has decreasing hemoptysis

  • Assess color, consistency, odor, amount of sputum

- Shows improving skin color
  - mobilizes lung secretions
  - SaO$_2$ WNL
  - paces activities and rest

  • Position in semi-Fowler's or high Fowler's

  • Assist/educate patient to TCDB q2-4h

  • Assist/educate patient to splint chest during coughing

  • Provide for frequent rest periods

  • Encourage fluid intake

  • Suction as needed

- Shows no evidence of organisms resistent to medications prescribed

  • Obtain cultures as ordered

RATIONALE: *The respiratory tract is the usual pathway of entry for tubercle bacilli. Retained secretions may cause atelectasis and impaired gas exchange.*

2 Altered Nutrition: Less than body requirements

r.t. loss of appetite, fatigue, and/or dyspnea

- Maintains adequate nutritional status
  - maintains, regains weight
  - normal serum electrolytes
  - albumin WNL

  • Obtain admission weight and monitor daily

  • Monitor serum electrolytes

  • Monitor albumin and lymphocyte values

- Takes, retains 80 percent of meals

  • Record percentage of meals eaten

  • Maintain high protein, high carbohydrate diet with small, frequent feedings

  • Place in semi-Fowler's position during meals

  • Encourage rest periods between meals

  • Consult with dietitian

MEDICAL

NURSING DIAGNOSES	OUTCOME CRITERIA	INTERVENTIONS
	• Patient/family demonstrate knowledge of diet	• Encourage significant other to bring patient's favorite foods
		RATIONALE: *Anorexia is a nonspecific effect of tuberculosis. Metabolic demands are increased while appetite and intake decreases.*
3 Sleep Pattern Disturbance *r.t. fever, night sweats, cough, fatigue*	• Approximates normal total sleep time and pattern • Demonstrates increased energy and decreased fatigue	• Offer cool bath/shower at bedtime and/or morning
	• Verbalizes feeling rested - absence of signs of sleep deprivation	• Organize nursing activities to allow for uninterrupted periods of sleep • Plan for rest periods during the day with family/significant other • Collaborate with patient and significant other to determine alternate comfort measures • Relate/educate duration of discomforting symptoms • Administer antipyretics as ordered
		RATIONALE: *The pulmonary symptoms of tuberculosis are usually aggravated at night and interfere with rest.*
4 Self-Esteem Disturbance *r.t. stigma associated with a contagious disease and isolation*	• Maintains adequate self-esteem - positive interactions with family/friends	• Encourage verbalization of feelings, concerns, thoughts, emotions: use active listening and clarification • Assist with management of aesthetic problems • Avoid unnecessary isolation precautions • Establish a trusting relationship through frequent positive contacts; identify strengths and support systems

NURSING DIAGNOSES	OUTCOME CRITERIA	INTERVENTIONS

• Verbalizes understanding of ability to return to normal activities

• Plan activities with patient and significant other as tolerated

• Work with patient and significant other to develop realistic, attainable goals/interventions

RATIONALE: *Restrictions on visitors, as well as need for isolation masks, can lead to feelings of guilt, lowered self-worth, and social isolation.*

5 Knowledge Deficit

r.t. lack of information about disease process, risk of infectious transmission, and home care maintenance

• Patient/family share attitudes, knowledge, concerns, questions
  - discuss pathophysiology of disease process, rationale for treatment
  - verbalize knowledge of complications
  - discuss expected course of recovery; ask appropriate questions
  - make realistic statements about expected course of recovery, prognosis

• Assess understanding of disease process, patient's readiness to learn and factors that affect learning
  - age
  - intelligence
  - education
  - physical health and well-being
  - anxiety, denial
  - past experiences
  - misconceptions
  - cultural attitudes toward disease
  - religious beliefs
  - motivation
  - locus of control

• Structure care plan based on assessment

• Explain nature of disease and purpose of treatment and procedures (include normal respiratory anatomy, pathophysiology, and communication of disease)

• Provide an environment conducive to learning
  - include family in teaching program
  - repeat as often as needed
  - simplify information
  - concentrate on vital aspects
  - reinforce learning with reading materials, written materials, and/or audiovisual aids
  - provide opportunity for questions
  - reduce environmental distractions

MEDICAL

NURSING DIAGNOSES	OUTCOME CRITERIA	INTERVENTIONS
	• Patient/family participate in care activities and comply with infection control precautions	• Explain importance of good hand-washing and good hygiene - coughing into tissues - use of mask if unable to physically follow directions - proper disposal of tissues - turn head when coughing - avoid direct contact with sputum - good housekeeping practices (sanitary procedures for care of dressings and urine at home) • Explain need to limit visitors first few weeks at home; private room is preferable initially • Explain importance of avoiding crowds and persons with URIs; avoid close contact with others until advised by physician
	• Patient/family demonstrate accurate knowledge of medications: dosage, schedule, effects, side effects	• Explain importance of continuing medications until stopped by physician (include instruction of medication actions, side effects, name, dosages, purposes, time of administration) • Stress need to avoid OTC medications without checking first with physician
	• Patient/family verbalize knowledge of follow-up appointments	• Discuss symptoms to report
	• Patient/family express commitment to consistent medical follow-up	• Explain importance of ongoing outpatient care

RATIONALE: *Education is needed to maintain and improve health as well as avoiding misconceptions and encouraging compliance.*

> **OTHER LESS COMMON NURSING DIAGNOSES:** *Impaired Gas Exchange;*
> *Ineffective Individual Coping; Powerlessness; Fluid Volume Deficit*

ESSENTIAL DISCHARGE CRITERIA

- Demonstrates effective breathing pattern
- Weight is stabilized
- Reports increased energy, decreased fatigue
- Verbalizes understanding of need for long-term medication therapy as directed by physician

- Displays positive interactions with family and friends
- Indicates ability to care for self at home
- Verbalizes knowledge regarding infectious process and prevention of transmission

MEDICAL

VENOUS INSUFFICIENCY (Leg Ulcers)

NURSING DIAGNOSES	OUTCOME CRITERIA	INTERVENTIONS
1 Impaired Tissue Integrity *r.t. venous insufficiency*	• Wounds are clean, debrided, and/or show reduction in size	• Assess for etiological factors associated with venous stasis wounds • Assess wound appearance, pain, itch, physical attributes of lower extremities • Perform debridement per physician order • Whirlpool/PT may be used for mechanical debridement • Perform topical application of enzyme and routine dressing changes • Provide damp-to-damp dressings, transparent dressings, hydrogels, or hydrocolloids

	• Participates in wound care program
	  - debridement
	  - topical treatment
		• Culture wound for signs of clinical infection or bone and joint involvement
		  - *after* necrotic tissue is removed and wound is irrigated with nonantimicrobial solution
		  - *before* antibiotics are started
		
		• Provide topical treatment
		  - cleanse wounds with solutions that do not impair fibroblast activity (sterile normal saline is appropriate)
		  - if wounds contaminated with staph, strep, or pseudomonas use diluted solutions of povidone-iodine, sodium hypochlorite, hydrogen peroxide, acetic acid
		  - choose dressings that provide moist healing environment
		  - provide for adequate absorption of wound drainage to promote development of granulation tissue, promote epithelial cell migration, and reduce pain

NURSING DIAGNOSES	OUTCOME CRITERIA	INTERVENTIONS
	• Discusses/demonstrates ways to optimize venous return	• Optimize venous return - keep legs higher than heart - discourage sitting with legs crossed - ambulate to tolerance - discourage constrictive clothing - provide pressure reduction for heels - provide measures to keep surrounding skin clean and pliable - use emollients to provide a barrier against irritants and to prevent xerosis - correctly fit and apply ace wraps, pressure gradient support stockings, sequential compression devices
		RATIONALE: *Topical wound therapy should be directed to removing all impediments to healing necrotic tissue, infection, and excessive exudate. Healing of venous leg ulcers and maintenance of skin integrity depend on venous return and delivery of oxygenated blood to peripheral tissues.*
2 Ineffective Individual Coping *r.t. changes in body image*	• Actively participates in wound management program	• Assess patient's past and present participation in wound management program
	• Expresses confidence in ability to manage wound	• Assess perception in body image regarding draining leg ulcers, odor • Assess coping styles/strategies • Assess available support systems • Assess perception of changes in lifestyle and social involvement • Reinforce and/or teach appropriate coping strategies to patient and/or caregiver
	• Resumes social activities and role-related responsibilities	• Encourage patient's expression of concerns/feelings regarding leg wounds and perceived effect on lifestyle
		RATIONALE: *Effective coping reduces stress and enables patient/family to deal more effectively with immediate issues and concerns.*

MEDICAL

NURSING DIAGNOSES	OUTCOME CRITERIA	INTERVENTIONS

3 Knowledge Deficit
 	
r.t. unfamiliarity with individual wound management program
	• Describes the wound management program
	• Demonstrates correct techniques of individual wound management program
		• Assess knowledge regarding current wound management program
		  - desired information
		  - learning ability, style
		  - previous method of wound management
		  - deficits that hamper learning (motivation, lifestyle, financial resources)

	• Describes preventative care and s/s of complications to report	• Provide individualized instructions regarding bathing, skin care, specific wound care procedure, s/s to report • Initiate referral to appropriate resources if needed
		RATIONALE: *To be effective, the care must be individualized based on the patient's knowledge, learning style, and need/readiness for information.*

OTHER LESS COMMON NURSING DIAGNOSES: *High Risk for Disuse Syndrome; Diversional Activity Deficit*

ESSENTIAL DISCHARGE CRITERIA

• Has clean wounds which show reduction in size

• Actively participates in wound management program

• Demonstrates correct techniques of individual wound management

WOUND INFECTION

NURSING DIAGNOSES	OUTCOME CRITERIA	INTERVENTIONS

1 Impaired Tissue Integrity
 	
r.t. wound infection
	• Becomes free of local or systemic infection
	  - normal VS, BP
	  - no odors or drainage around or through
	  - incision free of redness, drainage; edges are approximated
	  - normal CBC
	  - negative cultures
	  - no nosocomial infection
		• Monitor VS q4h
		• Assess the following wound parameters q4-8h
		  - size: length, width, and depth
		  - extent of tissue involvement: partial or full thickness
		• Assess the following wound parameters at dressing change or at least q4h
		  - type of tissue in wound base (viable versus nonviable granulation tissue, necrotic tissue)
		  - exudate: volume, color, consistency, and odor
		  - wound edges and surrounding skin: presence of epithelialization, maceration, induration, denudation, papules, pustules
		  - presence of foreign bodies: suture material, dressing material, etc.
		• Assess presence of pain in and around wound and medicate as indicated

	• Shows normal lab values
	  - albumin
	  - total protein
	  - electrolytes
	  - ABGs
	  - BUN
		• Monitor lab values that impact on wound healing and report abnormalities

	• Cultures are negative for aerobic and anaerobic bacteria	• Obtain wound culture (aerobic culture in open viable wounds, anaerobic culture in wounds with necrotic tissue or sinus tracts)
		  - flush wound with saline
		  - utilize a Ca alginate swab; swab the wound edges and the wound base
		  - use correct technique to minimize risk of further contamination

MEDICAL

203

NURSING DIAGNOSES	OUTCOME CRITERIA	INTERVENTIONS

	• Wound tissue shows progression through healing phases	• Provide appropriate environment for wound healing
		  - remove necrotic tissue on foreign bodies: consult with physician on methods of debridement of necrotic tissue or suture removal (loose debris may be removed by irrigation of the wound surface; hydrotherapy may also be used)
		  - if topical antibiotics are indicated based on wound culture, apply as ordered
		  - obliterate dead space in wound by using light packing
		  - choose a dressing that will absorb excess wound exudate
		  - choose a dressing that will maintain a moist environment over the wound surface
		  - secure dressing to encourage mobility

	• Cultures show no evidence of nosocomial infection	• Use aseptic technique when providing wound care; consult with the physician to determine if sterile or clean technique will be used
		  - sterile technique: use sterile gloves, instruments, and supplies
		  - clean technique: use clean gloves, sterile instruments, and clean supplies
		
		• Wear gloves when handling body fluids; hand-washing will be done prior to and after each patient contact; gowns and eye protection should be used if splashing of body fluids occurs

		RATIONALE: *Increased VS, abnormal laboratory cultures may be indicators of local or systemic infection. H&H and ABGs indicate volume and O_2 capacity to assist in healing. Albumin and total protein indicate nutritional parameters available to wound healing. Cleansing, debridement, and dressing remove a medium for bacterial growth. Viable, red, moist tissue is essential for wound healing to occur. Confining and containing body fluids prevent cross-contamination.*

NURSING DIAGNOSES	OUTCOME CRITERIA	INTERVENTIONS

2 Knowledge Deficit
 	
r.t. inability to demonstrate wound management skills
	• Patient/family correctly demonstrate knowledge of required care
	  - demonstrate wound care procedure
	  - accurately describe wound tissue condition
	  - correctly identifies s/s of infection
		• Determine if patient can do own wound care; involve family as back-up
		
		• Demonstrate correct wound care technique
		
		• Observe a return demonstration; continue with lessons until acceptable technique is demonstrated
		
		• Explain s/s of wound infection and how to describe tissue condition and ask for demonstration that information is understood
		
		• Provide printed information about s/s of infection, the steps of wound care, and whom to notify if wound condition deteriorates
		
		• Assess home situation and make referrals for appropriate home services as indicated

		RATIONALE: *A competent, knowledgeable patient/family member is likely to provide safe, effective wound care.*

3 Altered Nutrition: Less than body requirements
 	
r.t. increased metabolic need relative to intake
	• Maintains balanced I&O
	  - shows normal serum electrolytes
	  - has no vomiting or abnormal GI functioning
		• Monitor I&O levels; report discrepancies
		
		• Assess amount of wound drainage; include in output measures

	• Maintains, gains weight	• Weigh daily
	• Takes, retains at least 80 percent of required nutrients	• Consult with dietary staff to insure that adequate calories and vitamins are provided for tissue defense and wound repair
	• Patient/family demonstrate knowledge of nutritional requirements	• Assist family in planning high calorie, high protein meals • Assist to identify food preferences, including foods high in complex carbohydrates and protein

MEDICAL

205

NURSING DIAGNOSES	OUTCOME CRITERIA	INTERVENTIONS

RATIONALE: *Assessment of nutritional status and interventions to optimize nutritional status will promote tissue repair and wound healing.*

OTHER LESS COMMON NURSING DIAGNOSES: *Body Image Disturbance; Pain; Fluid Volume Deficit*

ESSENTIAL DISCHARGE CRITERIA

- Is free from s/s of wound infection; viable, healing tissue is present

- Patient/family verbalize/demonstrate correct knowledge of wound care and assessment

SURGICAL NURSING

SURGICAL

ADRENALECTOMY

NURSING DIAGNOSES	OUTCOME CRITERIA	INTERVENTIONS

See "Postoperative Care" care plan in General Section

1 Fluid Volume Deficit

r.t. altered fluid regulatory mechanisms

- Shows normal VS
- Has good skin turgor, moist mucous membranes
- Has no bleeding

- Monitor VS, CVP q1-2h until stable, then per post-op routine
  - assess effects of posture on BP; assist with ambulation when BP is labile
  - report to physician immediately: hypotension; rapid, weak pulse; and/or decreasing urinary output

---

- Maintains balanced I&O

- Monitor I&O
- Administer IV fluids, glucocorticoid preparations (IV/PO) and insulin as ordered

---

- Shows normal serum electrolytes

- Monitor serum electrolytes and blood glucose

- Maintains stable body weight

- Weigh daily

RATIONALE: *Removal of the adrenal gland diminishes the availability of glucocorticoids and mineral corticoids to regulate fluids during a stress response, so that post-op cardiovascular collapse and shock are more likely.*

---

2 Knowledge Deficit

r.t. unfamiliarity with surgical procedure and follow-up regimen

- Patient/family discuss physiology of disease process, rationale for treatment

- Instruct (patients having a bilateral adrenalectomy) regarding the lifelong requirement of glucocorticoid and mineral corticoid replacement
- Instruct (patients having a unilateral adrenalectomy) regarding glucocorticoid replacement requirement for approximately 2 years post-op

---

- Patient/family discuss knowledge of complications

- Describe early s/s of adrenal insufficiency

- Patient/family express concerns, questions

- Encourage questions and feedback

NURSING DIAGNOSES	OUTCOME CRITERIA	INTERVENTIONS
	• Patient/family participate in care activities	• Discuss need to wear or carry medical alert information
		RATIONALE: *Explaining the prescribed treatment and encouraging verbalization minimize stress and foster commitment to treatment regimen.*
3 High Risk for Infection *r.t. immunosuppression*	• Remains free of local infections - no odors or drainage around or through - incision is free of redness, drainage; edges are approximated	• Use strict surgical asepsis when changing wound dressings • Monitor for edema, redness, warmth • Instruct about wound care, hand-washing technique, and avoiding contact with those with URI
	• Remains free of systemic infection - normal CBC - negative cultures - no nosocomial infection - no fever	• Monitor WBCs, cultures
	• Mobilizes secretions	• Encourage coughing and deep breathing
		RATIONALE: *These measures are to monitor for and decrease the risk of infection in the immunocompromised patient.*

OTHER LESS COMMON NURSING DIAGNOSES: *Pain; Activity Intolerance; High Risk for Injury*

ESSENTIAL DISCHARGE CRITERIA

• Is adrenally sufficient

• Is free of infection

• Verbalizes knowledge of medications, complications, emergency treatment, and reportable s/s

SURGICAL

AMPUTATION

NURSING DIAGNOSES	OUTCOME CRITERIA	INTERVENTIONS

See "Postoperative Care" care plan in General Section

1 Impaired Physical Mobility

r.t. loss of limb

- Regains mobility after wound healing

  - Assist with ambulation 12-24 h post-surgery
  - If unable to walk, assist out of bed to wheelchair or chair 12-24 h after surgery
  - While in bed, elevate stump for 24 h
  - Assist with progressive mobility; assist out of bed to chair and progress to ambulation with crutches or walker

- Shows no evidence of contractures

  - Avoid pillow under stump after 24 h to prevent flexion contracture of the hip
  - Turn and position on side, back, and abdomen (after 24 h) to maintain ROM and prevent contractures
  - Perform ROM exercises q4h to unaffected extremities
  - Perform abduction and extension exercises to affected extremity q4h
  - Instruct and demonstrate upper body building exercises and use of trapeze

- Demonstrates use of adaptive devices to increase mobility

  - Provide and instruct in using ambulation devices: crutches, walker
  - Encourage use of good walking shoe
  - Maintain stump in relaxed, downward position when ambulating

  RATIONALE: *These measures encourage ambulation and independence as soon as possible and prevent complications due to immobility. They also foster a positive approach to the loss of a body part.*

NURSING DIAGNOSES	OUTCOME CRITERIA	INTERVENTIONS
2 High Risk for Injury *r.t. surgical intervention, infection, or prosthesis trauma*	• Incisional site remains clean, dry, and intact with no evidence of excessive bleeding or infection	• Monitor VS q2-4h for 24 h, then q8h or as indicated • Assess dressings and incision for color and amount of drainage • Assess stump for edema, proximal pulses, tissue perfusion, and pain • If drains in place, monitor color and amount of drainage • If cast in place, monitor CMS and bleeding • Assist in applying Ace bandages in circular eight technique or stump shrinker • Demonstrate and encourage stump massage as ordered • Obtain referral to orthotist for prosthetic follow-up as indicated
		RATIONALE: *These measures promote healing and prevent the development of complications.*
3 Pain *r.t. surgical amputation or phantom limb pain*	• Verbalizes/displays freedom from pain	• Assess character, intensity, location of pain
	• Reports relief following analgesia	• Administer analgesics and sedatives as ordered and use PCA when possible • Assess effectiveness of pain relief measures 30 min to 1 h after interventions
	• Identifies activities that reduce or aggravate discomfort	• Assist and encourage position changes • Assist with nonpharmacologic pain control methods (relaxation, music, imagery) • Pace activities and provide rest periods

SURGICAL

211

NURSING DIAGNOSES	OUTCOME CRITERIA	INTERVENTIONS
	• Describes any phantom sensations and/or pain; participates in managing pain	• Discuss and explain phantom sensations and/or pain • Encourage person to talk about feelings and concerns • Instruct on appropriate use of analgesics and comfort measures **RATIONALE:** *Pain control enables the person to focus on rehabilitative efforts and to conserve physical and psychic energy.*
4 Body Image Disturbance *r.t. limb loss*	• Expresses feelings; displays behaviors consistent with adaptive coping patterns - expresses feelings - shares feelings with family - identifies own strengths	• Assess meaning of the loss of limb for the patient • Assess patient's response to limb loss (denial, shock, anger, depression) • Encourage and provide time for expression of loss and grief • Assist in identifying positive coping behaviors • Encourage communication with significant other regarding feelings and concerns • Encourage participation in amputee support group
	• Participates in self-care	• Encourage patient to view stump • Promote independence in ADL and stump care • Praise accomplishment and review progress in coping **RATIONALE:** *Developing and utilizing effective coping strategies foster adaptation to body image changes.*

NURSING DIAGNOSES	OUTCOME CRITERIA	INTERVENTIONS
5 Knowledge Deficit *r.t. inexpereince with stump care and rehab program*	• Patient/family verbalize/ demonstrate ability to manage self-care at home and to follow rehab program - anatomy and physiology of amputation - reportable s/s: fever, inflammation of incision, prolonged phantom pain, increasing edema of the stump - wound, stump care - performing ADL	• Demonstrate dressing changes, incisional care, and skin care • Encourage independence in ADL and stump care as early as possible • Explain and provide list of s/s to report to physician
	• Expresses commitment to rehab follow-up	• Stress importance of rehabilitation program and reinforce physical therapy directives • Assess need for home healthcare referral
		RATIONALE: *Knowledge of what is expected on discharge assists the patient in adapting effectively to daily living and in avoiding complications which may require readmission to an acute care setting.*

> **OTHER LESS COMMON NURSING DIAGNOSES:** *Fluid Volume Deficit; High Risk for Impaired Skin Integrity; High Risk for Peripheral Neurovascular Dysfunction*

SURGICAL

ESSENTIAL DISCHARGE CRITERIA

- Maintains mobility at optimal level
- Reports pain is controlled
- Has clean, dry, and intact incisional area

- Demonstrates positive coping patterns
- Verbalizes/demonstrates understanding and competence for home care management and rehabilitation

APPENDECTOMY

NURSING DIAGNOSES	OUTCOME CRITERIA	INTERVENTIONS

See "Postoperative Care" care plan in General Section

1 Ineffective Breathing Pattern

r.t. painful respiratory effort

- Exhibits normal depth of respirations
- Exhibits unlabored RR, depth, and rhythm WNL

- Report rise in patient's temperature, RR, pulse

- Exhibits normal respiratory status
  - 12-20 breaths/min
  - SaO_2 WNL

- Monitor respirtory status q2-4h
- Encourage deep breathing exercises q2h
- Use incentive spirometer q2h
- Teach incision splinting to facilitate deep breathing exercises
- Perform pulmonary toileting as necessary
- Encourage early and frequent ambulation
- Administer O_2 therapy as ordered

RATIONALE: *Early detection and treatment of ineffective respiratory efforts promote recovery.*

---

2 Pain

r.t. tissue trauma

- Verbalizes/displays freedom from pain
  - no guarding of incision

- Note duration, location, and intensity of pain

- Reports comfort following analgesia

- Alleviate patient's anxiety regarding pain with adequate explanations and deep breathing exercises
- Note frequency of self-medication
- Educate in use of PCA pump as indicated

- Identifies medication or activity that reduces or aggravates discomfort

- Reinforce pre-op teaching: incisional splinting
- Administer narcotic analgesics to prevent pain

NURSING DIAGNOSES	OUTCOME CRITERIA	INTERVENTIONS
		RATIONALE: *Comfort facilitates coughing, deep breathing, ambulation, and early recovery.*
3 Knowledge Deficit *r.t. unexpected surgery*	• Has list of reportable s/s	• Instruct s/s to report to physician - fever, chills, or redness at incisional site - drainage or foul odor noted from suture line
	• Possesses emergency phone numbers	• Return to emergency department for fever
	• Verbalizes correct knowledge of follow-up care regimen	• Advance activity and ambulation gradually as advised by physician
		RATIONALE: *Knowledge of post-op regimen enhances self-care and recovery.*

> **OTHER LESS COMMON NURSING DIAGNOSES:** High Risk for Infection; Anxiety

SURGICAL

ESSENTIAL DISCHARGE CRITERIA

- Verbalizes comfort
- Ambulates freely with unlabored respirations

- Verbalizes correct knowledge of wound care, activity, medications, and follow-up regimen

ARTHROPLASTY, TOTAL JOINT REPLACEMENT

NURSING DIAGNOSES	OUTCOME CRITERIA	INTERVENTIONS

See "Postoperative Care" care plan in General Section

1 High Risk for Fluid Volume Deficit

r.t. highly vascular surgical area

- Does not present s/s of hypovolemia during postoperative phase
- *Hip:* shows no bleeding; wound drainage does not exceed 500 mL during first 24 h and does not exceed 100 mL second 24 h
- *Knee:* wound drainage during the first 8 h is about 200 mL, less than 25 mL by 48 h post-op
- Shows normal VS, BP

- Assess for potential hemorrhage by monitoring VS and wound drainage qh x 4h, q2h x 8h, then q8h until discharge

---

- Shows CRT < 3 sec

- Assess pedal pulses, CRT, s/s of early shock at same intervals as VS and wound drainage

---

- Has dry, intact dressing

- Inspect patency of drainage tubes and devices q2h

- H&H WNL

- Monitor H&H

- Urinary output WNL

- Monitor I&O q4-8h
- Reinfuse blood using autotransfusion method, as directed

RATIONALE: *Because fluid volume deficit results from an output that is greater than intake, these parameters are monitored to identify when fluid balance is re-established.*

---

2 Pain

r.t. tissue trauma

- Verbalizes/displays freedom from pain

- Assess level of pain (1-10 scale) q2-4h

- Reports comfort following administration of analgesia
- Exhibits signs of decreasing pain

- Provide prescribed analgesics before pain becomes severe; report if insufficient

---

- Identifies medication or activity that reduces or aggravates discomfort

- Maintain limb in proper position
- Move gently with sufficient assistance; maintain flexion, within limitations

NURSING DIAGNOSES	OUTCOME CRITERIA	INTERVENTIONS
	• Alternates periods of activity and rest	• Teach/provide supplementary pain control measures: distraction, diversion, imaging, relaxation exercises
		RATIONALE: *Alleviating pain minimizes the stress response and promotes healing, recovery, and patient satisfaction.*
3 High Risk for Impaired Skin Integrity *r.t. decreased mobility, pressure from appliances and wound drainage*	• Has clear and intact skin	• Assess all skin areas q4h
	• No excoriation around incisional area - dressings remain dry	• Monitor fade time • Turn q2h, unoperated side or 45° both sides (with specific order); use abduction pillow or two regular pillows between legs for hip replacement (no pillow under knee for knee replacement) • Provide mobility aids (trapeze or special mattress) as needed • Involve patient in position shifting routine by encouraging "shifts" using trapeze, q30 min or more often • Use heel and elbow protectors • Keep sheets, elastic wraps, bed clothing wrinkle-free
		RATIONALE: *Frequent turning prevents pressure against prominences. A special mattress or heel/elbow protectors also reduce pressure against affected areas.*
4 High Risk for Injury (external) *r.t. unsteady gait, weakness, pain*	• Remains free of injury	• Encourage use of trapeze for arm strength • Monitor H&H; if low, ambulate with caution or postpone • Encourage isometrics, gluteal exercises, abdominal exercises • Reinforce PT muscle exercises and teaching regarding transfer and ambulation • Provide walker, elevated toilet seat

SURGICAL

NURSING DIAGNOSES	OUTCOME CRITERIA	INTERVENTIONS
		• Assist/supervise each transfer, ambulation until agreed safe by PT • Provide additional analgesia 30 min prior to major moves or ambulation
		RATIONALE: *Developing arm, gluteal, and abdominal strength enhances free, balanced movement and steady gait. Supervision with assistive devices further reduces the risk of injury.*
5 Knowledge Deficit *r.t. home management of fatigue, pain, immobility*	• Patient/family demonstrate required care/skill - demonstrates safe transfer, ambulation	• Explain use of CPM for knee replacement as indicated • Collaborate with PT, discharge planner to mutually reinforce teaching of transfer, ambulation, assistive devices
	• Patient/family list reportable s/s	• Review reportable s/s: increasing pain, fever, tenderness in calf or thigh, sharp chest pain
	• Patient discusses relaxation, activity, diet	• Verify knowledge of follow-up care techniques, medications, diet, activity, rest, appointments
	• Patient/family verbalize knowledge of follow-up appointments	• Verify safe, realistic home care plan; assess need for assistive devices or healthcare visitor
		RATIONALE: *Providing essential information promotes self-care, family participation, and compliance with postoperative regimen and enhances recovery.*

> **OTHER LESS COMMON NURSING DIAGNOSES:** *High Risk for Injury (allergic reaction); High Risk for Injury (displacement of prosthesis); High Risk for Injury (fat embolism, thrombophlebitis); High Risk for Infection; Impaired Physical Mobility; Altered Tissue Perfusion; Constipation; Ineffective Airway Clearance*

ESSENTIAL DISCHARGE CRITERIA

- VS WNL; afebrile
- Exhibits no s/s of cardiopulmonary or peripheral vascular complications
- Exhibits no signs of joint dislocation
- Has clear, intact skin
- Controls pain with oral analgesia

- Transfers/ambulates, performs ADL with minimal assistance
- Demonstrates knowledge of weight-bearing, adduction, flexion precautions
- Accurately describes recommended diet, rest, physical therapy, follow-up activities
- Demonstrates safe use of assistive devices

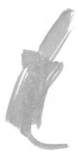

SURGICAL

BURNS AND GRAFTS

NURSING DIAGNOSES	OUTCOME CRITERIA	INTERVENTIONS

See "Postoperative Care" care plan in General Section

1 Pain

r.t. exposed nerve endings and edema due to burn injury

- Verbalizes/displays reasonable comfort

- Assess HR, BP, RR
- Assess the level of discomfort using a 0-10 point self-rating scale to obtain an objective measure

- Achieves, maintains sustained comfort

- Adminster ordered analgesia
  - medicate with maximal dose to break pain cycle as long as LOC, HR, BP are stable
  - instruct to ask for medication when pain begins and not to wait
  - re-evaluate pain medication 5 min after IV; 20 min after IM; monitor VS and behavior; ask patient to rate pain using scale
  - explain that until there is sustained relief, alternatives will be tried

- Reports reasonable comfort during dressing changes, PT

- Perform exercises, PT, or dressing changes shortly before peak of drug effects

- Actively participates in nonpharmacologic pain control techniques

- Explain other pain relief treatments (relaxation techniques, diversion, music therapy, or imagery)
- Position for comfort

- Maintains body temperature WNL; no episodes of chilling, shivering

- Maintain warm environment approximately 76-82°F to ensure comfort; monitor body temperature
- Consider referral for hydrotherapy

RATIONALE: *Pain causes many symptoms: increased BP, HR, RR, as well as pupillary dilation, diaphoresis, pallor, grimacing, clenching fists, and apprehension. Scheduling analgesia for peak effect at the time of activity or wound care prevents unnecessary pain.*

NURSING DIAGNOSES	OUTCOME CRITERIA	INTERVENTIONS
2 Fluid Volume Deficit *r.t. plasma loss and fluid shift into interstitium*	• Maintains balanced fluid volume; adequate tissue perfusion	• Record baseline weight; weigh at same time, same scale
	• Maintains VS, BP WNL - balanced I&O - CVP, Hct WNL - serum K, Na WNL after first 24-48 h - urinary sp. gr. WNL - PCWP/CVP WNL - no pulmonary edema after first 24-48 h - has a period of diuresis after first 24-48 h - palpable peripheral pulses - CRT < 3 sec	• Monitor HR, BP, RR, I&O temperature, urinary output, PCWP, and/or CVP if available qh during fluid resuscitation and acute phase, then q4-8h when stable • Monitor for hypothermia • Assess for signs of hypovolemia - restlessness - significant decrease in BP - significant increase in HR - rapid or labored respirations - decrease in urine output - decrease or absent peripheral pulses - CRT > 3 sec - CVP < 5 cm/H_2O • Start IV with large bore needle (size 18 or 16); maintain IV fluids per orders (crystalloids or colloids usually are ordered depending on physician preference)
	• Is free of fluid overload - no dyspnea, crackles - no increase in BP - no dysrhythmias	• Assess and report signs of excessive fluid replacement: dyspnea, crackles, increase in BP, CVP > 15 cm/H_2O
	• ECG WNL or normalizing	• Assess ECG for dysrhythmias that may result from hemodynamic instability and/or abnormal electrolytes • Monitor lab results; report abnormal results to physician • Assist with application of dressing to reduce evaporative fluid loss

RATIONALE: *Assessment of fluid volume status helps determine the effectiveness of fluid and electrolyte therapy.*

SURGICAL

NURSING DIAGNOSES	OUTCOME CRITERIA	INTERVENTIONS

3 Altered Tissue Perfusion (renal, cardio-pulmonary, gastrointestinal, peripheral)
 	
r.t. hypovolemia, peripheral edema
	• Maintains adequate systemic tissue perfusion
	  - unlabored respirations
	  - urinary output WNL
	  - no urinary hematuria or discoloration
	  - skin warm, dry
	  - palpable peripheral pulses
		• Assess and report any s/s of decreased tissue perfusion
		  - monitor VS q1-4h; report any significant decrease in BP, HR > 100 BPM, labored respirations
		  - monitor urinary output; report output < 30 mL/h
		  - observe for hematuria (or brownish-red, indicating intravascular hemolysis)
		  - monitor skin color; report cool, pale, mottled, or cyanotic skin in unburned areas

	• Shows no changes in baseline LOC	• Report any changes in LOC, restlessness, or confusion
	• Adjusts to position changes without dizziness, fainting	• Change patient's position slowly to allow time for autoregulatory mechanisms to adjust to position change • Maintain adequate fluid replacement • Maintain optimal mobility • Provide adequate nutrition
	• Peripheral edema diminishes	• Palpate peripheral pulses; report absence or decrease in quality (peripheral pulses should be marked and checked with Doppler flow meter qh for 48 h post-burn or until edema subsides) • Assess and record presence of edema; if present - elevate extremity above level of heart
	• Shows decrease in circumference of burned areas	• Measure circumference of burned area to determine if edema is increasing - assist with escharotomy or fasciotomy of circumferential burns
		RATIONALE: *Measures to optimize fluid, electrolyte, and nutritional balance help to maintain circulation, circulating volume, and promote tissue healing.*

NURSING DIAGNOSES	OUTCOME CRITERIA	INTERVENTIONS
4 High Risk for Infection *r.t. burn injury*	• Remains free of systemic or local infection - no signs of systemic infection - normal VS, BP - normal CBC - negative cultures - no nosocomial infection - no s/s of infection - afebrile	• Assess and record HR, respirations, BP, and temperature • Report any signs of local infection • Monitor for therapeutic and nontherapeutic effects of topical anti-infectives (silver sulfadiazine, mafenide acetate, silver nitrate) • Monitor WBCs; report persistent elevations and/or significant changes • Evaluate need for antibiotics, tetanus toxoid, and/or tetanus immune globulin • Practice good hand-washing; use mechanical friction, soap and water before/after care • Implement isolation precautions
	• Is free of bladder infection - no burning on urination - urine not cloudy or has foul odor - negative urine cultures	• Secure catheters to prevent piston movement • Place an occlusive sterile dressing over invasive catheters - transparent, occlusive dressing should be changed q72h or when integrity is disrupted - gauze dressing should be changed q48h or when integrity is disrupted • Eliminate all nonessential stopcocks on IV tubings • Select new anatomic site for tape each time catheter is inserted
	• Burn areas show no evidence of infection - show progressive phases of tissue healing - no purulent drainage, erythema, new swelling	• Change all dressings using sterile technique • Change dressing at graft and donor site per orders - donor sites are usually dressed with a hydrocolloid - graft sites are delicate and should not be dislodged; cover with large, occlusive bulky dressing to hold skin securely - evaluate sheet skin grafts for blebs which interfere with healing

SURGICAL

NURSING DIAGNOSES	OUTCOME CRITERIA	INTERVENTIONS

RATIONALE: *Measures that minimize tissue trauma, provide barriers to infection, and minimize entry of pathogens all reduce the risk of infection.*

5 Impaired Skin Integrity

r.t. partial thickness or full thickness burn

- Experiences no further skin impairment

- Assess skin q4h during acute phase and q8h thereafter; report any color changes of skin, mucous membranes, nail beds
- Turn q2h, or more often if bony prominences remain erythematous > 15 min after pressure is relieved (erythema unresolved within 15 min indicates tissue ischemia)
- Prevent skin shear and friction
  - allow feet to rest against footboard when HOB elevated
  - do not elevated HOB higher than 30° (to decrease sliding)
  - provide heel and elbow protectors
  - use lift sheet to reposition
- Apply tape without tension to prevent blistering
  - remove tape by peeling away while stabilizing skin, or use gauze or Montgomery straps
  - avoid use of adhesive
- Keep skin clean and dry
- Use aseptic technique for dressing changes

RATIONALE: *These measures help to prevent further skin breakdown, prevent pressure and trauma to injured tissue.*

> **OTHER LESS COMMON NURSING DIAGNOSES:** *Impaired Physical Mobility; Altered Nutrition: Less than body requirements; Body Image Disturbance; Ineffective Individual Coping; Knowledge Deficit; Hypothermia; Pain; Fluid Volume Excess; High Risk for Disuse Syndrome*

ESSENTIAL DISCHARGE CRITERIA

- Maintains physiological homeostasis
- Shows blood lab values WNL
- Has healing burn area, free of infection
- Verbalizes/displays reasonable comfort

- Patient/family verbalize/demonstrate understanding of burn healing and therapeutic regimen including wound care
- Patient/family recognize complications; identify when to notify physician

SURGICAL

CARDIAC SURGERY

NURSING DIAGNOSES	OUTCOME CRITERIA	INTERVENTIONS

See "Postoperative Care" care plan in General Section

1 Decreased Cardiac Output

r.t. blood loss, dysrhythmias, and compromised contractility

- Demonstrates stable hemodynamic parameters
  - CVP 0-8 mmHg
  - ECG, cardiac enzymes WNL
  - urinary output WNL
  - oriented to person, time, and place

- Monitor noninvasive hemodynamic parameters qh until stable, then as indicated
  - RR and temperature
  - observe for hemodynamic decompensation
  - auscultate heart and lungs q2-4h
  - monitor cardiac enzymes as indicated

- Achieves, maintains cardiac output sufficient for desired lifestyle
  - RR normalizing
  - CRT WNL
  - warm, moist skin; good turgor
  - pink mucous membranes
  - chest drainage decreasing; no frank bleeding

- Monitor cardiac output qh until stable
  - assess cardiac rhythm, neck veins, CRT, peripheral pulses
  - assess color and temperature of skin and skin turgor
  - observe chest tube drainage for amount, color, and consistency

- Shows no cardiac dysrhythmias

- Monitor ECG pattern for cardiac dysrhythmias q1-2h
  - determine pacemaker type and setting, if indicated
  - keep exposed pacemaker wires wrapped in sterile dressing
  - notify physician of any abnormal parameters or assessment

RATIONALE: *Effectiveness of cardiac output is determined by these assessment parameters. Prompt treatment of cardiac decompensation prevents complications from poor perfusion.*

2 Fluid Volume Deficit

r.t. surgical fluid loss and vasodilatation experienced during the rewarming period

- Achieves balanced I&O

- Monitor I&O q4h
- Administer blood and fluids as prescribed
- Reinfuse blood using autotransfusion method as indicated

- Shows stable hemodynamic parameters

- Monitor hemodynamic parameters qh until stable, then per post-op routine

NURSING DIAGNOSES	OUTCOME CRITERIA	INTERVENTIONS
	• Shows normal fluid and electrolyte balance	• Assess for postoperative hemorrhage and hemodynamic decompensation
		• Monitor BUN, Hct, K, and creatinine
	• Displays good skin turgor, moist mucous membranes	• Assess skin turgor and oral mucosa for hydration status
		RATIONALE: *Optimal circulation volume and fluids and electrolyte balance are essential for cellular repair and recovery.*
3 Ineffective Breathing Pattern *r.t. anatomical incision and splinting*	• Takes at least 12-20 deep, regular respirations/min	• Assess respiratory parameters: ABGs, RR, depth, and quality
	• Chest x-rays are clear	• Auscultate lungs
		• Suction prn
	• ABGs WNL	• Maintain ventilatory settings as ordered
		• Determine adequate endotracheal tube cuff inflation, if indicated
		• Administer analgesics, sedatives as needed to maintain ventilator control
	• Weans from ventilator	• Wean from ventilator when awake with adequate respiratory mechanics
		• Use tactile and vocal stimuli to increase breathing rate/depth
		• Encourage deep breathing
		• Provide aggressive pulmonary toilet following weaning from ventilator
		• Promote coughing, deep breathing, turning q2h
		RATIONALE: *Assessment of respiratory parameters and ventilatory interventions helps determine the adequacy of effectiveness of the breathing pattern. Effective breathing pattern is essential to O2 perfusion and cellular nutrition.*

SURGICAL

NURSING DIAGNOSES	OUTCOME CRITERIA	INTERVENTIONS
4 Altered Tissue Perfusion (cardio-pulmonary) *r.t. decreased cardiac output*	• Has palpable pulses; normal CRT	• Assess peripheral pulses and document characteristics (symmetry, rate, weak, bounding)
	• Maintains urinary output WNL	• Monitor urinary output • Assess for peripheral edema
	• Maintains HR 60-100 beats/min	• Use Doppler pulses if necessary • Provide for passive and active exercises • Apply elastic stockings
	• Exhibits warm, dry skin	• Assess skin for color, temperature and symmetry • Measure both calves; assess for tenderness, redness, edema
		RATIONALE: *Injury can occur if perfusion is inadequate.*
5 Impaired Gas Exchange *r.t. altered ventilation/perfusion ratio*	• Exhibits balanced ventilation/perfusion ratio - achieves, maintains normal (for patient) RR, HR, rhythm - neurobehavioral abnormalities absent, reduced - cyanosis resolved - ABGs WNL	• Monitor RR, HR qh until stable • Assess neurobehavioral characteristics q1-2h - level of restlessness/calm - orientation to time, place, person • Maintain CT patency and function • Maintain O_2 supplement at recommended level • Limit suction duration < 15 sec • Implement airway clearance techniques • Assist with technological support of arterial oxygenation (mechanical ventilation, incentive spirometry) • Monitor ABGs, Hb as indicated
		RATIONALE: *Interventions to clear airway improve ventilation/perfusion ratio.*

NURSING DIAGNOSES	OUTCOME CRITERIA	INTERVENTIONS
6 Pain *r.t. surgical interruption of body structure, flatus, and immobility*	• Verbalizes/displays freedom from pain	• Monitor self-reports of pain q2-4h • Assess for angina
	• Reports comfort following analgesia	• Provide routine analgesic dosing; observe for effects
	• Identifies medication or activity that reduces or aggravates discomfort	• Position to alleviate pressure, stretch, or strain
	• Alternates periods of activity and rest	• Promote uninterrupted rest periods • Provide sensory and procedural information before potentially painful techniques • Provide emotional support; listen, give positive feedback • Instruct about nonpharmacological methods of pain control (imagery, progressive muscle relaxation, and distraction)
		RATIONALE: *Pain relief promotes healing by minimizing the energy demands associated with the stress response.*

7 Impaired Verbal Communication
 	
r.t. presence of endotracheal tube
	• Transmits messages through alternative methods (written communication, flip chart)
	• Demonstrates increased ability to understand
	  - affirms caregiver responses to messages
	  - responds appropriately to care
	• Demonstrates decreased frustration with communication; displays calm body posture, social expressions
		• Provide alternative methods of communication (pad and pencil, flash cards, flip chart, pantomime)

		RATIONALE: *Successful communication reduces sensory overload, anxiety, and stress response.*

SURGICAL

NURSING DIAGNOSES	OUTCOME CRITERIA	INTERVENTIONS

8 High Risk for Infection

r.t. inadequate primary defenses and invasive procedures

- Remains free of local/systemic infections
  - incision is free of redness, drainage; edges are approximated
  - is afebrile; normal VS
  - no nosocomial infection

- Reduce entry of organisms into individuals
  - meticulous hand-washing
  - aseptic technique for dressing changes and endotracheal suction
- Teach patient/family about s/s of infection
- Restrict invasive devices (IVs, central lines, Foley catheters)

RATIONALE: *These actions minimize entry of pathogens and maximize the immune response.*

9 Altered Nutrition: Less than body requirements

r.t. increased nutritional requirements for wound healing

- Maintains/regains weight
- Shows normal lab values

- Monitor body weight, I&O, total proteins, albumin qd

- Has no vomiting

- Eliminate/modify etiologies/related factors where possible (pain, nausea, fluid volume deficit)
- Provide nutrition that supplies adequate protein and calories

- Takes/retains 80 percent of meals

- Serve frequent small meals
- Serve favorite foods
- Assist with feedings
- Administer oral hygiene after meals and in morning and evening
- Consult dietitian

RATIONALE: *Optimal nutritional status promotes cellular repair.*

NURSING DIAGNOSES	OUTCOME CRITERIA	INTERVENTIONS
10 Self-Esteem Disturbances *r.t. lifestyle change and body image*	• Identifies positive aspects of self - makes positive self-reports - asserts self	• Assess and mobilize current support system
	• Expresses a positive outlook for the future	• Assist in identifying and expressing feelings
	• Analyzes own behavior and its consequences	• Assist in identifying positive self-evaluations
	• Identifies ways of exerting control and influencing outcomes	• Examine and reinforce positive abilities, traits • Help to identify negative thoughts • Refer to community resources as indicated
		RATIONALE: *Exploring feelings and effective coping mechanisms enhance self-esteem.*
11 Altered Family Processes *r.t. surgical outcomes and disruption of roles in the family system*	• Family members freely express feelings to each other	• Assist family with appraisal of the situation; give positive support to openness among family members • Create a private and supportive hospital environment for family
	• Family participates in care of the ill family member	• Acknowledge strengths to family when appropriate
	• Family facilitates patient's change from sick role to well role	• Discuss meaning of role transition and how it can be fostered
	• Maintains functional mutual support system • Seeks appropriate external resources when needed	• Make referrals to support networks as needed (pastoral care, social services)
		RATIONALE: *A strengthened family support system enhances compliance with the medical regimen, post-op recovery, and quality of life.*

SURGICAL

NURSING DIAGNOSES	OUTCOME CRITERIA	INTERVENTIONS
12 Altered Health Maintenance *r.t. insufficient knowledge of incisional care, pain management, s/s of complications, pharmacological care, risk factors, stress management, and follow-up care*	• Discusses lifestyles that will promote health	• Assess knowledge of primary prevention (diet, weight control, avoid alcohol and tobacco, regular exercise) • Assess home resources
	• Identifies, describes health behaviors needed to manage condition	• Determine knowledge to manage condition (wound care, medications, risk factors, restrictions, follow-up care) • Teach importance of secondary prevention (physical exams)
	• Describes reason for reporting s/s of complications: fever, weakness, dyspnea, coughing, edema, lethargy	• Teach reportable s/s; explain reasons • Determine need for referrals

RATIONALE: *Interventions to reduce risk factors will contribute to the success of surgical intervention.*

OTHER LESS COMMON NURSING DIAGNOSES: *Dysfunctional Ventilatory Weaning Response; Relocation Stress Syndrome; Sleep Pattern Disturbance; Knowledge Deficit; Altered Thought Processes*

ESSENTIAL DISCHARGE CRITERIA

• Maintains oxygenation and cardiac output sufficient for desired lifestyle

• Shows stable hemodynamic parameters

• Maintains stable body weight

• Controls pain with oral analgesia

• Shows no evidence of infection

• Patient/family verbalize understanding of follow-up regimen and reduction of risk factors

CHOLECYSTECTOMY

NURSING DIAGNOSES	OUTCOME CRITERIA	INTERVENTIONS

See "Postoperative Care" care plan in General Section

1 Ineffective Breathing Pattern

r.t. decreased lung expansion

- Takes at least 12-20 deep, regular respirations/min
  - has clear lungs bilaterally
  - remains afebrile

- Perform TCDB q2h
- Assist to TCDB 30 min after analgesia
- Splint incision with pillow, binder, or hands
- Dangle, ambulate as indicated
- Administer analgesia; assess effects

RATIONALE: *Chest and body mobility with splinting and analgesia expands chest without undue pain.*

2 Impaired Skin Integrity

r.t. surgical incision, skin irritation from bile salts, altered nutrition

- Has clean incision; edges well-approximated
  - surrounding tissue free from irritation

- Record T-tube drainage
- Keep T-tube unclamped with collection bag below waist level
- Anchor tubes
- Observe, record color, type, amount of drainage, stools
- Change dressings frequently; use Montgomery's straps if possible

- Reports minimal discomfort from pruritus

- Wash incisional skin with mild soap and water; apply Vaseline gauze, zinc oxide, Karaya powder, or other protective paste, as necessary

RATIONALE: *Protection from kinks or tension prevents tissue injury. Special products provide moisture (if necessary), minimize itching, and shield the skin from further impairment.*

SURGICAL

233

NURSING DIAGNOSES	OUTCOME CRITERIA	INTERVENTIONS
3 Knowledge Deficit *r.t. home care needs*	• Lists reportable symptoms	• Review reportable symptoms: jaundice; pruritus; clay-colored stools; dark urine; foul-smelling, dark brown or green drainage from wound or around T-tube; increasing T-tube drainage; chronic heartburn; bloating
	• Demonstrates safe wound and T-tube care	• Demonstrate wound and T-tube care; give rationale for procedures
	• Lists medications, dosages, effects, and side effects	• Review medications, dosages, effects, and side effects
	• Selects appropriate dietary items from list; reports correct rationale	• Provide written instructions regarding diet instructions and restrictions

RATIONALE: *Providing the necessary information facilitates patient involvement, promotes self-care, and improves compliance with the treatment plan.*

OTHER LESS COMMON NURSING DIAGNOSES: *High Risk for Fluid Volume Deficit; Impaired Physical Mobility; High Risk for Infection; Altered Nutrition: Less than body requirements*

ESSENTIAL DISCHARGE CRITERIA

- Is afebrile
- Shows no signs of wound infection
- Demonstrates wound and T-tube care (if applicable)

- Describes s/s of wound infection
- Lists reportable symptoms
- Correctly selects both prescribed and contraindicated foods from list

CHOLELITHIASIS, LITHOTRIPSY

NURSING DIAGNOSES	OUTCOME CRITERIA	INTERVENTIONS

See "Postoperative Care" care plan in General Section

1 Anxiety

r.t. insufficient knowledge of lithotripsy procedure

- Verbalizes understanding of procedure

- Demonstrates effective, appropriate coping mechanisms in managing anxiety

- Determine level of understanding of procedure
- Reinforce physician's explanation of procedure

- Provide instruction on general information regarding post-op routine
- Include reasons for activities, oral dissolving agents, and their importance
- Provide brochures and/or educational video
- Evaluate effectiveness of teaching and need for further reinforcement or support
- Suggest relaxation techniques and diversional activities to use while waiting for procedure

RATIONALE: *Maladaptive coping strategies and moderate to severe anxiety interfere with the learning process.*

2 Pain

r.t. lithotripsy procedure

- Reports level of pain

- Verbalizes increased comfort in response to treatment

- Assess location, severity, and duration of pain
- Observe for nonverbal s/s of pain

- Observe for symptoms of biliary colic
- Administer analgesics and assess effectiveness
- Utilize nonpharmacologic pain control methods as appropriate (positioning, relaxation, diversion, etc.)

RATIONALE: *These measures promote comfort and detect symptoms of biliary obstruction.*

SURGICAL

235

NURSING DIAGNOSES	OUTCOME CRITERIA	INTERVENTIONS

3 Knowledge Deficit
 	
r.t. post-procedure expectations/discharge instructions
	• Verbalizes appropriate follow-up instructions
	  - pathophysiology of disease
	  - reportable s/s
	  - expected course of recovery
	  - follow-up appointments
		• Explain symptoms of potential complications (biliary colic/obstruction) and appropriate follow-up
		
		• Review discharge instructions with patient and/or family
		
		• Provide clear written discharge instructions

		RATIONALE: *Enhanced knowledge alleviates anxiety and promotes compliance.*

> **OTHER LESS COMMON NURSING DIAGNOSES:**
> *Altered Nutrition: Less than body requirements; Fear*

ESSENTIAL DISCHARGE CRITERIA

• Reports minimal pain/discomfort

• Demonstrates minimal anxiety

• Verbalizes understanding of discharge instructions

COLON RESECTION

NURSING DIAGNOSES	OUTCOME CRITERIA	INTERVENTIONS

See "Postoperative Care" care plan in General Section

1 Fluid Volume Deficit

r.t. acute ischemic event

- Exhibits normalizing fluid and electrolyte balance
  - Assess for severe fluid/electrolyte loss, metabolic acidosis, hypovolemic shock

- Shows normal VS, BP, CVP
  - has no bleeding
  - Monitor post-op VS, CVP, NGT q1-4h
  - Measure abdominal girth q8h

- Displays good skin turgor, moist mucous membranes
  - Assess mucous membranes, skin turgor

- Maintains balanced I&O
  - Maintain strict I&O

- Shows normal fluid and electrolyte balance
  - normal urinary sp. gr.
  - Monitor serum electrolytes, urinary sp. gr.
  - Replace IV fluids, electrolytes, blood, and plasma as ordered
  - Notify physician of change in status

- Maintains stable body weight
  - Monitor weight qod

RATIONALE: *If perforation occurs, gas and fluids will accumulate, causing distention, sepsis, and fluid/electrolyte and acid/base imbalance.*

2 Pain

r.t. acute ischemia and surgical trauma

- Experiences sustained comfort
  - verbalizes, displays freedom from pain; reports reasonable comfort
  - displays behaviors consistent with comfort (relaxed body posture; no guarding of surgical area)
  - reports comfort following administration of analgesia
  - has normal bowel sounds; no rigidity of abdomen
  - identifies medication or activity that reduces/aggravates discomfort
  - alternates periods of activity and rest

- Assess abdomen for signs of peritonitis, ileus (but limit palpation), increased severity and diffuseness of pain, rebound tenderness, guarding
- Provide narcotic, NSAIDs as prescribed
- Position for comfort, but limit sudden movement

SURGICAL

NURSING DIAGNOSES	OUTCOME CRITERIA	INTERVENTIONS

| | | **RATIONALE:** *Successful interventions to prevent pain perception will reduce anxiety and stress response, will prevent complications, and promote recovery.* |

3 Altered Nutrition: Less than body requirements

r.t. major resection

- Maintains adequate nutritional status
  - maintains normal GI function
  - regains weight
  - shows normal serum electrolytes
  - has no vomiting

- Assess GI function; auscultate for returning bowel sounds, which should return 2-4 d post-op
- Maintain NGT function; remove when ordered
- Provide parenteral nutrition if ordered
- Introduce clear liquids and enteral nutrition slowly, then solids

- Patient/family demonstrate knowledge

- Provide discharge instructions to patient/family concerning TPN management; consult Home Health
- Consult with dietitian as indicated

RATIONALE: *Gradual introduction of enteral nutrients prevents accumulation of gas and fluids and promotes GI tolerance to feedings.*

4 Altered Tissue Perfusion (gastrointestinal)

r.t. interruption of arterial flow

- Shows improved tissue perfusion
  - stoma is cherry red
  - no retraction or prolapse into the abdomen

- Assess stoma color and integrity
- Inspect stomal dressing, if any, for irritation, drainage, bleeding

RATIONALE: *Frequent assessment determines adequacy of tissue perfusion to new stomal site.*

NURSING DIAGNOSES	OUTCOME CRITERIA	INTERVENTIONS

5 Knowledge Deficit
 	
r.t. unfamiliarity with postoperative course and treatment regimen
	• Patient/family discuss pathophysiology of disease process, rationale for treatment
	• Patient/family verbalize knowledge of complications
		• Provide patient/family education
		  - potential post-op complications (bleeding, infection)
		  - presence of diarrhea caused by rapid transit for up to 6 months post-op

	• Patient/family list reportable s/s	• Review reportable s/s: change in wound/stoma appearance, complications
	• Patient/family demonstrate required care skills	• Teach colostomy care (should start functioning 2-4 d post-op; encourage patient to look at stoma and touch apparatus) and plans for later surgical closure, as indicated • Consult with enterostomal therapist as indicated
	• Patient/family express commitment to consistent medical follow-up • Patient/family discuss relaxation, activity, diet	• Review prescribed diet, medications, activity, relaxation
	• Patient/family possess phone numbers of emergency medical help	• Verify and provide information for routine and emergency help
		RATIONALE: *Providing essential information will promote patient/family involvement and enhance compliance with the post-op regimen.*

SURGICAL

> **OTHER LESS COMMON NURSING DIAGNOSES:** *Diarrhea; Body Image Disturbance; Impaired Skin Integrity; High Risk for Infection; Ineffective Management of Therapeutic Regimen*

ESSENTIAL DISCHARGE CRITERIA

- Returns to normal hydration levels
- Reports control over pain with oral analgesia
- Verbalizes understanding of medications/diet to decrease bowel transit time

- Returns to normal body weight or has plans for TPN follow-up at home
- Demonstrates correct colostomy care as indicated

FACIAL FRACTURES

NURSING DIAGNOSES	OUTCOME CRITERIA	INTERVENTIONS

See "Postoperative Care" care plan in General Section

1 Pain
r.t. facial fractures

- Verbalizes pain relief 30 min after receiving pain medicine

- Order pain medicine as ordered
- Keep HOB elevated
- Offer other relaxation techniques such as imagery, distraction, or breathing techniques

RATIONALE: *Comfort measures reduce anxiety and promote healing.*

---

2 Altered Nutrition: Less than body requirements

r.t. pain from facial fractures, difficulty chewing, and lack of appetite

- Maintains weight

- Weigh daily

- Shows normal lab values

- Monitor CBC, albumin, electrolytes, and vitamins

- Takes, retains 80 percent of meals

- Assess ability to chew and swallow
- Consult with dietitian for soft diet
- Encourage nutritious snacks and shakes
- Provide atmosphere that is conducive to comfortable eating
- Offer pain medicine before meals

- Affirms the need to eat high protein diet

- Explain need for protein, vitamins to enhance healing

RATIONALE: *Facial manipulation (wired jaws), loss of taste and smell, the inability to chew, and a blenderized diet can contribute to weight loss.*

---

3 Ineffective Breathing Pattern

r.t. facial edema, wiring

- Takes at least 12-20 deep, regular breaths/min

- Assess RR, rhythm, and depth q2-4h

RATIONALE: *Treatment for facial fractures often compromises the airway.*

NURSING DIAGNOSES	OUTCOME CRITERIA	INTERVENTIONS
4 Body Image Disturbance *r.t. facial disfigurement*	• Shows awareness of change or loss	• Assist in the expression of feelings by providing privacy and support
	• Expresses grief	• Communicate acceptance of feelings • Offer social opportunities with persons who have had similar experiences
	• Acknowledges change	• Provide education about condition, prognosis, rehab services, and care
	• Demonstrates an interest in appearance and own care	• Praise small accomplishments • Encourage visits from family and friends • Involve patient and family in care
		RATIONALE: *Facial trauma can lead to temporary or permanent facial changes to which the patient may need to adjust.*
5 Sensory Alteration (visual, olfactory, gustatory) *r.t. facial fractures*	• Demonstrates understanding of sensory changes	• Assess the effect this change has on the nutritional status and on time perception • Educate as to the senses affected by the injury • Alter environmental factors to provide meaningful stimuli • Maintain verbal and eye contact and touch • Give clear, concise explanations of environment, treatments, etc.
	• Is free from injury	• Provide for safety: rails up, call light in reach, uncluttered room
		RATIONALE: *If the patient is unable to see, smell, or taste the food, this will affect nutrition; if the patient is not able to see, the visual loss may affect time and space orientation.*

SURGICAL

241

NURSING DIAGNOSES	OUTCOME CRITERIA	INTERVENTIONS
6 Impaired Verbal Communication *r.t. pain, surgical manipulation, immobility of facial structures*	• Communicates needs and wants easily, using both nonverbal communication and other means	• Assess the level of ability of communication • Provide paper, pens, chalk board, or a picture board for communication • Be aware of the limitations and provide ample time to listen and understand • Keep call bell within reach to minimize anxiety --- **RATIONALE:** *A wired jaw and swollen lips, tongue, and pharynx all contribute to unclear speech.*

OTHER LESS COMMON NURSING DIAGNOSES: *Altered Oral Mucous Membranes; High Risk for Infection (CSF Leak); Knowledge Deficit; Ineffective Airway Clearance; Impaired Swallowing; Altered Tissue Perfusion*

ESSENTIAL DISCHARGE CRITERIA

- Controls pain
- Maintains weight
- Has full and easy respirations
- Experiences no difficulty swallowing

- Communicates needs
- Begins to verbalize acceptance of altered body image

FEMOROPOPLITEAL BYPASS

See "Postoperative Care" care plan in General Section

1 Altered Tissue Perfusion (peripheral) *r.t. vascular obstruction*	• Maintains neurovascular integrity to the extremity	• Perform neurovascular assessment q2-4h • Document and report immediately any evidence of neurovascular compromise
	• Reports/displays absence of pain	• Assess for pain
	• Displays no pallor, cyanosis	• Observe color of skin
	• Has palpable peripheral pulses	• Palpate pulses using marked areas for consistent assessment
	• Shows no evidence of paresthesia or paralysis	• Monitor for evidence of paraesthesia and absence of or decreased sensation, including 2-point discrimination • Observe for paraesthesia of anterior surface of affected leg, dorsum of foot and great toe, and inability to dorsiflex foot/extend toes • Position affected extremity with slight knee flex • Avoid pressure over peroneal nerve
	• Shows no edema	• Observe for presence and amount of edema
	• Extremities are of equal warmth	• Compare temperatures of both extremities
	• CRT is < 3 sec	• Observe capillary filling after compression of arteries of extremity • Elevate extremity to level of heart until edema is controlled, but not above the patient's CVP

SURGICAL

243

NURSING DIAGNOSES	OUTCOME CRITERIA	INTERVENTIONS
	• Patient/family discuss potential complications; have list of reportable s/s	• Instruct patient/family about s/s of peripheral neurovascular compromise • Emphasize importance of notifying nurse/physician immediately of numbness or tingling, increasing pain, increased swelling, or change in color
		RATIONALE: *Failure of circulatory return to extremity when pressure is released indicates arterial injury. The best check for sensitivity is 2-point discrimination. The primary concern of neurovascular dysfunction is impairment of nerves or blood vessels distal to the area of surgery. Early detection of neurovascular compromise can avoid irreversible and permanent damage. Permanent and irreversible damage resulting in paresis, paralysis, or amputation can occur rapidly, even over a period of hours. Elevating the extremity aids venous return to decrease edema, but elevating the extremity above the patient's CVP impedes arterial flow and increases edema rather than decreases it. Pressure on the peroneal nerve can result in permanent foot drop.*
2 High Risk for Infection *r.t. surgical incision*	• Incision is free of redness, drainage; edges are approximated	• Assess surgical site q8h and with dressing changes; report any changes/abnormal findings
	• Shows normal VS; is afebrile	• Monitor temperature; report elevation
	• Shows normal CBC, WBC count, differential	• Monitor results of CBC and report WBC/differential abnormalities • Utilize appropriate precautions to prevent infections - aseptic technique - avoid invasive procedures • Teach patient/family about appropriate aseptic practice
	• Shows negative cultures	• Obtain cultures per order and report abnormalities

NURSING DIAGNOSES	OUTCOME CRITERIA	INTERVENTIONS
	• Takes, retains at least 80 percent of required diet	• Provide diet high in protein and calories to promote healing
		RATIONALE: *Patients with one or more infection symptoms or risk factors are considered high risk. High calorie, high protein, and high vitamin foods promote cellular repair and regeneration.*

3 Knowledge Deficit
 	
r.t. unfamiliarity with treatment regimen
	• Patient/family discuss, demonstrate required care of extremity	• Instruct patient/family to protect peripheral circulation
		  - keep legs level with or slightly lower than heart to promote arterial circulation
		  - avoid prolonged exposure to cold environment
		  - avoid pressure on extremities by use of protective devices
		  - change positions at least every hour
		  - avoid leg crossing
		  - encourage ROM exercises
		  - avoid standing or sitting with legs dependent for long periods of time

	• Patient/family discuss required rest, activity, diet; affirm need to reduce risk factors	• Explain, provide exercise program or active/passive ROM to extremities q2h as appropriate
		
		• Teach about modifying lifestyle to reduce risk factors
		  - smoking
		  - high fat diet
		  - sedentary lifestyle
		  - hypertension
		  - stress

	• Patient/family discuss, have list of reportable s/s
	  - cuts
	  - rashes
	  - ulcers
	  - reddened areas
	  - increased pain
		• Instruct about s/s to report to physician; explain significance of these complications

		RATIONALE: *Exercise promotes adequate circulation and formation of collateral blood vessels. Knowledge of how to prevent vascular occlusion will optimize success of surgical intervention.*

SURGICAL

> **OTHER LESS COMMON NURSING DIAGNOSES:** Activity Intolerance; Chronic Pain; Impaired Physical Mobility

ESSENTIAL DISCHARGE CRITERIA

- Neurovascular assessment WNL
- Shows no s/s of infection

- Patient/family affirm need to prevent further peripheral vascular occlusion

FEMUR FRACTURE

See "Postoperative Care" care plan in General Section

1 Pain

r.t. trauma, muscle spasm, and surgery

- Verbalizes/displays reasonable comfort

- Assess location, duration, severity of pain; identify precipitating or relieving factors

---

- Identifies medication or activity that reduces or aggravates discomfort

- Reposition in proper alignment q2h
- Massage back and buttocks
- Provide an orthopedic bedpan

- Reports comfort following analgesia

- Administer prescribed narcotic analgesic q3-4h for 3-5 days or use PCA, if prescribed
- Administer non-narcotic analgesics as prescribed

RATIONALE: *Muscle spasm, trauma, and surgery result in nerve and tissue injury that causes pain. Optimal alignment reduces pressure on nerves and tissue and decreases strain on muscles.*

2 Impaired Physical Mobility

r.t. fractured femur and soft tissue trauma

- Demonstrates progressive ability to move in bed, ambulate, and transfer self without bearing weight on affected extremity

- Perform neurovascular assessment q2-4h on affected extremity
- Keep on bed rest for prescribed period of time; explain purpose of bed rest and gradual increase in mobility
- Explain use of trapeze bar and use of unaffected foot flat on bed with knee bent to move upward in bed or to lift buttocks
- Support joints of injured extremity
- Teach quadriceps, buttocks, and triceps setting exercises
- Assist with transfer from bed to chair without weight bearing on affected leg as prescribed
- Supervise use of assistive devices, i.e., crutches, walker

SURGICAL

NURSING DIAGNOSES	OUTCOME CRITERIA	INTERVENTIONS
		RATIONALE: *Bed rest promotes healing by tissue requirements. Support of joints and affected extremity prevents additional injury and relieves pressure and pain.*
3 Body Image Disturbance *r.t. temporary loss of independence*	• Expresses positive statements about self	• Assess patient's concerns regarding self-concept and body image • Encourage verbalization of feelings about altered level of functioning and dependency • Give realistic feedback about changes in level of functioning and expected outcome
	• Readily participates in treatment and care activities	• Allow participation in all therapeutic modalities offered in treatment • Allow independence in self-care to the extent possible
		RATIONALE: *A feeling of being listened to and understood contributes to a positive mental attitude. Participation in care fosters positive feelings of control and autonomy.*

OTHER LESS COMMON NURSING DIAGNOSES: *Altered Peripheral Tissue Perfusion; Altered Tissue Perfusion, Cardiopulmonary; Impaired Skin Integrity; High Risk for Infection; Knowledge Deficit*

ESSENTIAL DISCHARGE CRITERIA

- Controls pain with oral analgesia
- Demonstrates transfer techniques and use of ambulatory assistive devices without weight bearing on affected extremity

- Discusses restrictions to follow at home

GASTRIC RESECTION/GASTROSTOMY

NURSING DIAGNOSES	OUTCOME CRITERIA	INTERVENTIONS

See "Postoperative Care" care plan in General Section

1 Knowledge Deficit (pre-op)

r.t. surgery, anesthesia, potential lifestyle adjustments, anticipated pain

- Patient/family discuss anatomy of disease process; rationale for surgery
  - Assess for understanding of surgical events

- Patient/family discuss expected course of recovery; ask appropriate questions
  - Explain postoperative care (NGT, IVs)
  - Allow time for questions and clarification

- Patient/family discuss relaxation, activity, diet
  - Describe postoperative care activities (TCDB, leg exercises, diet)

- Patient/family discuss medication
  - Describe and discuss use of narcotics
  - Administer preoperative medicines as ordered

- Patient/family participate in care activities
  - Involve significant others in preoperative care

RATIONALE: *Preoperative knowledge deficits have negative impacts on postoperative pain and compliance. Including significant others in postoperative care may aid compliance with postoperative regimens. (Note: This surgery is often done on an emergency basis, which would require an alteration of this plan.)*

2 Pain

r.t. incision, NGT

- Verbalizes/displays freedom from pain
  - Assess for verbal and nonverbal pain

- Reports comfort following analgesia
  - Administer pain medications regularly, as ordered

- Identifies medication or activity that reduces or aggravates discomfort
  - Determine noninvasive pain relief measures previously utilized
  - Teach, encourage commonly used noninvasive techniques (e.g., relaxation)

SURGICAL

249

NURSING DIAGNOSES	OUTCOME CRITERIA	INTERVENTIONS
		• Promote frequent turning for comfort
		• Use gastric suction to remove liquids, gas, and blood from stomach
		RATIONALE: *Pain can cause guarding with movement, leading to complications of immobility. Anxiety and gastric distension can increase pain.*
3 **Altered Nutrition: Less than body requirements** *r.t. disruption of normal bowel function and gastrostomy feedings*	• Maintains homeostasis of fluids and electrolytes	• Auscultate for bowel sounds • Monitor I&O
	• Exhibits no s/s of gastric dilatation	• Monitor for NGT dysfunction (note: manipulation of the NGT not generally done) • Monitor for early satiety and regurgitation • Measure NGT drainage to accurately determine F&E corrections • Report s/s of abdominal pain, hypotension, or tachycardia
	• Describes dietary regimens to reduce occurrences of dumping syndrome	• Monitor weight daily when feedings begin • Give blenderized food at room temperature • Clamp tube between feedings • Report s/s of dumping syndrome • Encourage moderate amount of fat, low carbohydrate
	• Identifies means to correct B_{12}, folic acid, and iron deficiencies	• Teach need for permanent parenteral administration of B_{12}, folic acid, iron supplements
		RATIONALE: *When bowel sounds return, carefully graduated feedings provide nutrition.*

NURSING DIAGNOSES	OUTCOME CRITERIA	INTERVENTIONS

4 Ineffective Breathing Pattern
 	
r.t. post anesthesia, incisional pain, decreased mobility
	• Exhibits improving respiratory status
	  - 12-20 deep, regular respirations/min
	  - baseline amount, color of secretions
	
	• ABGs, SaO2 WNL
		• Assess RR and depth; auscultate for adventitious breath sounds
		• TCDB q2h or more frequently until fully ambulatory
		• Encourage use of incentive spirometer q2h while awake
		• Position to promote chest expansion
		• Monitor ABGs and pulse oximetry

	• States minimal or no discomfort during postoperative pulmonary toilet	• Administer pain relief medications 30 min prior to activity • Teach splinting of incision during TCDB exercises • Administer O2 as ordered
		RATIONALE: *Anesthesia, immobility, high abdominal incisions, and pain prevent optimal breathing pattern.*

5 High Risk for Aspiration
 	
r.t. gastrostomy feedings
	• Exhibits no evidence of aspiration
	  - has clear breath sounds
	  - is afebrile
		• Assess for changes in RR, development of adventitious breath sounds
		• Monitor for temperature spike
		• Avoid stress before and after meals
		• Provide rest after each meal
		• Place in high Fowler's position during and 1 h following feedings
		• Increase intake gradually from clear liquids to blenderized feedings
		• Change to continuous feedings if indicated

		RATIONALE: *A frequent complication of gastrostomy feedings is aspiration pneumonia.*

SURGICAL

NURSING DIAGNOSES	OUTCOME CRITERIA	INTERVENTIONS
6 High Risk for Impaired Skin Integrity *r.t. presence of gastrostomy*	• Skin remains intact around gastrostomy	• Assess site around gastrostomy for evidence of redness and breakdown
	• Initiates appropriate skin care measures	• Keep skin clean and dry • Use protective barriers as needed
		RATIONALE: *Gastric secretions are irritating to the skin.*
7 Knowledge Deficit *r.t. long-term lifestyle adjustments and feedings via a gastrostomy tube*	• Patient/family discuss anatomy of surgery, rationale for post-op care • Patient/family list reportable s/s	• Teach s/s of potential complications (pain, persistent diarrhea, tarry stools, vomiting)
	• Patient/family participate in care activities	• Provide privacy during feedings • Encourage client to sit with family during meals
	• Patient/family express concerns, questions	• Allow expression of feelings
		RATIONALE: *Eating is a highly social activity. Changes in normal eating patterns may lead to depression. Include family in teaching activities to aid in successful lifestyle adjustments.*

> **OTHER LESS COMMON NURSING DIAGNOSES:** *Diarrhea; High Risk for Fluid Volume Deficit; Altered Oral Mucous Membrane; Impaired Social Interaction; Social Isolation; Impaired Adjustment; High Risk for Activity Intolerance; Body Image Disturbance; Altered Tissue Perfusion*

ESSENTIAL DISCHARGE CRITERIA

• Has clear lungs with no s/s of aspiration pneumonia

• Shows stabilized weight

• Tolerates gastrostomy feedings

• Controls pain with oral analgesics

• Displays intact skin around gastrostomy

• Patient/family reiterate s/s of potential complications

NURSING DIAGNOSES	OUTCOME CRITERIA	INTERVENTIONS

See "Postoperative Care" care plan in General Section

NURSING DIAGNOSES	OUTCOME CRITERIA	INTERVENTIONS
1 Pain *r.t. tissue trauma secondary to surgical incision*	• Verbalizes/displays freedom from pain	• Assess type, character, and location of pain • Administer analgesia routinely - assess effectiveness

	• Displays no nonverbal pain behaviors (i.e., moaning, crying, grimacing)	• Provide noninvasive pain relief
		  - distraction
		  - relaxation techniques
		  - comfort measures

	• Displays no guarding behaviors	• Anchor all tubes and drains securely to prevent pulling
	• Mobilizes secretions with minimal discomfort	• Encourage to use splinting techniques
		RATIONALE: *Pain is real to and is based on the individual's perception of it. Relief of pain allows performance of postoperative respiratory and mobility exercises.*

2 Ineffective Airway Clearance
 	
r.t. secretions
	• Clears secretions effectively
	  - usual rate/depth of respirations
	  - clear lung sounds
	  - absence of cough
	  - afebrile
	  - usual skin color
		• Assess for symptoms of ineffective airway clearance q4h (adventitious breath sounds, cough, dyspnea, fever, cyanosis)
		• Teach to perform
		  - deep breathing exercises q2h
		  - coughing q2h
		  - use of incentive spirometer q2h
		  - splinting with movement and breathing exercises
		• Obtain satisfactory return demonstration of respiratory exercises
		• TCDB q2h
		• Encourage ambulation as prescribed
		• Encourage fluids to 2500 mL/d to help liquify secretions, unless contraindicated

SURGICAL

NURSING DIAGNOSES	OUTCOME CRITERIA	INTERVENTIONS
		RATIONALE: *Respiratory exercises and early ambulation are done postoperatively to prevent atelectasis due to mucous plugs, excessive secretions, and/or shallow breathing.*
3 High Risk for Fluid Volume Deficit *r.t. decreased oral intake and excessive fluid losses*	• Shows normal VS, BP	• Monitor VS per post-op routine
	• Displays good skin turgor, moist mucous membranes	• Monitor for s/s of fluid volume deficit - poor skin turgor, dry mucous membranes
	• Shows normal serum electrolytes	• Monitor electrolytes qd
	• Achieves, maintains balanced I&O	• Monitor I&O balance qd • Observe amount, type, and color of NG drainage q4h as indicated • Monitor amount of oral feeding taken when prescribed • Administer prescribed IV fluids
	• Has stable body weight	• Weigh daily
		RATIONALE: *Patients with drainage tubes (i.e., NG, chest tubes) are at risk for dehydration and electrolyte imbalances.*
4 Anxiety *r.t. unfamiliar routines of hospitalization*	• Recognizes anxiety and uses effective coping mechanisms - verbalizes decrease in anxiety - demonstrates ability to learn postoperative teaching required	• Explain all procedures to patient • Provide reassurance and comfort • Make frequent visits to patient • Decrease sensory stimulation • Assist patient to identify his usual coping mechanisms • Encourage patient to verbalize his anxieties and needs
		RATIONALE: *Anxiety varies with the individual depending on the severity of the threat and can effect the patient's ability to cope with hospitalization.*

NURSING DIAGNOSES	OUTCOME CRITERIA	INTERVENTIONS
5 Knowledge Deficit *r.t. unfamiliarity with post-op follow-up care*	• Patient/family list medications	• Instruct how to take and monitor effects, side effects of all medications
	• Patient/family participate in care activities	• Instruct patient to inspect wound daily for - redness - swelling - drainage - warmth
	• Patient/family list reportable s/s	• Report any s/s of wound infection or elevated temperature to physician
	• Patient/family discuss diet activity	• Instruct patient to prevent gastric distention by - eating slowly - limiting gas-producing foods (i.e., beans, cabbage) - eating small meals • Instruct to not bend or lift heavy objects or drive for the period of time prescribed by physician
	• Patient/family verbalize knowledge of follow-up appointments	• Instruct to keep all follow-up appointments

RATIONALE: *Teaching should be done when patient faces new and unfamiliar situations regarding his/her health. Teaching will help patient reach and maintain his/her optimum level of health.*

SURGICAL

OTHER LESS COMMON NURSING DIAGNOSES: Pain; Impaired Gas Exchange; Altered Nutrition: Less than body requirements

---

ESSENTIAL DISCHARGE CRITERIA

- Is afebrile
- Tolerates diet
- Shows VS, Hct, and electrolytes WNL

- Verbalizes comfort
- Exhibits clear lungs
- Verbalizes/demonstrates knowledge regarding wound care, diet, activity limitations, and medications

HIP PIN (PROSTHESIS)

NURSING DIAGNOSES	OUTCOME CRITERIA	INTERVENTIONS

See "Postoperative Care" care plan in General Section

1 Pain

r.t. trauma and muscle spasms

- Verbalizes/displays freedom from pain or reasonable comfort
  - relaxed body posture, facial expressions
  - no guarding

- Evaluate pain: location, quality, onset, duration, causative factors, relieving factors; rate pain on a scale from 1-10
- Appraise and evaluate for sudden increase in pain, muscle spasms, changes in joint mobility, position, chest pain, SOB, restlessness, changes in LOC

- Reports comfort following analgesia

- Evaluate effect of prescribed analgesia before complaints; report if insufficient relief

- Identifies medication or activity that reduces or aggravates pain

- Employ collaborative interventions
  - epidural infusions
  - narcotics, analgesics
  - muscle relaxants
  - NSAIDs
  - thermal treatment
  - PT
  - continuous passive ROM devices
  - other exercising devices and early ambulation/activity
- Maintain limb in proper position; move gently with sufficient assistance
- Furnish accurate information to reduce fear of addiction, cause of pain, and therapeutic regimen
- Educate about alternative pain control such as distraction, diversion, imaging, relaxation exercises, breathing exercises, therapeutic touch

RATIONALE: *These measures relieve surgical pain, reduce anxiety, and reduce muscle spasms. Early recognition prompts immediate intervention and associated prevention of complications.*

NURSING DIAGNOSES	OUTCOME CRITERIA	INTERVENTIONS

2 Altered Tissue Perfusion (peripheral)
 	
r.t. decreased mobility, positioning, and surgical intervention
	• Displays increased perfusion
	  - warm/dry, peripheral pulses present/strong (3 = normal on a scale from 1-4)
	  - VS WNL
	  - alert, oriented to date, place, time
	  - balanced I&O
	  - absence of edema
	  - no increased redness
	  - absence of ecchymosis
	  - absence of drainage
	  - wound approximated
	  - free of pain or discomfort
		• Monitor VS frequently for s/s of hypovolemia, shock, infection, or sepsis
		• Watch for changes in mental status, pallor, SOB, VS, orthostatic pressure changes, signs of fluid and electrolyte imbalances
		• Monitor diagnostic tests as appropriate such as CBC, PT, PTT
		• Evaluate for any s/s of bleeding or DIC
		• Evaluate for s/s of infection and no increase of positive signs of REEDA
		• Assess for pain: onset, duration, quality, intensity, site, and radiation
		• Inspect for positive Homans' sign
		• Inspect for patency of drainage devices, tubes, drains
		• Observe and monitor for s/s of compartment syndrome such as increased pain, swelling, changes in color and warmth by measuring thigh
		• Medicate as appropriate
		• Encourage early ambulation if not contraindicated
		• Avoid standing or lying for long periods of time
		• Encourage TCDB q2h

	• Experiences early detection, timely intervention for complications	• Inspect and report any s/s of pulmonary emboli such as sudden onset of pain, cyanosis, respiratory distress, hemoptysis, diaphoresis, hypoxia, anxiety, restlessness
		• Employ collaborative interventions: PT, thermal treatment, medications as prescribed (anti-inflammatory agents, narcotics, antibiotics)
		• Consider high risk for complications
		  - formation of thrombus/emboli
		  - fractures
		  - respiratory compromise
		  - diabetes
		  - bleeding

SURGICAL

NURSING DIAGNOSES	OUTCOME CRITERIA	INTERVENTIONS
		• Use elastic stockings, automated pneumatic hose, Ace bandages to improve circulation
		RATIONALE: *Identify problems early before complications occur by reducing pressure and keeping proper alignment and elevation. These measures decrease swelling and improve circulation.*
3 Impaired Physical Mobility *r.t. surgical procedure, decreased ROM, decreased muscle strength, pain, restrictive therapeutic regimen*	• Demonstrates knowledge and compliance with treatment regimen	• Monitor for circulation and nerve function of affected body part; note any changes in warmth, color, and perfusion • Monitor VS per post-op routine • Monitor diagnostic tests as ordered • Monitor for AAO to time, place, and person • Monitor for PERRLA • Assess for causative factors r.t. immobility • Assess for increased pain with mobility and mediate at least 30 min prior to movement • Assess and provide for adequate nutritional support • Assess for age-related musculoskeletal changes • Position for optimum comfort and alignment of affected joint • Instruct in use of safety devices (crutches, walkers, trapeze bars, chairs, etc.) • Observe for adequate intake and output • Observe for elimination bowel and bladder problems

NURSING DIAGNOSES	OUTCOME CRITERIA	INTERVENTIONS
	• Demonstrates increased strength and use of affected extremity	• Maintain adequate exercise program: have patient participate in prescribed ROM, ambulation, and PT activities and use isometric or passive ROM devices as ordered • TCDB q2h • Provide for medications as prescribed • Provide for daily ADL as per ability to assist • Encourage family to be involved in care
		RATIONALE: *Proper alignment, early mobilization, medication, and assistance with ambulation and positioning prevent complications and promote healing.*
4 High Risk for Infection *r.t. surgical procedure, implantation of prosthetic devices*	• Exhibits adequate wound healing and no s/s of systemic or local infection	• Assess and document for s/s of infection (decreased skin integrity, redness, swelling) • Monitor VS and watch for s/s of sepsis (fever, chills, diaphoresis, altered LOC, positive cultures) • Utilize aseptic techniques when treating patient (hand-washing, wound sterility, cleanse and change dressing as prescribed) • Encourage TCDB • Provide regular skin and catheter care as needed • Handle drains with sterile technique when emptying and repositioning • Assist with ADL as needed • Administer medications as prescribed (anti-infectants, antibiotics, etc.) • Educate patient about aseptic technique; care of wound and drain

SURGICAL

NURSING DIAGNOSES	OUTCOME CRITERIA	INTERVENTIONS
		RATIONALE: *Aseptic and sterile techniques reduce chances of nosocomial infection. Early assessment prevents complications.*

5 Knowledge Deficit
 	
r.t. lack of previous experiences with this surgery
	• Patient/family discuss anatomy of surgery and rationale for treatment	• Assess knowledge level and readiness to learn
		  - encourage support and participation from significant others
		  - determine physical and psychosocial needs and prioritize to meet learning needs
		
		• Review disease process, surgical procedure, and therapeutic regimen

	• Patient/family participate in care activities • Patient/family demonstrate required skill in use of transfer devices	• Collaborate with physical therapist, discharge planner to mutually reinforce transfer, ambulation, and use of devices
	• Patient/family verbalize knowledge of s/s of complications	• Review reportable s/s such as increasing pain, fever, numbness and tingling in extremity, pain and redness in calf, sharp chest pain
	• Patient/family discuss medications, relaxation, activity, diet	• Validate knowledge of follow-up care techniques, medications, diet, activity, rest
	• Patient/family discuss expected course of recovery, ask appropriate questions; have follow-up appointments	• Confirm safe environment, realistic plans for home care, and meeting follow-up appointments • Stress the importance of continuing therapeutic regimen and participation in rehabilitation period
		RATIONALE: *Knowledge promotes independence, self-care, participation in care, and informed choices.*

> **OTHER LESS COMMON NURSING DIAGNOSES:** *Body Image Disturbance; Anxiety;*
> *Self-Care Deficit; Constipation; Impaired Skin Integrity; Ineffective Management of Therapeutic*
> *Regimen; Fear; Altered Nutrition: Less than body requirements; High Risk for Fluid Volume Deficit*

ESSENTIAL DISCHARGE CRITERIA

- Shows stable VS; is afebrile
- Exhibits no cardiopulmonary or peripheral vascular complications
- Incision is healing without infection
- Has clear, intact skin
- Takes oral medications for analgesia and anticoagulation therapy
- Demonstrates knowledge of weight-bearing, abduction, adduction, flexion precautions

- Takes prescribed fluids, diet
- Bowel and urinary elimination patterns WNL
- Accurately describes diet, rest, PT, follow-up activities
- Demonstrates safe use of assistive devices
- Describes safe home environment for care
- Identifies long-term needs and who is responsible for actions to be taken
- Identifies available resources; possesses specific referrals

SURGICAL

HYSTERECTOMY

NURSING DIAGNOSES	OUTCOME CRITERIA	INTERVENTIONS

See "Postoperative Care" care plan in General Section

1 High Risk for Fluid Volume Deficit

r.t. postoperative bleeding, NPO

- Maintains balanced I&O

- Shows VS, blood counts stable, WNL

- Exhibits no s/s of shock

- Assess for s/s of fluid volume deficit: low BP, elevated HR, pallor, slow CRT, low H&H, low urinary output

- Administer IV fluids as ordered if PO intake and bowel sounds are absent

- Monitor pad count, amount, and color of discharge

RATIONALE: *Frequent monitoring prompts early detection, management of deficits.*

2 Altered Urinary Elimination

r.t. temporary bladder atony

- Voids within 6-8 h after discontinuation of urinary catheter

- Assess for bladder distention and absence of urinary output
- Monitor and record I&O
- Insert indwelling catheter, as ordered, if bladder atony is suspected

RATIONALE: *Anesthesia-related bladder atony can produce retention/distention. Early detection/prevention of retention prevents overdistention.*

3 High Risk for Injury

r.t. bed rest, decreased mobility, venostasis

- Is free of s/s of thromboembolism, DVT
  - Homans' sign
  - calf tenderness
  - sudden chest pain
  - sudden onset of dyspnea

- Assess for s/s of DVT, PE, or thromboembolism
- Apply antiembolic and/or pneumatic stockings
- Instruct patient on leg pumping exercises, ROM, early ambulation, and to avoid high Fowler's position and pressure under the knees
- Instruct to report any s/s of thromboembolism

NURSING DIAGNOSES	OUTCOME CRITERIA	INTERVENTIONS
		RATIONALE: *Pelvic surgery creates tissue trauma and swelling that reduces active venous flow from legs. Exercises and antiembolic stockings foster venous return.*
4 Pain *r.t. incisional discomfort*	• Reports reduced pain; tolerates increased activity	• Assess pain level and tolerance using pain scale • Administer analgesia as ordered; evaluate and record effects • Provide alternate comfort measures: turning, relaxation, massage, distraction
		RATIONALE: *Analgesia and other comfort measures combine to produce sustained pain control.*
5 High Risk for Infection *r.t. wound contamination, invasive lines and tubes, atelectasis, and pneumonia*	• Exhibits normal VS	• Monitor temperature frequently and record
	• Displays no redness, swelling around IV sites	• Assess IV sites, indwelling catheter output for signs of infection
	• Is free of urinary cloudiness or foul odor	• Utilize aseptic technique when changing dressings and performing site care
	• Exhibits normal breath sounds	• Assess breath sounds q shift and prn; monitor for lung congestion • Initiate early ambulation and periodic turning while on bed rest • Instruct to TCDB q2h when awake
		RATIONALE: *Frequent monitoring for signs of infection, combined with preventative techniques, reduces the risk for bacterial invasion.*

SURGICAL

NURSING DIAGNOSES	OUTCOME CRITERIA	INTERVENTIONS
6 Body Image Disturbance *r.t. perceived rejection by significant other, loss of feminine identity*	• Makes positive statements about self and relationship with significant other	• Assess understanding of body changes after hysterectomy • Assess for the need for follow-up, psychosocial support, and/or counseling • Allow expression of grief over loss of reproductive organ(s) and threats to feminine identity
	• Asks questions; seeks clarifications	• Clarify misconceptions about structural and physiologic changes
		RATIONALE: *Expression of concerns and accurate perceptions of reality in presence of supportive person(s) foster positive self-appraisal.*
7 Anxiety *r.t. misconceptions after hysterectomy*	• Verbalizes understanding of sexual adjustment related to hysterectomy - hormones are replaced synthetically - normal intercourse can resume when post-op healing is complete	• Assess the level of understanding of both patient and significant other about sexual functioning after hysterectomy
	• Patient/partner display physical closeness, support, caring	• Encourage physical closeness between partners; initiate discussion of fears, emotions, and sexual functioning
	• Patient/partner discuss fears; acknowledge accurate information	• Clarify misconceptions about sexual functioning • Provide reading materials on hysterectomy and sexual functioning; encourage discussion between partners
		RATIONALE: *Clarifying misconceptions about post-hysterectomy sexuality reduces inappropriate fears.*

NURSING DIAGNOSES	OUTCOME CRITERIA	INTERVENTIONS

8 Knowledge Deficit
 	
r.t. plan of care, post-discharge care
	• Verbalizes accurate understanding of self-care after discharge
	  - diet
	  - activity
	  - medications
	  - reportable s/s
	  - wound, perineal care
	  - follow-up appointments
		• Assess level of understanding of plan of care: diet and activity progression, postoperative care, and expectations
		
		• Assess readiness to learn aspects of hysterectomy self-care at home
		
		• Implement patient teaching plan as appropriate on the following
		  - post-op plan of care (diet, activity, I&O, monitoring)
		  - surgical menopause
		  - hormonal replacement therapy
		  - structural changes after hysterectomy
		  - discharge planning
		  - reportable s/s after discharge
		  - wound and perineal care
		  - follow-up appointments

RATIONALE: *A knowledgeable, competent patient is likely to manage a safe and uneventful recovery at home.*

OTHER LESS COMMON NURSING DIAGNOSES: *Altered Tissue Perfusion; Ineffective Breathing Pattern; Impaired Skin Integrity; Constipation; Knowledge Deficit*

ESSENTIAL DISCHARGE CRITERIA

- Returns to preoperative physiologic levels
- Performs ADL, rest, activity, and ambulates without assistance
- Performs safe wound care
- Verbalizes freedom from pain
- Regains normal urinary elimination pattern

- Discusses dosages, effects, side effects, and drug/food interactions of medications
- Discusses emotional and sexual adjustment to changes in body's structure and function
- Possesses written follow-up appointments and list of s/s to report to physician

SURGICAL

LAPAROTOMY

NURSING DIAGNOSES	OUTCOME CRITERIA	INTERVENTIONS

See "Postoperative Care" care plan in General Section

1 Pain
r.t. surgical incision

- Verbalizes/displays freedom from pain

- Assess pain on 1-10 pain rating scale
- Position patient comfortably
- Teach splinting of incision with folded blanket, pillow, or hands when moving or coughing

- Reports comfort following administration of analgesia

- Administer analgesics and monitor for effectiveness

- Identifies activities that reduce or aggravate discomfort

- Utilize nonpharmacologic pain management strategies
- Notify physician of persistent pain if not responding to interventions

RATIONALE: *Frequent assessment of pain, anticipatory analgesia, and comfort measures produce sustained levels of comfort.*

2 High Risk for Infection
r.t. break in skin integrity

- Exhibits no s/s of local infection
  - exhibits no odors or drainage around/through incision
  - incision edges are approximated

- Assess incision for redness, warmth, and drainage q4h and prn
- Change dressing prn using sterile technique
- Teach patient not to touch dressing or incision site

- Exhibits no s/s of systemic infection
  - remains afebrile
  - shows normal VS, BP
  - shows normal CBC

- Monitor VS per post-op routine; report elevated temperature
- Monitor lab values; report critical values as indicated

- Experiences no adverse effects of antibiotics

- Administer antipyretics and antibiotics as ordered

RATIONALE: *The body's primary body defense mechanism is disrupted by the surgical incision. Protection from bacterial invasion is essential.*

NURSING DIAGNOSES	OUTCOME CRITERIA	INTERVENTIONS

3 Ineffective Breathing Pattern
 	
r.t. location of incision, pain, abdominal distention
	• Exhibits improving respiratory status
	  - lungs clear
	  - 12-20 deep, regular breaths/min
		• Auscultate lungs q4h
		• Assess breathing pattern and rate q4h
		• Place in semi-Fowler's position while in bed
		• Encourage TCDB q2h prn
		• Assist with incentive spirometry as ordered
		• Teach splinting of incisional area
		• Ambulate qid
		• Provide analgesia prior to activities

		RATIONALE: *Coughing, deep breathing, exercises, and ambulation improve lung expansion and tissue aeration, preventing pneumonia and promoting healing.*

4 High Risk for Fluid Volume Deficit
 	
r.t. fluid loss associated with bleeding, drainage
	• Exhibits adequate circulating volume
	  - normal LOC
	  - brisk CRT
	  - moist mucous membranes; good skin turgor
	  - normal serum electrolytes
	  - no excess drainage, bleeding
		• Assess LOC, CRT, mucous membranes, skin turgor, pallor, and cyanosis with VS
		• Monitor lab values; report critical values
		• Assess abdominal dressing for excess drainage q4h

	• Achieves, maintains balanced I&O	• Support circulating volume
		  - administer replacement IVF as ordered
		  - consult physician regarding type and cross-match blood as needed
		  - administer blood products as ordered

		RATIONALE: *Early detection of internal bleeding and excess drainage prompt the timely management of fluid volume deficits.*

SURGICAL

| **OTHER LESS COMMON NURSING DIAGNOSES:** Urinary Retention; Constipation |

ESSENTIAL DISCHARGE CRITERIA

- VS WNL
- Has clean, dry, and well-approximated incision

- Maintains comfort with oral analgesia
- Ambulates with minimal respiratory effort

LARYNGECTOMY (TOTAL OR PARTIAL)

NURSING DIAGNOSES   OUTCOME CRITERIA   INTERVENTIONS

See "Postoperative Care" care plan in General Section

NURSING DIAGNOSES	OUTCOME CRITERIA	INTERVENTIONS
1 Ineffective Airway Clearance *r.t. inability to remove airway secretions*	• Exhibits respiratory effort, rate, and pattern WNL - 12-20 deep, regular breaths/min	• Auscultate breath sounds • Monitor RR and pattern with VS
	• ABGs WNL	• Monitor ABGs • Encourage deep breathing • Administer O_2 as ordered
	• Respiratory secretions are cleared by coughing or suctioning	• Encourage the client to cough without dislodging the tracheostomy tube • Use sterile suction if necessary • Perform tracheostomy care
	• Mucous production decreases	• Increase fluid intake to 2-3 L/d unless contraindicated by cardiac or renal complications • Increase humidity in the environment
		RATIONALE: *Lack of O_2 due to respiratory secretions results in decreased O_2 and increased carbon dioxide in the blood. Adventitious breath sounds occur due to air moving over secretions in the tracheobronchial tree. Increasing humidity and hydration helps to liquify secretions.*
2 Pain *r.t. surgical incision*	• Verbalizes/displays freedom from pain	• Ask the client to describe the pain on a scale of 1 to 10 • Monitor objective data such as guarding, withdrawal, altered thought process, moaning, crying, pacing, facial expression, change in BP, pulse, RR, diaphoresis
	• Reports comfort following analgesia	• Administer pain medications as ordered when pain first starts and prior to activities that precipitate pain; assess the response

SURGICAL

NURSING DIAGNOSES	OUTCOME CRITERIA	INTERVENTIONS
	• Identifies medication or activity that reduces or aggravates discomfort	• Provide accurate information regarding surgical procedure and pain medication to reduce fear and enhance trust • Remove odors, excessive light, and noise from the environment • Teach use of distraction • Instruct and promote relaxation techniques • Use application of heat and cold when appropriate • Use cutaneous stimulation such as massage
		RATIONALE: *Pain response may result in autonomic or physical responses, as well as subjective statements. Pharmacological agents interfere with the pain response in the nervous system. Treating pain early will decrease the response.*
3 Altered Nutrition: Less than body requirements *r.t. difficult swallowing from edema and pain at incision*	• Maintains/regains weight	• Monitor weight
	• Shows normal serum electrolytes	• Monitor serum electrolytes and CBC • Monitor oral intake and output
	• Swallows, retains 80 percent of feedings	• Offer small frequent feedings • Offer thick liquid or soft foods • Place patient in upright position 60 min after eating • Perform oral hygiene before and after eating
	• Has no vomiting	• Eliminate noxious stimuli and provide for socialization • Stay with client during meals and offer support • Monitor choking or possible aspiration; use suction if indicated

NURSING DIAGNOSES	OUTCOME CRITERIA	INTERVENTIONS
		• In case of supraglottic laryngectomy, teach patient to perform a Valsalva maneuver when swallowing
		RATIONALE: *Small feedings and soft foods with a thick consistency are easier to swallow. Oral hygiene and environmental factors affect appetite. Upright position will use gravity to help expand the thorax and facilitate swallowing. Aspiration of vomitus may precipitate pneumonia. Choking may occur due to edema. Patient may not swallow due to fear of choking. Valsalva maneuver exaggerates normal swallowing process and facilitates movement of food down esophagus.*
4 Body Image Disturbance *r.t. artificial opening in neck*	• Verbalizes feelings regarding change in body image	• Establish a therapeutic nurse/client relationship • Encourage patient to discuss his/her feelings in a climate of acceptance • Utilize therapeutic touch • Encourage to experiment with various stoma coverings • Give positive support to patient's efforts to compensate
	• Verbalizes and demonstrates acceptance of changed body image	• Encourage patient to make decisions as appropriate • Provide support and encouragement as patient establishes him/herself in the new role or new self-image
		RATIONALE: *Discussion of feelings facilitates resolution of the grieving process. Success in small decisions builds self-confidence and helps patient adapt to role and body image changes.*

SURGICAL

271

NURSING DIAGNOSES	OUTCOME CRITERIA	INTERVENTIONS
5 Impaired Verbal Communication *r.t. removal of vocal cords*	• Communicates verbally	• Anticipate client's needs • Allow expressions of frustration • Establish temporary means of communicating: use of "word cards," note pad for writing, or pointing to objects • Make a referral to a support group such as The Lost Cord Club or I Can Cope
	• Demonstrates familiarity with prosthetic devices for artificial speech	• Make a referral to a speech pathologist • Discuss the use of devices and techniques such as a voice prosthesis, esophageal speech, and an electrolarynx
		RATIONALE: *Support groups and verbalization provide a means of decreasing frustration. Temporary communication techniques provide for the patient's needs at present. Prosthetic devices can become a satisfactory alternative to speech loss.*

6 Knowledge Deficit
 	
r.t. lack of information
	• Patient/family verbalize/demonstrate understanding of self-care	• Teach aspects of stoma care
		  - suctioning, cleaning laryngectomy tube
		  - care of voice prosthesis
		  - situations that require covering stoma
		  - symptoms that indicate complications
		  - what to do in emergencies
		• Make referral to home health services for follow-up care

		RATIONALE: *Teaching with assessment of learning and follow-up care provide information needed for self-care.*

OTHER LESS COMMON NURSING DIAGNOSES: *Impaired Home Maintenance Management;
Anxiety; Altered Tissue Perfusion; High Risk for Infection; Hopelessness*

ESSENTIAL DISCHARGE CRITERIA

- Is afebrile
- Has clear chest sounds
- Maintains pre-op body weight

- Shows no evidence of redness, swelling, or discharge around stoma
- Cares for stoma and communicates effectively

SURGICAL

MAMMOPLASTY

NURSING DIAGNOSES	OUTCOME CRITERIA	INTERVENTIONS

See "Postoperative Care" care plan in General Section

1 Anxiety

r.t. change in body image

- Verbalizes a decrease in anxiety
- Exhibits no palpitations
- Shows normal respiratory and pulse rates

- Assess verbal and physiological response, i.e., palpitations, increased respirations and pulse rates

- Displays no more than mild to moderate anxiety

- Determine level of anxiety (mild, moderate, severe) observing behaviors such as restlessness, insomnia, crying, startle reaction, and inability to relax

- Patient and family interact regarding treatment and prognosis

- Encourage a social support system (e.g., family, friends, clergy)
- Encourage verbalization of fears and acknowledge patient's feelings; be a listener

RATIONALE: *Changes in VS may indicate the degree of anxiety experienced. High levels of anxiety impede learning and distort perception of the situation. Anxiety can be reduced or controlled when support from others is given. Listening establishes rapport and promotes expression of concerns which helps the patient to make appropriate decisions regarding care.*

2 Impaired Skin Integrity

r.t. surgical reconstruction of breast

- Is free of infection and necrosis along incision line
  - no bloody or purulent drainage
  - no edema, erythema, discoloration
  - no increasing pain
  - CRT WNL

- Monitor and record output from drains, noting amount and character
- Assess dressing/incision for drainage, edema, erythema, foul odor, increased pain, discoloration, CRT, and firm fibrous capsule
- Avoid taking BP, administering injections, venipuncture, or IVs in affected arm
- Administer antibiotics as ordered
- Encourage wearing a brassiere unless contraindicated by the physician

NURSING DIAGNOSES	OUTCOME CRITERIA	INTERVENTIONS
		• Encourage wearing loose fitting clothing or nonconstrictive jewelry (i.e., watch, bracelet) on affected arm
	• Describes s/s of infection; needs to report to physician	• Teach patient signs of infection (i.e., unrelieved pain, temperature change, increased drainage, or edema)
		RATIONALE: *Excessive amounts of drainage (bloody or purulent) can indicate early signs of complications. Drainage of these fluids promotes healing. Frequent assessment of the incision area prompts early detection of infection, tissue ischemia, or rejection of implant. Protecting the affected arm from constriction or punctures prevents additional tissue trauma and portals of entry for bacteria and maintains implant position and alignment. It also minimizes pressure on tissues and promotes circulation/healing.*
3 Pain *r.t. surgery*	• Verbalizes/displays freedom from pain	• Assess pain symptoms, location, duration, intensity (0-10 scale), and precipitating factors
	• Reports comfort following analgesia	• Assess RR, degree of pain relief, presence of numbness or paralysis in lower extremities q2h, if epidural analgesia used • Administer pain medication as prescribed; evaluate effectiveness
	• Identifies medication or activity that reduces or aggravates discomfort; identifies source of comfort	• Reposition patient slowly on back or on unaffected side • Support affected areas during coughing and deep breathing exercises • Encourage diversional activity such as relaxation techniques, guided imagery, or therapeutic touch

SURGICAL

NURSING DIAGNOSES	OUTCOME CRITERIA	INTERVENTIONS
		RATIONALE: *Frequent pain assessment and consistent pain management produce sustained relief. Careful positioning avoids injury or pressure to incision. Analgesics alter pain perception which fosters increased activity and required arm exercises. Diversion reduces pain and anxiety by refocusing thoughts away from source of pain.*

4 Altered Tissue Perfusion (breast area) *r.t. implant rejection or inadequate blood supply*	• Exhibits adequate tissue perfusion
	  - no pallor or cyanosis
	  - shows intact skin
	  - has controllable pain
		• Assess breast area (nipple, areola if possible) for discoloration (pallor or cyanosis), edema, blebs, or hematoma; notify physician of any complications
		
		• Position patient with head and knees elevated, but relaxed

		RATIONALE: *Frequent inspection of breast area prompts timely interventions, reducing risk of tissue necrosis or implant rejection.*

> **OTHER LESS COMMON NURSING DIAGNOSES:** *Ineffective Individual Coping; Knowledge Deficit; Body Image Disturbance; High Risk for Fluid Volume Deficit; Impaired Physical Mobility*

ESSENTIAL DISCHARGE CRITERIA

• Expresses confidence in treatment and prognosis

• Shows no tissue cyanosis or wound infection

• Verbalizes sense of reasonable comfort

• Shows adequate circulation of breast without implant rejection

MASTECTOMY

See "Postoperative Care" care plan in General Section

1 Knowledge Deficit (pre-op)

r.t. breast cancer and treatment

- Patient/family discuss pathophysiology and surgical anatomy of disease, treatment

  - Assess patient's/family's learning abilities
  - Initiate open and supportive communication with patient/family
  - Provide explanation of significant terms, procedures, treatment, and aftercare principles

- Patient/family express concerns, ask questions

  - Follow up with teaching materials from American Cancer Society and National Cancer Institute
  - Review all information
  - Seek feedback from patient/family that affirms their understanding of information and materials

- Patient/family express commitment to consistent medical follow-up

  - Provide phone numbers for further resources (support groups: Reach to Recovery, Cancersearch, and I Can Cope)

RATIONALE: *Information and materials facilitate positive adjustment because the woman and her family have more knowledge and have more choices, and thus feel more in control.*

2 Anxiety

r.t. breast cancer diagnosis

- Verbalizes anxieties related to diagnosis, surgery, and treatment; demonstrates positive coping behaviors

  - Assess fears and anxieties relating to the cancer diagnosis, the work-up procedures, and surgery
  - Allow/encourage her to vent her frustrations, concerns; maintain open and supportive communication
  - Reassess her anxiety and review information, feelings as needed

RATIONALE: *Decreased anxiety promotes positive psychological healing and fosters adjustment to the cancer experience.*

SURGICAL

NURSING DIAGNOSES	OUTCOME CRITERIA	INTERVENTIONS
3 Impaired Skin Integrity *r.t. breast and axillary node dissection, incision sites*	• Incision sites show healing without s/s of infection - no bleeding - no swelling, redness - no purulent drainage - no increase in pain	• Assess dressing and surrounding site for bleeding, redness, swelling, color, purulent drainage, and pain q4h for first 24 h and q shift thereafter
	• Has decreasing amounts of drainage with decreasing bleeding and no cloudiness	• Monitor suction drainage; note color, amount
	• Participates in own wound care - uses sterile, clean techniques - lists s/s of infection	• Teach wound care with first dressing change; seek verbal feedback • Teach s/s of infection; seek verbal feedback affirming accurate understanding • Provide teaching materials about incision care and infection prevention
		RATIONALE: *Information and ongoing assessment by patient and nurse reinforce teaching. Information promotes patient autonomy in self-care of incision sites.*
4 Pain *r.t. breast surgery*	• Verbalizes/displays consistent levels of comfort; presents no contradicting pain behaviors	• Assess for pain q2-4h • Instruct about pain control measures, both pharmacological and behavioral • Medicate for pain RTC rather than as needed
	• Reports comfort following analgesia	• If medication is ineffective, obtain order to increase dosage or scheduling to produce sustained comfort
	• Identifies medication or activities that reduce or aggravate discomfort	• Encourage distraction, diversional and physical activity for pain control; premedicate to increase activity levels
		RATIONALE: *Pain must first be addressed in order to establish trust and to promote the patient's ability to participate in self-care.*

NURSING DIAGNOSES	OUTCOME CRITERIA	INTERVENTIONS
5 Impaired Physical Mobility *r.t. breast surgery*	• Verbalizes accurate understanding of extent of altered mobility	• Assess affected arm for numbness, tingling, and other sensory changes • Premedicate as needed to encourage movement of arm • Teach initial post-op exercises to maintain ROM (limited movement needed for simple ADL such as hair combing, putting on clothes)
	• Demonstrates postoperative exercises to improve mobility of affected arm	• Instruct about prevention of swelling (elevating arm, ROM exercises) • Explain long-term care to affected arm such as avoidance of BPs, venipuncture, and tight clothing, and weight-lifting restrictions
		RATIONALE: *These measures (teaching, mediating, ROM, activity) reduce susceptibility for immobility of affected arm. This promotes self-care and appropriate progression toward normal function.*
6 Ineffective Individual Coping *r.t. grief and body image disturbance*	• Demonstrates successful coping strategies	• Assess coping mechanisms • Discuss, reinforce positive coping strategies • Encourage patient to verbalize feelings; allow time for validation of these feelings • Explain grief process • Encourage patient to visualize incision and verbalize her feelings about loss of breast
	• Identifies and affirms need to seek supportive person, groups	• Explore/identify appropriate community resources that are available (American Cancer Society groups, support groups, Reach to Recovery) • Review options to assist with decreased body image such as night bra and specialty shops that have clothing tailored to women with mastectomies

SURGICAL

NURSING DIAGNOSES	OUTCOME CRITERIA	INTERVENTIONS

RATIONALE: *Early assessment and promotion of coping strategies facilitate emotional healing and allow the woman to adapt to loss of her breast.*

OTHER LESS COMMON NURSING DIAGNOSES: *High Risk for Injury; Social Isolation; Sexual Dysfunction; Spiritual Distress; Decisional Conflict; High Risk for Fluid Volume Deficit*

ESSENTIAL DISCHARGE CRITERIA

- Has wound healing without complications
- Displays reduced anxiety and positive coping behaviors
- Demonstrates increased participation in self-care activities

- Controls pain with oral analgesia
- Verbalizes accurate knowledge of healing process, activity regimen, potential complications, follow-up appointments

NURSING DIAGNOSES	OUTCOME CRITERIA	INTERVENTIONS

See "Postoperative Care" care plan in General Section

1 Pain

r.t. surgery

- Reports comfort following analgesia

- Give pain medication before meals and prn as ordered
  - monitor for effectiveness

RATIONALE: *Medication reduces perception of pain from inflammation and trauma.*

2 High Risk for Fluid Volume Deficit

r.t. fluid volume loss

- Shows normal VS, BP, H&H

- Assess VS per post-op routine
- Monitor H&H

- Shows no bleeding

- Monitor for excessive bleeding on nasal packing/dressing q15 min for 1 h and prn; record time and amount
- Monitor for vomiting bright red blood
- Check back of throat using penlight if client swallows frequently; if bleeding is present, notify physician immediately
- If packing comes out, do not cut; call physician and stay with patient
- Instruct patient to avoid Valsalva maneuvers; use laxatives and antiemetics as indicated

- Maintains balanced I&O and electrolytes

- Offer PO fluids frequently, accommodating patient preferences; avoid hot fluids

RATIONALE: *Frequent monitoring produces early detection, correction of bleeding from surgical site. Frequent intake of fluid helps maintain fluid volume balance.*

SURGICAL

NURSING DIAGNOSES	OUTCOME CRITERIA	INTERVENTIONS

3 Ineffective Breathing Pattern
 	
r.t. mouth breathing
	• Exhibits improving respiratory status
	  - takes 12-20 deep, regular respirations/min
		• Perform measures to improve breathing pattern
		  - encourage patient to breathe through mouth
		  - monitor for dyspnea from nasal obstruction and/or edema
		  - place in semi-Fowler's position
		  - minimize anxiety

		RATIONALE: *Positioning, airway clearance, and tension reduction combine to facilitate the patient's own efforts toward achieving normal respiratory rhythm and depth.*
4 High Risk for Aspiration *r.t. nasal drainage*	• Experiences no episodes of aspiration	• Encourage to expectorate, not swallow blood or secretions • Perform oral hygiene q2h • Apply ice to nose to minimize swelling and bleeding
		RATIONALE: *Expectoration and oral hygiene eliminate secretions. Ice to nose contracts venous vessels, reducing bleeding.*

5 Knowledge Deficit
 	
r.t. unfamiliarity with post-op regimen
	• Patient/family verbalize and demonstrate knowledge of self-care techniques
	  - reportable s/s
	  - prevention of bleeding
	  - medications: dosages, effects, side effects
		• Teach self-care techniques
		  - if fever, excessive pain, or bleeding occurs, call surgeon
		  - if nasal packing is in place, it is to be removed by the surgeon, not the patient
		  - avoid blowing nose until 48 h after the packing is removed
		  - do not strain, cough, or have a bowel movement until several days after the packing is removed
		  - bowel movements may have a tarry appearance several days after surgery
		  - take and finish all of antibiotics as ordered

		RATIONALE: *A knowledgeable, competent patient is likely to perform safe self-care techniques at home.*

| **OTHER LESS COMMON NURSING DIAGNOSES:** |
| *Altered Nutrition: Less than body requirements; Anxiety* |

ESSENTIAL DISCHARGE CRITERIA

- Displays no s/s of excessive bleeding from nose
- Experiences no aspiration

- Controls pain with oral analgesics
- Demonstrates understanding of self-care instructions

SURGICAL

NECK SURGERY, RADICAL

NURSING DIAGNOSES	OUTCOME CRITERIA	INTERVENTIONS

See "Postoperative Care" care plan in General Section

---

1 Ineffective Airway Clearance

r.t. excessive or thick secretions, edema, obstructed tracheostomy

- Remains oxygenated per patent airway
  - VS stable, normal
  - normal LOC
  - normal ABGs, SaO$_2$, Hb
  - clear chest x-rays

- Assess for restlessness, increased pulse, and change in depth, character, and rate of respirations every 15 min immediately postoperatively, then according to institutional standards

- Monitor ABGs, SaO$_2$ levels, Hb, chest x-rays, neurologic indicators of pain, and/or hypoxia

---

- Mobilizes secretions

- Monitor sputum for amount, odor, and consistency

- Encourage fluid intake, up to 3000 mL/d

- Turn and reposition q2h

- Encourage to cough and deep breathe q2h; vigorous coughing may cause bleeding

- Postural drainage, percussion, and vibration q4h as ordered

- Provide 4x4s and paper bag for removal of sputum expectoration

- Provide adequate humidification as ordered (mist collar or bedside humidifier)

- Suction tracheostomy as indicated, at least hourly initially; use sterile saline to liquify secretions

- Administer O$_2$ as ordered

- Elevate HOB 30-45°

- Encourage use of incentive spirometer q2h while awake

- Perform tracheostomy care q8h and prn or per institutional guidelines; includes change of inner cannula, ties, and dressing and check of tube position

NURSING DIAGNOSES	OUTCOME CRITERIA	INTERVENTIONS

	• Patient/family participate in care activities	• Teach patient/family
		  - self-suctioning, may use mirror
		  - tracheostomy care, including cleansing of tube, application of clean dressing and ties
		  - covering of stoma prior to proximity with foreign objects, such as application of facial, hair, or powder products or when bathing, shaving or in dusty/smoky environments
		  - no swimming
		  - no smoking

	• Identifies, has list of reportable s/s	• Teach to notify physician for increased resistance when replacing tracheostomy tube, presence of lump in throat, dysphagia, bleeding, increased temperature, new pain
		RATIONALE: *Prevent pooling of secretions that interfere with oxygenation.*
2 Altered Nutrition: Less than body requirements *r.t. NPO status, nausea, anorexia, or inability to swallow*	• Maintains/regains weight	• Weigh patient 2-3 x per week

	• Swallows/retains feedings	• Administer tube feedings when ordered
		  - keep HOB elevated at least 45° during feedings and for 30 min after
		  - keep tracheostomy cuff inflated during feeding and for 30 min after

	• Takes at least 80 percent of required nutrition	• Begin oral feedings when ordered
		  - perform oral care and, if prescribed, viscous lidocaine before meals
		  - start with water and advance as tolerated
		  - explore patient preferences
		  - encourage selection of soft foods
		  - offer warm rather than cold foods
		  - stay with patient during meals at first; ensure privacy
		
		• Have suction equipment available during meals; observe for choking, dyspnea, cyanosis, gastric fullness, regurgitation, diarrhea, bowel sounds

SURGICAL

NURSING DIAGNOSES	OUTCOME CRITERIA	INTERVENTIONS
		• Observe suture line and tracheal aspirate for leakage of food contents during and after feedings
		• Record food intake
		• Consult with dietitian to plan adequate caloric intake
	• Patient/family demonstrate competence with required feeding techniques	• Teach family and patient to administer tube feedings, if patient will be discharged with tube
		• Teach patient/family oral feeding techniques, such as proper positioning, tipping head forward to avoid aspiration, removing leftover food particles from oral cavity
		RATIONALE: *Adequate nutrition is necessary for wound healing and recovery.*
3 Body Image Disturbance *r.t. change in appearance and function of body parts*	• Acknowledges change in body image	• Communicate with patient to assess awareness of body changes, emotional responses, coping patterns, and level of self-esteem
	• Expresses positive feelings about self	• Accept patient's perception of self and expression of negative emotions
		• Assess readiness to view and touch self postoperatively; assist to cleanse hands and touch reconstructed area
		• Maintain calm, reassuring manner
		• Reassure that perceptions will change with time
		• Encourage support from significant others; assist in significant others' adjustment; aid family in treating patient as a person, not an invalid
		• Prepare visitors for patient's appearance and suggest therapeutic comments that they might verbalize to the patient
		• Encourage to look in mirror at surgical area
		• Perform therapeutic touch with patient's consent

NURSING DIAGNOSES	OUTCOME CRITERIA	INTERVENTIONS
		• Provide for contact with other persons having similar surgical experiences, if desired by patient

RATIONALE: *When confronting bodily changes, ventilation of feelings with emotional support enhances development of new body image.*

---

4 Impaired Verbal Communication

r.t. possible removal of vocal cords, laryngeal edema, tracheostomy

• Communicates effectively

• Identify preference for method of nonverbal communication such as pen and paper, magic slate, communication board, gestures, flash cards, lip reading

• Communicate preference to all healthcare personnel

• Answer call light promptly and in person; alert unit staff that patient is unable to speak

• Reinforce preoperative teaching of use of selected communication method

• Visit patient frequently; anticipate needs

• Initiate conversation; do not alter your speaking manner, since ability to understand is not affected

• Allow time for communication; acknowledge feelings

• If patient will be writing, keep dominant hand free of intravenous access

• Reinforce strategies introduced by speech therapist

• Reassure that speech will return if total laryngectomy was not performed

RATIONALE: *Patient's communication needs can be met by alternate methods that can be supported by nursing interventions.*

SURGICAL

NURSING DIAGNOSES	OUTCOME CRITERIA	INTERVENTIONS
5 Knowledge Deficit *r.t. lack of information regarding postoperative self-care*	• Patient/family participate in care activities	• Assess anxiety level related to surgery and condition; assess readiness for decision-making • Give choices and encourage patient to participate actively in self-care • Encourage usual grooming habits

	• Patient/family discuss anatomy of surgery, rationale for treatment, expected course of recovery, s/s to report	• Teach patient/family
		  - anatomical changes
		  - purpose of tracheostomy; arrange for patient to handle tracheostomy tube
		  - neck range of motion with or without resistance when ordered
		  - how to contact community resources
		
		• Provide repeated explanations as needed
		
		• Provide written directions for future reference

	• Identifies plan for emergency communication; has emergency phone numbers	• Encourage wearing of identification tag/bracelet labeled "neck breather" • Design means of emergency communication at home
		RATIONALE: *Self-care increases sense of control and promotes self-concept. Planning for emergencies at home increases sense of confidence, security.*

OTHER LESS COMMON NURSING DIAGNOSES: *Impaired Swallowing; High Risk for Fluid Volume Deficit; High Risk for Infection; Altered Oral Mucous Membranes; Ineffective Individual Coping; Altered Tissue Perfusion (peripheral); Impaired Skin Integrity; Improved Physical Mobility*

ESSENTIAL DISCHARGE CRITERIA

- Shows stable VS; afebrile
- Has clear breath sounds
- Maintains stable weight
- Patient/family demonstrate appropriate feeding techniques

- Communicates thoughts and feelings related to new body image
- Demonstrates use of effective alternative speech methods
- Identifies community resources to assist with post-op adjustment

NURSING DIAGNOSES	OUTCOME CRITERIA	INTERVENTIONS

See "Postoperative Care" care plan in General Section

1 Ineffective Breathing Pattern

r.t. pain with breathing and coughing secondary to location of incision

- Exhibits improving respiratory status
  - clear breath sounds bilaterally

- Cooperates with breathing and ambulation activities

- Auscultate lung fields q8h and prn for diminished and abnormal breath sounds

- Institute an incentive spirometer device/deep breathe and cough q2h while the patient is awake

- Encourage self-turning/splinting; have side rails in an upright position to assist self-turning

- Turn side to side q2h if self-turning is not possible

- Encourage early and frequent ambulation

RATIONALE: *Deep breathing exercises, incentive spirometer, and early ambulation promote ventilation and help to prevent atelectasis*

2 Altered Tissue Perfusion (peripheral)

r.t. post-surgical volume depletion

- Shows BP and HR WNL

- Hb WNL

- Shows brisk CRT < 3 sec
- Has warm extremities

- Has urinary output WNL

- Monitor VS per post-op routine

- Review CBC and report abnormal findings to physician

- Monitor CRT q8h and prn

- Document I&O q8h; notify physician if below normal

- Assess dressing at surgical site q2-4h for s/s of bleeding

- Administer IV fluids, blood products as ordered

RATIONALE: *A nephrectomy is a very vascular surgery and may lead to excessive fluid loss resulting in a decrease in cardiac output and peripheral perfusion.*

SURGICAL

NURSING DIAGNOSES	OUTCOME CRITERIA	INTERVENTIONS
3 Altered Urinary Elimination *r.t. use of catheters*	• Maintains balanced I&O - urinary output WNL - urine shows no bright red bleeding	• Monitor urinary output via the catheter or other drainage tube and record each tube's drainage separately • Observe and monitor the color and consistency of the urine (urine should be pink or dark red initially) • Determine urinary output at least q1-2h in the immediate post-op phase
		RATIONALE: *A patent catheter prevents urinary stasis/retention and subsequent infection. Increased amounts of mucus, sediment, or blood in the urine may occlude the drainage tubing or catheter.*
4 Pain *r.t. surgical incision*	• Verbalizes/displays freedom from pain - reports comfort following analgesia - identifies medications or activities that reduce or aggravate discomfort	• Assess level of pain using a predetermined scale for objective data • Give analgesics at least q3-4h as ordered for 24-48 h, post-op • Give analgesics for breakthrough pain prior to activity; evaluate effectiveness
		RATIONALE: *A nephrectomy is an extensive surgical procedure involving muscles, nerves, and excessive tissue, which may cause severe postoperative pain. Comfort facilitates earlier mobility, healing, and recovery.*

NURSING DIAGNOSES	OUTCOME CRITERIA	INTERVENTIONS
5 Knowledge Deficit *r.t. inexperience with post-op home care and fear of adequacy of one kidney*	• Describes potential adequacy of one kidney; expresses feelings about loss of kidney	• Provide information, answer questions, listen to concerns • Explain mechanism of kidney function
	• Describes and demonstrates satisfactory wound care	• Teach wound care
	• Correctly lists reportable s/s	• Teach s/s of complications - low output, fever, general illness - hematuria - flank pain unoperated side, unexplained weight gain
	• Possesses schedule for outpatient visits to physician	• Obtain correct feedback from patient/family regarding follow-up care - when to call physician - outpatient schedule - activity and work plan

RATIONALE: *Provide, through teaching/learning, the knowledge and skills needed for self-care, which increases compliance.*

SURGICAL

OTHER LESS COMMON NURSING DIAGNOSES: *Fluid Volume Deficit; Impaired Skin Integrity; High Risk for Infection*

ESSENTIAL DISCHARGE CRITERIA

- Expresses adequate pain control
- Maintains balanced I&O
- Shows normal VS and temperature

- Is free of pulmonary complications
- Verbalizes understanding of post-op regimen
- Verbalizes and demonstrates knowledge of follow-up regimen: wound care, activity, follow-up appointments

PELVIC FRACTURE

NURSING DIAGNOSES	OUTCOME CRITERIA	INTERVENTIONS

See "Postoperative Care" care plan in General Section

1 Pain
r.t. pelvic fracture

- Verbalizes/displays freedom from pain

- Assess q2h for pain, intensity, location, and characteristics

- Reports comfort following administration of analgesia

- Maintain proper body alignment
- Administer narcotic analgesics routinely to prevent pain

- Identifies medication or activity that reduces discomfort

- Assist in exploring methods for alleviation or control of pain

RATIONALE: *Pain alleviation promotes early healing and recovery.*

2 Altered Tissue Perfusion (peripheral)

r.t. interruption of blood flow

- Demonstrates increased perfusion
  - peripheral pulses present/strong
  - VS WNL
  - H&H WNL

- Assess color, temperature, CRT, and pulses involved extremity q2-4h
- Check for calf tenderness (Homan's sign), swelling, redness, and temperature
- Monitor clotting time, H&H
- Alternate or reduce pressure on the skin's surface with possibility of an air mattress

RATIONALE: *These measures detect and prevent venous stasis and tissue injury.*

3 High Risk for Impaired Skin Integrity

r.t. pelvic traction (immobility)

- Remain free of pressure ulcers

- Frequently inspect areas of the skin in contact with the traction apparatus for erythema and blanching
- Provide measures to eliminate chafing or rubbing in these areas
- Encourage upper and lower body range of motion
- Assess nutritional status and consult dietitian if needed

NURSING DIAGNOSES	OUTCOME CRITERIA	INTERVENTIONS
		• Provide optimum nutrition and increased protein intake to provide a positive nitrogen balance
		RATIONALE: *Protection and nutrition promote tissue healing and prevent pressure ulcers.*
4 Constipation *r.t. immobility (pelvic traction)*	• Re-establishes normal pattern of bowel functioning - character, frequency of stools return to baseline - bowel sounds are present	• Compare usual pattern of elimination with present pattern (note color, odor, consistency, amount, and frequency of stools) • Auscultate abdomen for presence, location, and characteristics of bowel sounds • Encourage PO fluids as tolerated • Review diet and offer foods high in fiber and bulk, unless contraindicated • Administer stool softener, mild stimulants, or bulk-forming agents as ordered
		RATIONALE: *Early detection and management alleviate constipation.*
5 Powerlessness *r.t. immobility (pelvic traction)*	• Demonstrates interest in care and surroundings - participates in care - asks questions, seeks clarification - initiates suggestions for comfort, diversion	• Explain pelvic traction and include in care • Allow time to fully answer questions • Keep patient informed and involved with condition and schedule treatments • Determine individual attitude about condition (e.g., cultural values) • Keep needed items within reach (call bell, urinal, tissues, or selected personal items) • Refer to support groups, counseling, or therapy, if indicated
		RATIONALE: *Providing control helps reduce the patient's feelings of powerlessness.*

SURGICAL

NURSING DIAGNOSES	OUTCOME CRITERIA	INTERVENTIONS

6 High Risk for Infection (urinary tract)
 	
r.t. immobility (pelvic traction)
	• Is free of UTI
	  - WBC count, serum electrolytes WNL
	  - urine clear, no foul odor
	  - no retention
	  - balanced I&O
		• Monitor WBC count and serum electrolytes
		• Assess for urinary frequency, color, burning, or foul odor
		• Assess frequently for bladder distention
		• Monitor I&O
		• Encourage PO fluids as tolerated

RATIONALE: *Pooling of urine can contribute to bacterial growth and lead to UTIs.*

OTHER LESS COMMON NURSING DIAGNOSES: *Impaired Physical Mobility; High Risk for Disuse Syndrome; Impaired Home Maintenance Management; Self-Care Deficit*

ESSENTIAL DISCHARGE CRITERIA

• Maintains sustained comfort with oral analgesia

• Is free from venous stasis and tissue injury

• Shows no evidence of infection or constipation

PORTAL SHUNT

NURSING DIAGNOSES	OUTCOME CRITERIA	INTERVENTIONS
1 High Risk for Fluid Volume Deficit *r.t. loss of fluid into interstitial space, loss of ascitic fluid when abdomen is surgically opened, loss of lymphatic fluid during surgery, and blood loss related to pre-existing problems with clotting mechanisms*	• Shows VS WNL (especially BP) • Shows hemodynamic parameters WNL for patient: CVP, PAP, PCWP	• Monitor VS and/or hemodynamic parameters q1-2h until stable and then q4h, or per post-op routine
	• Maintains urinary output WNL • Has palpable peripheral pulses • Electrolytes WNL	• Monitor for excessive amounts of draining from the NGTs or operative site
	• Shows balanced I&O	• Maintain parenteral fluids at constant rate
	• Displays skin color, temperature, and turgor WNL	• Monitor skin color, temperature, turgor, and integrity
		RATIONALE: *Perioperative fluid loss requires the frequent monitoring and management of circulating fluid volume.*
2 Fluid Volume Excess *r.t. decreased plasma colloidal pressure, Na retention associated with pre-existing decrease in osmotic pressure*	• Shows VS WNL	• Monitor VS
	• Exhibits no respiratory distress - RR, depth, and pattern normal - no adventitious breath sounds - no edema or neck vein distention - stable weight	• Monitor for s/s of volume overload - increased abdominal girth - rales - peripheral edema, altered hemodynamic parameters - weight gain
	• Hemodynamic parameters WNL - CVP - PAP - PCWP	• Administer medications as ordered to decrease fluid volume (diuretics)
	• Shows balanced I&O • Shows urinary sp. gr. WNL	• Monitor I&O q4h; sp. gr. as needed
	• Electrolytes WNL • Serum albumin WNL • H&H WNL	• Monitor serum electrolytes, BUN, H&H
	• Stabilizes or decreases abdominal girth	• Monitor skin integrity, especially in the areas of edema

SURGICAL

NURSING DIAGNOSES	OUTCOME CRITERIA	INTERVENTIONS
	• Has minimal or no ascites	• Monitor abdominal girth q4-8h • Assess skin for discoloration • Administer therapies as ordered to increase intravascular osmotic pressure (salt poor albumin) • Institute a dietary regime (low Na, fluid restriction) • Change position q2h and assess skin especially at bony prominences
		RATIONALE: *Frequent monitoring for signs of fluid volume excess prompts early detection and management to reverse fluid retention.*
3 Ineffective Breathing Pattern *r.t. splinting from incisional pain, diaphragmatic elevation from ascites, and cerebral depression from anesthetics*	• Shows no evidence of adventitious sounds on lung auscultation	• Auscultate lungs q4h and before/after each pulmonary toilet effort
	• Displays free chest expansion bilaterally	• Monitor chest wall movement watching for symmetry, use of accessory muscles, and intercostal retractions
	• Exhibits normal RR, depth, pattern, rhythm, and effort	• Monitor respiratory status with VS
	• Shows ABGs WNL	• Monitor ABGs as ordered
	• Cooperates with pulmonary toilet without undue resistance	• Assess level of incisional pain and treat appropriately
	• Mentation WNL for patient	• Monitor for restlessness, increased anxiety, and air hunger • Elevate HOB 30-45°
	• Verbalizes accurate knowledge of why pulmonary toilet is important; actively participates in carrying it out	• Assist and teach patient the pulmonary toilet - turn - cough - deep breathing • Teach how to splint incision during coughing

NURSING DIAGNOSES	OUTCOME CRITERIA	INTERVENTIONS
		• Assist patient to a comfortable position that promotes optimal chest expansion
		RATIONALE: *Frequent pulmonary monitoring and aggressive TCDB and positioning are required to counteract the effects of splinting and shallow respiration associated with a high incision.*
4 Pain *r.t. invasive surgical procedure*	• Expresses feeling of comfort	• Assess for type, intensity, and location of pain
	• Appears rested and relaxed	• Observe for nonverbal clues of discomfort
	• Carries out pain control measures in a timely fashion	• Assess the effectiveness of pain relief measures • Maintain a quiet and restful environment • Consider cultural influences on pain response • Administer analgesics as ordered • Change the patient's position frequently to promote comfort

	• Participates in care-related activities with minimal discomfort	• Administer other comfort measures
		  - back rubs
		  - relaxation techniques
		  - cold/heat therapy
		• Incorporate significant others in the pain relief modality, if possible

		RATIONALE: *A coordinated combination of analgesia and comfort measures produces sustained relief of pain.*

SURGICAL

NURSING DIAGNOSES	OUTCOME CRITERIA	INTERVENTIONS
5 Altered Nutrition: Less than body requirements *r.t. pre-existing impaired absorption of nutrients and fat-soluble vitamins, increase in metabolic demands of surgery/healing, and NPO status*	• Maintains stable weight	• Weigh daily at same time
	• Electrolytes WNL	• Monitor serum electrolytes, BUN, and creatinine
	• Serum protein, albumin, H&H WNL	• Monitor serum albumin, total protein, H&H
	• Consumes required calories/day	• Observe and record oral intake
	• Tolerates oral, enteral, or IV feedings without adverse effects	• Administer parenteral nutrition as ordered and monitor for complications - aspiration - hyperglycemia - HHNK - fluid overload • Administer enteral nutrition as ordered • If administering enteral nutrition - keep HOB elevated 30° - monitor residuals q4h - auscultate bowel sounds q4h
		RATIONALE: *Highly nutritive feedings, orally or parenterally, are required to meet the increased metabolic demands of the postoperative healing process.*
6 High Risk for Infection *r.t. invasive surgical procedure, pre-existing impaired immune response, and presence of indwelling catheters*	• Shows evidence of progressive incisional healing - pink - approximated - granulation tissue present - incisional drainage is serous and nonpurulent	• Observe wound for s/s of infection - redness, tenderness, warmth - purulent drainage - separating suture line

NURSING DIAGNOSES	OUTCOME CRITERIA	INTERVENTIONS

	• Remains free of infection
	  - temperature WNL
	  - WBC WNL
	  - negative blood cultures
	  - respiratory secretions remains clear, odorless, and negative on cultures
	  - urine remains clear, odorless, free of sediment, and negative on cultures
	  - skin is clear, intact
		• Monitor WBC count and differential
		• Monitor cultures
		• Inspect respiratory secretions q4h
		• Inspect urine q4h
		• Inspect skin q8h

	• Patient/family comply with infection prevention requirements	• Teach patient regarding the need to wash hands • Offer oral hygiene q4h • Maintain good pulmonary toilet q4h • Provide tissues and disposal bag for expectorated sputum • Promote good nutritional intake especially of protein and vitamin C • Provide appropriate skin care to edematous areas
		RATIONALE: *Consistent monitoring of these parameters provides for early detection and treatment of infection. Other interventions help prevent entry of pathogens.*
7 **Altered Protection** *r.t. alterations in clotting mechanisms associated with pre-existing liver dysfunction and malnutrition*	• Is free of petechiae, melena, hematuria, fever, redness, drainage	• Assess for signs of bleeding: tarry stool, bloody urine, bloody NG aspirate, bruising, oozing from puncture sites, orifices, bleeding mucous membranes
	• Shows VS WNL	• Monitor VS per post-op routine, or as indicated
	• Shows PT, PTT, platelet counts WNL	• Monitor PT, PTT, platelets, and FSP
	• Maintains personal cleanliness, clean environment	• Promote personal and environmental cleanliness • Institute safety precautions

SURGICAL

NURSING DIAGNOSES	OUTCOME CRITERIA	INTERVENTIONS
	• Shows no signs of bleeding and hemorrhage of skin or mucous membranes	• Avoid IM injections and arterial sticks; if necessary, use the smallest gauge needle possible • Maintain pressure for several minutes over venipuncture sites • Use electric shaver rather than straight razor • Use soft-bristled toothbrush or oral swabs for oral hygiene • Avoid skin shearing; handle patient gently during movement
		RATIONALE: *Frequent monitoring and prevention of trauma or abrasion reduce risk of bleeding and hemorrhage.*
8 Impaired Skin Integrity *r.t. tissue edema*	• Has clean incision with edges approximated	• Inspect condition of surgical incision as appropriate
	• Shows no peripheral edema, swelling • Has palpable peripheral pulses	• Observe extremities for color, warmth, swelling, pulses, texture, edema, ulceration
	• Has clean, moist mucous membranes	• Inspect mucous membranes for redness, extreme warmth, drainage
	• Has intact skin with no shearing or breakdown	• Monitor for areas of redness and breakdown • Monitor for discoloration, bruising, rashes, abrasions, excessive dryness • Monitor for sources of pressure, friction • Restrict use of soap to baths only; follow with lotion • Use eggcrate or other low pressure mattress • Maintain dry, clean linen • Use paper or transparent tape instead of adhesive
		RATIONALE: *Friable, edematous skin requires careful monitoring and prevention of pressure and abrasions.*

NURSING DIAGNOSES	OUTCOME CRITERIA	INTERVENTIONS
9 Anxiety *r.t. threat of injury or death*	• Reports feeling of decreased anxiety • Experiences few physical symptoms associated with anxiety (nail biting, twitching, etc.) • Identifies cause of anxiety	• Maintain awareness and sensitivity to threat of death; provide opportunities for expressing/ verbalizing fears and worries

	• Uses support systems to cope with anxiety	• Encourage significant others to participate in care
		• Teach stress reduction techniques
		  - meditation
		  - imagery
		  - relaxation
		• Involve patient in care-related decisions

	• Expresses feeling of safety	• Use a calm, reassuring approach • Explain all procedures • Stay with patient during anxiety-producing episodes • Listen attentively and maintain eye contact • Acknowledge dependence • Anticipate needs
		RATIONALE: *Being present, encouraging verbalization of feelings, and enhancing effective coping strategies will lower anxiety to a tolerable level.*

10 Knowledge Deficit
 	
r.t. lack of information regarding disease process, surgical intervention, home management
	• Patient/caregiver verbalizes/demonstrates competency with home care
	  - dietary regime
	  - potential complications
	  - surgical procedure
	  - medication regime
	  - s/s of infection and poor healing
		• Determine degree of insight; clarify any misconceptions
		• Provide and review written dietary instructions
		• Demonstrate, observe return demonstration of incisional care, abdominal girth measurement, and stool testing for occult blood
		• Discuss prescribed activities and limitations
		• Provide, discuss written instructions regarding medications, purpose, dosage, effects, adverse effects

SURGICAL

NURSING DIAGNOSES	OUTCOME CRITERIA	INTERVENTIONS
		• Provide, discuss list of reportable s/s to include: decreased mental ability, increased abdominal girth/weight, peripheral edema, fever, nausea, vomiting, tarry stools, hematuria, purulent drainage from wound
		• Encourage to incorporate learned skills into daily routine while in hospital

RATIONALE: *A knowledgeable, competent patient and caregiver are likely to manage a safe and uneventful recovery period at home.*

OTHER LESS COMMON NURSING DIAGNOSES: *Impaired Gas Exchange; Impaired Physical Mobility; Sleep Pattern Disturbance; Bathing/Hygiene, Dressing/Grooming, Toileting Self-Care Deficits; Body Image Disturbance; Altered Thought Processes*

ESSENTIAL DISCHARGE CRITERIA

- Exhibits effective breathing pattern; adequate oxygenation and ventilation
- Is afebrile; no local infection
- Maintains balanced fluids and electrolytes
- Shows baseline coagulation factors
- Shows baseline serum protein

- Maintains sufficient nutritional intake
- Is alert, oriented
- Expresses satisfaction with level of pain control
- Demonstrates knowledge/skill regarding home care activities, therapy regimes, wound care

PROSTATECTOMY, TUR

NURSING DIAGNOSES	OUTCOME CRITERIA	INTERVENTIONS

See "Postoperative Care" care plan in General Section

1 Pain

r.t. bladder spasms, clots in tubing, surgical trauma

- Verbalizes, displays freedom from pain

- Displays no rigidity of abdomen

- Avoids activity that aggravates discomfort

- Reports comfort following analgesia

- Assess bladder spasms: pain, leakage around catheter, contraction of bladder

- Irrigate catheter prn for patency
- Examine abdomen for bladder distention

- Instruct to avoid straining to void

- Control pain: analgesia prn, distraction, relaxation exercises; evaluate

RATIONALE: *To maximize pain treatment, bladder spasms should be treated and distention avoided.*

2 High Risk for Injury

r.t. highly vascular surgical area, irritation of catheter, and surgical trauma

- Shows no evidence of active bleeding
  - no bright red urine or clots in urine
  - normal VS, BP
  - normal H&H, platelets, coagulation times

- Affirms need to avoid lifting, straining per instructions

- Observe urine for bright bleeding, clots in tubing and around catheter

- Monitor VS per post-op routine

- Monitor H&H, platelets, coagulation times

- Maintain catheter traction as directed

- Teach to avoid lifting, straining for 6 weeks

RATIONALE: *Early detection, protection prompt timely management of hemorrhage.*

SURGICAL

303

NURSING DIAGNOSES	OUTCOME CRITERIA	INTERVENTIONS

3 High Risk for Infection
 	
r.t. surgical instrumentation, indwelling catheter
	• Is free of s/s of systemic infection
	  - afebrile
	  - no redness, odors, drainage around incision, catheter
	  - urine is free of cloudiness, foul odor
		• Monitor body temperature q4h
		• Observe for confusion, restlessness, behavior change
		• Assess for s/s of UTI
		• Observe for purulent drainage from urethra, incision
		• Examine urine for turbidity, foul smell
		• Encourage fluids to 3000 mL/d unless contraindicated
		• Use aseptic technique for catheter care q8h

		RATIONALE: *Monitoring prompts early detection and management of infection.*
4 Altered Urinary Elimination (retention, incontinence) *r.t. edema, clots, or trauma to urinary sphincter or perineal nerves*	• Denies urgency or full bladder	• Monitor continuous bladder irrigation, if used; otherwise, irrigate with 30-60 mL of N/S as necessary per orders • Assess for s/s of suprapubic distention, discomfort q4h • Measure urinary residual per orders postcatheter removal
	• Balanced I&O by post-op day 2	• Monitor I&O
	• Voids with minimal difficulty postcatheter removal	• Teach perineal exercises • Teach to be alert for urethral stricture up to 6 months post-op • Teach to void upon urge or at least q2-3h
		RATIONALE: *These measures facilitate return to normal urinary elimination.*

NURSING DIAGNOSES	OUTCOME CRITERIA	INTERVENTIONS
5 Knowledge Deficit *r.t. anxiety about bleeding, incontinence, post-op activity restrictions, retrograde ejaculation, erectile dysfunction, and infertility*	• Demonstrates post-op wound care prn	• Explain, demonstrate wound care if required

	• Has list of s/s to report to physician	• Teach reportable s/s
		  - clots
		  - burning
		  - frequency
		  - retention
		  - loss of bladder control
		  - bladder distention
		  - increasing pain
		  - cloudy urine
		  - foul-smelling urine
		  - persistent incontinence

	• Describes recommended activity, diet, medications, follow-up appointments	• Review activity limitations: avoid straining, lifting for 6 weeks • Review diet, activity, medications, self-care, follow-up appointments

RATIONALE: *Providing essential information facilitates patient/family involvement and promotes self-care.*

OTHER LESS COMMON NURSING DIAGNOSES: *Sexual Dysfunction; Body Image Disturbance; High Risk for Impaired Skin Integrity*

SURGICAL

ESSENTIAL DISCHARGE CRITERIA

- Is afebrile
- Shows no urinary obstruction, retention
- Shows no major new bleeding or clots in urine
- Is voiding qs
- Pain is controlled with oral analgesia

- Describes effects, side effects of surgery
- Verbalizes accurate knowledge about pathologic findings
- Describes/demonstrates recommended, safe self-care, follow-up plans, and appointments

RECTAL SURGERY

NURSING DIAGNOSES	OUTCOME CRITERIA	INTERVENTIONS

See "Postoperative Care" care plan in General Section

1 Pain
r.t. rectal irritation and pressure

- Verbalizes/displays freedom from pain

- Assess location, characteristics, and intensity of post-op pain q2-4h
- Assess acceptable level of pain for patient

- Reports comfort following analgesia

- Medicate regularly for pain relief with prescribed analgesics and monitor results

---

- Identifies medication or activity that reduces or aggravates discomfort

- Collaborate with patient to determine what methods may be used to reduce pain
- Explore nonpharmacological interventions which provide pain relief, i.e., relaxation, positioning, distraction
- Provide sitz bath for comfort

RATIONALE: *Careful analysis of pain characteristics aids in the differential diagnosis of pain. Treatment of pain minimizes the stress response and enhances recovery.*

---

2 Colonic Constipation
r.t. pain during elimination

- Has normal stool consistency and frequency

- Monitor dietary and fluid intake
- Suggest drinking fruit juice (such as prune juice) and water before breakfast, unless contraindicated
- Encourage high fiber diet, eliminating foods that cause diarrhea or constipation
- Medicate with stool softeners, only as ordered

RATIONALE: *High fiber diet and good hydration keep stool soft and moist.*

NURSING DIAGNOSES	OUTCOME CRITERIA	INTERVENTIONS
3 Knowledge Deficit *r.t. unfamiliarity with home care of rectal wound*	• Patient/family list reportable s/s	• Discuss s/s to report to physician: bleeding, persistent diarrhea, constipation, weight loss

	• Patient/family demonstrate required care skills	• Discuss wound management
		  - expect tissue sloughing 7-10 d post-op
		  - report bleeding, necrosis, or wound/urinary infection
		  - take medications
		
		• Provide patient with information on natural methods for relieving and preventing constipation or diarrhea (i.e., high fiber diet, fluid intake of 2 L/d); avoid using toilet tissue (use cotton wipes)

	• Patient/family discuss required activity	• Encourage activity, but avoid long standing, sitting
		RATIONALE: *A knowledgeable, competent patient is likely to manage a safe and uneventful recovery.*

OTHER LESS COMMON NURSING DIAGNOSES:
Altered Urinary Elimination; High Risk for Injury

ESSENTIAL DISCHARGE CRITERIA

- Achieves acceptable pain relief with oral medications
- Verbalizes understanding of home wound management
- Returns to normal bowel and urinary elimination pattern

SURGICAL

RETINAL DETACHMENT

NURSING DIAGNOSES	OUTCOME CRITERIA	INTERVENTIONS
1 High Risk for Injury (external) *r.t. visual limitations and presence of bilateral eye patches postoperatively*	• Remains free of physical injury/trauma throughout hospitalization - no bleeding or injury - no episodes of sudden, severe pain	• Orient patient to surrounding environment upon admission and as needed throughout hospitalization • Modify environment to reduce potential safety hazards - keep needed items within patient's reach - remove items and equipment from patient's path - keep 4 side rails in upright position at night (the bottom side rails *may* be down during the day depending on patient's level of understanding and compliance with safety precautions) • Report sudden, severe pain
	• Complies with positioning, bed rest, activity as ordered	• Position patient as ordered • Supervise bed rest/activity as ordered • Avoid measures that would increase intraocular pressure (coughing, sneezing) • Administer antiemetics as ordered
		RATIONALE: *Familiarizing the patient with his/her surroundings and modifying them reduces the risk of injury.*
2 Anxiety *r.t. loss of vision and lack of knowledge about perioperative care*	• Verbalizes feelings regarding visual loss	• Encourage patient/family to verbalize concerns and fears - potential post-op vision loss (90 percent of surgical repairs are successful) - possible role changes - financial stability
	• Verbalizes accurate knowledge of pre-, intra-, and postoperative care routines	• Give simple, accurate information about care routines; clarify any misinformation • Reassure patient of normal responses to visual loss and fears

NURSING DIAGNOSES	OUTCOME CRITERIA	INTERVENTIONS

RATIONALE: *Encouraging communication of fears and concerns allows the nurse to assess support systems, correct any misinformation, and assist patient/family in recognizing possible role changes. Accurate information and appropriate teaching enhance the patient's understanding of perioperative events. Validating that the patient's anxiety is a normal response promotes self-esteem.*

---

3 High Risk for Infection

r.t. increased susceptibility from interruption of body surfaces

- Remains free of local and systemic infection
  - no drainage or red, swollen areas around eye
  - normal CBC
  - no s/s of infection
  - no fever
  - negative cultures

- Assess for s/s of infection q6-8h
  - reddened, edematous eyelids
  - purulent drainage from the eye
  - elevated body temperature
  - elevated serum electrolytes, WBC count, and abnormal eye culture and sensitivity

- Use aseptic technique with all aspects of eye care, especially the installation of ophthalmic drops
  - wash hands before and after all patient care
  - avoid contamination of eye dropper through contact with skin and other surfaces
  - follow handling and storage instructions of eye medications (as well as other eye care equipment, patches, or shield)
  - instruct patient/family about aseptic technique

- Promote wound healing
  - provide adequate rest and proper nutrition and fluid intake
  - instruct about use of an eye patch during day and eye shield at night

- Notify physician promptly for any evidence of infection

SURGICAL

RATIONALE: *Prompt and continuous assessments alert to early signs of infection. Aseptic technique significantly reduces the risk of infection. Adequate rest and proper nutrition and fluid intake combine to foster general health. Use of an eye patch or shield significantly reduces or prevents strain and irritation of the suture line.*

NURSING DIAGNOSES	OUTCOME CRITERIA	INTERVENTIONS
4 Altered Health Maintenance (high risk for) *r.t. insufficient knowledge of permitted activities, complications, medication, restrictions, and follow-up care*	• Patient/family verbalize, demonstrate accurate knowledge of activity restrictions	• Reinforce activity restrictions as prescribed by physician
	• Patient/family discuss, demonstrate correct knowledge of medications	• Explain information regarding each prescribed medication - name, purpose, action - dosage schedules - medication administration - drug interactions including food/drug interactions, special medication, precautions, and side effects
	• Patient/family identify reportable s/s	• Instruct about s/s to be reported - eye pain - loss of vision - vision abnormalities - redness, elevated body temperature, increased drainage
	• Patient/family identify specific modifications for care at home	• Assist to identify potential postdischarge problems and plan accordingly - home environment/safety - cooking and shopping - transportation - medications - ADL
	• Possess schedule for follow-up appointments	• Reinforce need for adequate follow-up care and stress importance of compliance with post-discharge regimen

RATIONALE: *Knowledge about and compliance with activity, medication, and home care regimens prevent or reduce the risk of complications. Patients are more likely to comply with follow-up care if they understand the importance of careful follow-up in the prevention of complications.*

OTHER LESS COMMON NURSING DIAGNOSES: Pain; Diversional Activity Deficit

ESSENTIAL DISCHARGE CRITERIA

- Vision approximates previous acuity (or patient adjusts to partial or complete loss of vision)
- Remains free of injury and infection

- Experiences reduced level of anxiety
- Demonstrates knowledge of care regimen

SURGICAL

SHOULDER SEPARATION

NURSING DIAGNOSES	OUTCOME CRITERIA	INTERVENTIONS

See Care Plan: "Postoperative Care" in General Section

---

1 Pain

r.t. disarticulation of shoulder joint

- Verbalizes/displays reasonable comfort
  - displays behaviors consistent with comfort (relaxed body posture)
  - reports comfort following administration of analgesia
  - does not guard surgical area
  - identifies source of comfort
  - identifies medication or activity that reduces/aggravates discomfort
  - alternates periods of activity and rest

- Ask patient to describe the pain on a scale of 1-10
- Remind to keep arm immobilized with sling, clavicle harness, immobilizer, or other device as ordered
- Instruct to not lie on affected side
- Administer narcotic and non-narcotic analgesics routinely; encourage adjunct use of relaxation techniques

RATIONALE: *Assessment of the degree of pain is enhanced by specific description from the patient. Immobilization decreases muscle spasms, keeps bone ends in alignment, and decreases swelling, thus decreasing pain. Pain is increased by pressure caused by lying on the injured joint.*

---

2 Altered Tissue Perfusion (peripheral)

r.t. edema or pressure from tight immobilizer

- Shows improved peripheral tissue perfusion in affected arm, hand
  - warmth of fingers of affected arm
  - no edema of finger
  - brisk CRT
  - palpable peripheral pulses

- Monitor skin color and presence of edema of fingers; compare with fingers of unaffected arm
- Monitor warmth of fingers of affected arm
- Test for CRT
- Check rate and strength of peripheral pulse
- Ask patient to move fingers frequently

RATIONALE: *Constriction of blood vessels results in decreased perfusion and is demonstrated by pale or cyanotic color, cold skin, or presence of edema. It is also manifested by decreased CRT and decreased or absent peripheral pulse. Movement of fingers increases circulation.*

NURSING DIAGNOSES	OUTCOME CRITERIA	INTERVENTIONS

3 High Risk for Injury
 	
r.t. pressure on peripheral nerves from constricting immobilizer
	• Remains free of injury with intact neuromuscular status
	  - no impairment of finger movement
	  - no impairment of finger sensation
		• Monitor numbness and ability to move fingers of affected extremity
		• Ask patient to hyperextend the thumb, wrist and four fingers
		• Abduct (fan out) all fingers
		• Have the patient touch the thumb to the small finger
		• Test ability of fingers to respond to pinprick, pressure, heat, cold, and touch; test distal fat pad of small finger, distal surface of the index finger, and the web space between thumb and finger
		• Monitor for numbness, tingling in fingers
		• Test vascular and neurologic status qh for 4 h, q4h for 24 h, then q8h until discharge

		RATIONALE: *Pressure on peripheral nerves causes decreased movement or decreased perception of feeling or pain.*
4 Knowledge Deficit *r.t. need for alignment of bone, vascular or neurologic complications, need for mobility of unaffected joints, and need for wariness of side effects of medications*	• Demonstrates understanding of need to maintain immobilizer and arm position	• Instruct how to check for proper position of sling or immobilizer • Palpate bone ends for swelling or malalignment • Instruct to keep upper arm parallel with the side of body, elbow bent at 90° angle, and lower arm across chest (as if wearing arm sling) when both standing and lying
	• Maintains full ROM of unaffected joints	• Perform ROM of unaffected joints, fingers
	• Performs own inspection of affected fingers for color, motion, edema, temperature of skin, feeling, movement	• Inspect and teach patient to check fingers for changes in color, temperature, edema • Inspect affected fingers for decreased movement, decreased sensitivity to pain or pressure, tingling; report problems to physician

SURGICAL

NURSING DIAGNOSES	OUTCOME CRITERIA	INTERVENTIONS
	• Performs own inspection of peripheral pulse, CRT in affected fingers and wrist	• Assess rate and strength of peripheral pulse in affected wrist • Inspect and teach patient to check for CRT in affected fingers and to report any changes
	• Reiterates correct knowledge of pain medication administration	• Instruct regarding administration of pain medications: purpose, dosages, side effects
		RATIONALE: *Immobility of bone ends is essential for healing. Swelling and pain indicate malalignment. Proper positioning of immobilizer and arm provides immobility of joint and promotes healing. Vascular changes cause pale or cyanotic changes, swelling, and cool skin, and pressure on peripheral nerves may cause changes in sensation and movement. Early detection is essential. Impairment of circulation results in decreased or absent peripheral pulse and increased CRT. Pain medications may cause gastric or neurologic symptoms that should be reported.*
5 Feeding, Bathing/Hygiene, Toileting, Self-Care Deficits *r.t. immobility of arm*	• Feeds self with one arm	• Teach how to cut up meat and feed with one arm and hand
	• Demonstrates feasible technique for toileting, bathing, combing hair, and brushing teeth with one arm	• Teach techniques for toileting, bathing, combing hair, and brushing teeth with one arm
	• Dresses self or has assistance at home	• Describe how to dress (using clothing with alternate fasteners); verify availability of assistance at home as needed
		RATIONALE: *Providing assistance in gaining skills in self-care is important in maintaining self-esteem. It is important to explore self-care prior to dismissal from the health facility.*

> **OTHER LESS COMMON NURSING DIAGNOSES:** Anxiety; Impaired Physical Mobility;
> Ineffective Management of Therapeutic Regimen; Impaired Home
> Maintenance Management; High Risk for Disuse Syndrome

ESSENTIAL DISCHARGE CRITERIA

- Verbalizes, displays freedom from pain
- Shows satisfactory peripheral tissue perfusion
- Maintains arm position of immobility

- Remains free of neuromuscular injury
- Demonstrates feasible self-care techniques (or has assistance) and is aware of symptoms of complications that should be reported

SURGICAL

SPLENECTOMY

See Care Plan "Postoperative Care" in General Section

1 High Risk for Infection

r.t. impaired skin integrity, decreased immune response after splenectomy

• Remains free of systemic and local infections	• Assess for factors that identify the patient at high risk for infection (age, procedures, disease conditions, medications, nutrition)
• Incision is free of redness, drainage; edges are approximated	• Inspect incision site for redness, swelling, drainage, pain, or discharge
• Shows normal VS, BP	• Assess VS per post-op routine • Auscultate breath sounds q8h
• Shows normal CBC	• Monitor CBC, amylase and lipase levels for increases
• Shows negative cultures	• Admit patient to an isolation room, if appropriate

• Screen all visitors and restrict those who have been exposed to an infection

• Obtain culture specimens when ordered; report results

• Decrease entry of organisms
  - meticulous hand-washing
  - maintain aseptic technique for all procedures (catheters, IV, wound dressing changes)
  - if able, limit unnecessary procedures

• Reduce risk of infection
  - instruct patient to balance activity with rest periods
  - encourage a diet high in protein and calories
  - assess for adequate immunizations against childhood diseases, bacterial and viral infections
  - administer polyvalent pneumococcal vaccine within 72 h after splenectomy and routine immunizations against influenza
  - monitor therapeutic and nontherapeutic effects of anti-infectives, if administered (superinfection)

NURSING DIAGNOSES	OUTCOME CRITERIA	INTERVENTIONS
	• Patient/family discuss and demonstrate required self-care, knowledge, and skills	• Instruct regarding infection prevention - teach patient and significant others about the infectious process - instruct patient to monitor incision site and have patient verbalize s/s of possible infections - administer prophylactic antibiotics for invasive procedures (dental work) - report to the physician immediately any flulike symptoms or nonspecific complaints (chills, fever, megalgias) - wear medic alert bracelet to notify medical personnel of possible post-splenectomy sepsis
		RATIONALE: *All of these measures combine to decrease susceptibility to infection, abscess formation, and pancreatitis while maintaining or increasing antibody titers.*
2 High Risk for Disuse Syndrome *r.t. immobility and increased platelet count*	• Is free of s/s of DVT - no localized warmth, redness in calves - no complaints of pain in legs - negative Homans' sign - palpable peripheral pulses	• Assess for s/s of DVT q4h
	• Exhibits adequate hydration - balanced I&O - normal electrolyte values - normal urinary sp. gr.	• Monitor hydration status q4h
	• Shows normal blood coagulation values	• Monitor blood coagulation studies qd
	• Actively cooperates with and discusses preventative measures	• Encourage to carry out active leg exercises unless contraindicated • Elevate the affected leg/legs above the level of the heart • Collaborate with the physician regarding the use of anti-embolic stockings or sequential pressure devices • Encourage the patient to decrease or avoid smoking

SURGICAL

NURSING DIAGNOSES	OUTCOME CRITERIA	INTERVENTIONS
	• Shows no signs of bleeding	• Administer anticoagulants as ordered by physician • Inspect for s/s of bleeding such as hematuria, bleeding gums, epistaxis, and ecchymosis
		RATIONALE: *These measures help to prevent complications of thromboembolism associated with the temporary increase of RBCs and platelets following splenectomy.*
3 High Risk for Fluid Volume Deficit *r.t. intravascular hypovolemia*	• Shows normal VS, BP	• Monitor VS for signs of shock q2-4h • Measure abdominal girth q shift • Inspect incision site for bleeding q4h
	• Shows no s/s of dehydration - skin warm, dry - normal peripheral pulses - alert, oriented - urinary output WNL	• Monitor for symptoms of shock q2-4h
	• Achieves balanced I&O • Shows normal fluid and electrolyte balance	• Monitor I&O q shift
	• H&H WNL	• Monitor H&H counts • Administer IV fluids, blood, or blood products, as ordered • If s/s of shock occurs - elevate legs with patient in supine position, if able - insert IV line as ordered - initiate emergency protocols for shock • Collaborate with physician regarding further replacement of fluid losses • Provide emotional support and simple explanations of treatment measures to decrease anxiety

NURSING DIAGNOSES	OUTCOME CRITERIA	INTERVENTIONS
		RATIONALE: *These measures detect changes in fluid status while preventing blood loss and complications of hypovolemic shock.*

4 Ineffective Breathing Pattern
 	
r.t. abdominal surgery and location of incision
	• Exhibits improving respiratory status
	  - stable VS
	  - clear breath sounds
	  - 12-20 deep, regular breaths/min
		• Monitor VS
		• Auscultate breath sounds q shift
		• Encourage coughing and deep breathing q2h and incentive spirometry; inspect sputum color
		• Provide respiratory therapy treatments, per orders
		• Maintain O_2 therapy, per orders
		• Position in a mid or high Fowler's
		• Increase fluids per orders

	• Shows improving skin color	• Monitor for cyanosis of lips and oral mucosa • Monitor for SOB on ambulation
	• Maintains SaO_2 WNL	• Monitor pulse oximeter and ABGs • Monitor chest x-ray; report results
		RATIONALE: *These measures foster prevention of potential respiratory complications and hypoxemic episodes.*

SURGICAL

OTHER LESS COMMON NURSING DIAGNOSES: *Pain; Impaired Physical Mobility*

ESSENTIAL DISCHARGE CRITERIA

- Exhibits no signs of systemic or local infection
- Shows stable VS WNL
- Has no bleeding

- Shows lab values WNL
- Has clear breath sounds
- Exhibits no signs of DVT

THORACOTOMY

NURSING DIAGNOSES	OUTCOME CRITERIA	INTERVENTIONS

See Care Plan: "Postoperative Care" in General Section

1 Ineffective Breathing Pattern

r.t. painful respiratory effort

- Exhibits improving respiratory status
  - 12-20 deep, regular respirations/min
  - clear breath sounds bilaterally

- Assess for s/s of pulmonary embolism
- Observe chest wall movement
- Monitor RR, depth, and quality
- Auscultate breath sounds q2-4h
- Assess for mediastinal shift
- Assess for s/s of respiratory distress, dyspnea
- Encourage coughing and deep breathing exercises q2h
- Encourage use of incentive spirometer q2h
- Teach incisional splinting to facilitate deep breathing exercises
- Perform pulmonary toileting exercises
- Encourage early and frequent ambulation

- Maintains patent drainage system

- Monitor status of closed chest drainage system
- Keep chest tube clamp at bedside at all times
- Maintain functioning of system by ensuring all connections are tightened and proper water seal levels are in effect, and by attaching closed chest drainage system to appropriate suction
- Maintain level of closed chest drainage system below level of chest
- Monitor CT for kinks and/or obstructions
- Maintain a sterile occlusive dressing
- Milk CT q2h at discretion of physician
- Document level of drainage q2h

NURSING DIAGNOSES	OUTCOME CRITERIA	INTERVENTIONS
	• Shows ABGs, chest x-ray WNL	• Monitor ABGs as ordered • Administer O₂ as ordered • Administer IPPB as ordered • Turn and position q2h
		RATIONALE: *Surveillance of respiratory functions provides for early detection of fluid accumulation or pressure shift in thorax and prompts timely interventions. Breathing exercises and ambulation foster pulmonary air exchange and reduce risk of embolism by improving peripheral circulation.*
2 High Risk for Injury (internal) *r.t. spontaneous pneumothorax secondary to sudden change in chest pressure*	• Exhibits intact neurologic status	• Monitor for sudden changes in mental status
	• Exhibits no evidence of hypoxia	• Assess for chest pain, cyanosis, dyspnea • Provide care related to mechanical ventilation as indicated
		RATIONALE: *Early detection and treatment of ineffective respiratory efforts prompt vigorous ventilatory assistance if needed and foster independent ventilatory efforts.*
3 Pain *r.t. tissue trauma*	• Verbalizes/displays freedom from pain	• Note duration, location, intensity of pain
	• Reports comfort following analgesia	• Administer narcotic analgesics regularly to prevent pain • Monitor for depressant effects of narcotic analgesics • Administer analgesics prior to coughing and deep breathing to alleviate breakthrough pain; assess the effects
	• Identifies medication or activity that reduces or aggravates discomfort	• Educate patient/family in PCA use

SURGICAL

NURSING DIAGNOSES	OUTCOME CRITERIA	INTERVENTIONS
		• Alleviate anxiety regarding pain with adequate explanations
		• Position for comfort
		• Reinforce pre-op teaching, i.e., splinting of incision

RATIONALE: *Comfort enhances coughing, deep breathing, and ambulation, which promote early recovery.*

4 High Risk for Fluid Volume Deficit *r.t. blood loss, excessive drainage, dehydration*	• Maintains balanced I&O	• Monitor I&O q8h
	• Shows normal VS, BP • Has good skin turgor, moist mucous membranes	• Assess VS q30 min for 1 h, qh for 2 h, q4h for 24 h; inspect skin, mucous membranes at same intervals
	• Shows normal fluid and electrolyte balance	• Monitor electrolytes, BUN, H&H, and creatinine
	• Shows no evidence of bleeding	• Monitor for excessive bleeding • Inspect CT and insertion site q4h for bleeding; note sudden onset of increased drainage • Notify physician of abnormal labs, s/s of hypovolemic shock

RATIONALE: *Surveillance of circulating volume provides early detection of excessive fluid loss and prompts timely fluid replacement interventions.*

NURSING DIAGNOSES	OUTCOME CRITERIA	INTERVENTIONS

5 Knowledge Deficit
 	
r.t. unfamiliarity with disease process, operative procedure, follow-up care
	• Patient/family discuss pathophysiology of disease process, rationale for treatment
	  - have list of reportable s/s
	  - have phone numbers for emergency medical help
	  - discuss relaxation, activity, diet
	  - participate in and discuss care activities
		• Instruct about required knowledge and care
		  - notify physician of fever, chills, redness, or drainage from operative site
		  - report to physician or emergency department for fever
		  - correctly describe how and why he/she needs to move and ambulate frequently, advancing activities gradually
		  - continue prescribed regimen of coughing, deep breathing, and ROM exercises

RATIONALE: *Knowledge of treatment regimen enhances self-care and post-op recovery while preventing complications.*

OTHER LESS COMMON NURSING DIAGNOSES: High Risk for Infection; Ineffective Airway Clearance; Fatigue; Impaired Gas Exchange; Impaired Verbal Communication

ESSENTIAL DISCHARGE CRITERIA

• Is free of respiratory difficulties, pain, and complications

• Shows temperature, WBC count, fluid and electrolyte balance WNL

• Patient/family verbalizes an understanding of follow-up care

SURGICAL

THYROIDECTOMY

NURSING DIAGNOSES	OUTCOME CRITERIA	INTERVENTIONS

See Care Plan: "Postoperative Care" in General Section

1 Ineffective Airway Clearance

r.t. respiratory obstruction resulting from laryngeal nerve damage, hemorrhage, or tetany

- Demonstrates normal RR, depth, and rhythm; minimal or absent hoarseness

- Assess for dyspnea, hoarseness, or weak voice
- Observe for dyspnea, crowing sound
- Keep tracheostomy set at bedside

- Shows no bleeding on pillow or dressing

- Observe pillow and dressings behind neck for bleeding

- Reports swallowing with minimal difficulty

- Monitor for increased difficulty swallowing or choking sensation
- Observe for sensation of dressing becoming tighter

- HR is within 20 bpm of baseline, BP WNL

- Have O_2 and suction equipment readily available
- Loosen dressing and remove clips/sutures, as ordered
- Elevate HOB 45° and call for medical help immediately, if needed

- Serum Ca WNL; no signs of deficiency are present
  - early signs: tingling around mouth or toes, fingers
  - late signs: positive Chvostek's and Trousseau's signs, grand mal seizures

- Observe for Ca deficiency (tetany)
- Administer calcium chloride or calcium gluconate, as ordered

RATIONALE: *Hoarseness is the first sign of laryngeal nerve damage, resulting in vocal cord spasm and respiratory obstruction. Tracheal compression from hemorrhage can cause respiratory obstruction. Ca deficiency can result in contraction of the glottis, respiratory obstruction, and death.*

NURSING DIAGNOSES	OUTCOME CRITERIA	INTERVENTIONS
2 Pain *r.t. surgical procedure*	• Verbalizes/displays freedom from pain	• Document subjective and objective evaluation of pain according to a standard scale • Teach patient to support the head and neck when coughing or turning by placing hands behind neck • Once clips/sutures are removed, teach patient to perform gentle ROM for the neck
	• Reports comfort following administration of analgesia	• Administer prescribed analgesics, as indicated, and assess effectiveness
		RATIONALE: *Pain and inactivity delay healing and recovery.*
3 Altered Nutrition: Less than body requirements *r.t. impaired swallowing resulting from edema or laryngeal nerve damage*	• Exhibits/maintains adequate nutritional status - maintains weight - takes 80 percent or more of meals	• Obtain baseline weight and weigh daily • Start soft foods as soon as tolerated • Encourage high-protein, high-carbohydrate diet
		RATIONALE: *Adequate intake promotes adequate healing and nutrition.*
4 Knowledge Deficit *r.t. need for lifelong thyroid replacement hormone (if total thyroidectomy)*	• Affirms need for lifelong hormone replacement therapy; describes dosage, schedule, effects, side effects	• Teach about the medication/ hormones required as replacement therapy
		RATIONALE: *Sustained hormone replacement prevents s/s of hypothyroidism.*

SURGICAL

> **OTHER LESS COMMON NURSING DIAGNOSES:** *Hyperthermia; Activity Intolerance; Decreased Cardiac Output; Ineffective Individual Coping; Anxiety; Sleep Pattern Disturbance; Body Image Disturbance; Impaired Home Maintenance Management; Impaired Verbal Communications*

ESSENTIAL DISCHARGE CRITERIA

- Has no hoarseness or dyspnea
- Displays no difficulty swallowing
- Verbalizes relief of pain or that it is well controlled with oral analgesics

- Maintains stable weight
- Affirms/describes need for lifelong thyroid replacement hormone therapy as indicated

URETERAL LITHOTRIPSY

NURSING DIAGNOSES	OUTCOME CRITERIA	INTERVENTIONS

1 High Risk for Infection
r.t. instrumentation of urinary tract
	• Is free of s/s of systemic infection
	  - no chills, fever
	  - negative UA
	  - normal H&H
	  - CBC WNL
	  - VS WNL
		• Monitor for chills
		• Monitor UA, H&H, CBC, VS

	• Is free of s/s of local infection
	  - denies chills, backache
	  - no severe bladder spasms
	    or urethral discharge
	  - incision is free of redness, drainage
	  - no urinary cloudiness, foul odor
		• Notify physician if patient shows any indications of infection
		  - chills
		  - fever
		  - flushed skin
		• Perform appropriate aseptic care of indwelling catheter
		• Maintain accurate I&O

		RATIONALE: *Surveillance is necessary because bacteremia can occur after any instrumentation of the urinary tract.*
2 Pain *r.t. postoperative procedure*	• Verbalizes, displays freedom from pain	• Observe patient and obtain information about pain q2-4h • Use a flow sheet to monitor pain (quality, intensity, duration, effect of narcotic(s), and comfort measures)
	• Reports comfort following analgesia	• Administer narcotic analgesic as appropriate • Provide patient/family with verbal/written accurate information about narcotic analgesics • Collaborate with physician to establish a regular schedule for administration of parenteral/oral narcotics
	• Identifies medication or activity that reduces or aggravates discomfort - identifies source of discomfort	• Provide nonpharmacologic pain measures (guided imagery, relaxation techniques) • Determine source of pain which may be related to the catheter or the surgical manipulation

SURGICAL

NURSING DIAGNOSES	OUTCOME CRITERIA	INTERVENTIONS
		RATIONALE: *Pain from different sources usually requires different intervention. Fear, loneliness, depression, and numerous other conditions may be sources of extreme discomfort for patients who may translate unconsciously their feelings into pain.*
3 Altered Urinary Elimination *r.t. removal of indwelling catheter and/or presence of stone fragments*	• Resumes normal voiding pattern - balanced I&O - absence of dysuria - no s/s of complication	• Measure I&O q24h • Monitor for complications - onset of fever, chills, hematuria, general aching - flank pain, sensation of bladder fullness • Strain all urine and send any stone fragments for analysis
	• Takes required fluids; maintains output equal to intake - clear urine - no retention	• Encourage (unless contraindicated) a fluid intake of at least 2.5 L/d • Measure all voidings and cumulative I&O; report signs of urinary retention • Encourage ambulation • Provide patient with verbal and written information
		RATIONALE: *UTI must be completely eradicated to remain free from urinary calculi. Ambulation and increased fluid intake help with elimination of fragments.*
4 Knowledge Deficit *r.t. lack of information regarding follow-up instructions, what to report to physician*	• Patient/family list reportable s/s	• Teach s/s warranting notification of physician - severe kidney or shoulder pain unrelieved by prescribed medication - inability to urinate - temperature > 38.5°C (101°F)
	• Patient/family demonstrate required care skills	• Teach to strain urine and retrieve stone for analysis

NURSING DIAGNOSES	OUTCOME CRITERIA	INTERVENTIONS
	• Patient/family discuss activity, diet, fluids	• Instruct to avoid heavy lifting • Encourage ambulation • Instruct patient to drink 2500 mL/d, unless contraindicated

RATIONALE: *A knowledgeable patient is likely to make timely notification of s/s of complications.*

> **OTHER LESS COMMON NURSING DIAGNOSES:** *Fluid Volume Deficit; Altered Tissue Perfusion; Ineffective Management of Therapeutic Regimen*

ESSENTIAL DISCHARGE CRITERIA

- Shows no s/s of UTI or hemorrhage
- Verbalizes relief of pain
- Demonstrates normal urinary elimination pattern
- Verbalizes knowledge of s/s to report to physician and how to strain urine

SURGICAL

URETEROLITHOTOMY

NURSING DIAGNOSES	OUTCOME CRITERIA	INTERVENTIONS

See Care Plan: "Postoperative Care" in General Section

1 High Risk for Infection

r.t. urinary stasis, invasive tubes/drains, and surgical incision

- Displays no s/s of localized or generalized infection
  - drainage is nonpurulent, diminishes in amount
  - no clots, obstructions of tubes, drains
  - clear, amber urine

- Monitor temperature q4h and notify physician of elevation
- Assess amount of drainage through drains and tubes, noting presence of clots/obstructions
- Assess appearance, color, odor of urine, and presence of any sediment
- Cleanse exterior of indwelling catheter per protocol
- Maintain drainage bag below level of bladder
- Employ aseptic technique when opening closed drainage urinary system devices
- Keep all dressings dry and intact
- Note characteristics of drainage on dressings
  - monitor incision site for swelling, redness, warmth, or presence or exudate
- Maintain total fluid intake of 2000-3000 mL for 24 h unless contraindicated (e.g., CHF, renal failure)
- Administer antibiotics as ordered; monitor effect and therapeutic levels when indicated

RATIONALE: *Early detection and prompt intervention augment the body's defenses against infection.*

2 High Risk for Fluid Volume Deficit

r.t. post-op hemorrhage and abnormal fluid loss secondary to surgical therapies

- Demonstrates stable hemodynamic parameters and fluid balance
  - VS WNL
  - fluid and electrolytes WNL
  - balanced I&O
  - H&H WNL
  - good skin turgor, moist mucous membranes
  - no pallor, cyanosis
  - stable body weight

- Assess VS and RR per post-op routine
- Evaluate electrolytes, BUN, creatinine, H&H, noting significant patterns; report abnormal values
- Monitor I&O and evaluate for negative fluid balance

NURSING DIAGNOSES	OUTCOME CRITERIA	INTERVENTIONS
		• Check skin turgor and mucous membranes
		• Evaluate complaints of thirst; provide oral care as needed
		• Note presence of restlessness, pallor, or cyanosis
		• Compare and evaluate pre- and post-op weights
		• Monitor frequency of dressing saturations; note characteristics, i.e., color, amount of drainage
		• Maintain oral intake of 2000-3000 mL for 24 h
		• Notify physician if urine output < 50 mL/h

RATIONALE: *Homeostatic mechanisms maintain fluid, electrolyte, and blood volume balances. Surgical interventions interrupt normal balance. Implement specific nursing interventions to counteract fluid and electrolytes and intracellular, extracellular, and vascular fluid imbalances.*

3 Pain *r.t. inflammation and surgical incision*	• Remains comfortable when performing ADL and when increasing level of activity during recovery period	• Encourage analgesics prior to increasing activity; allow enough time for medication to take effect
		• Instruct in use of splinting technique over incisional site
		• Provide general comfort measures, i.e., positioning, pillow supports, and splints
		• Utilize measures to reduce anxiety, i.e., explanations, listening, anticipating needs
		• Allow adequate rest periods

RATIONALE: *Social, environmental, and personal factors influence an individual's perception of pain and pain tolerance level. Nursing interventions address these factors to promote the use of adaptive techniques for effective pain control.*

SURGICAL

NURSING DIAGNOSES	OUTCOME CRITERIA	INTERVENTIONS

4 **Ineffective Breathing Pattern**

r.t. immobility, effects of anesthesia, and increased pain with movement

- Maintains adequate respiratory function without complications - takes 12-20 deep, regular respirations/min

- Monitor rate and quality of respirations
- TCDB at least q2h
- Assist in use of inspiratory spirometry q2h
- Encourage and assist with early ambulation
- Instruct to splint over incisional site when coughing and deep breathing
- Elevate HOB at least to a 30° angle
- Auscultate lung fields q4-8h
- Instruct in proper body mechanic technique for changing from a lying to a sitting position
- Utilize side rails as extra support when moving in bed

RATIONALE: *Adequate respiratory function requires synchronous movement of the walls of the chest and abdomen. Coughing clears the lungs of stagnant secretions by the use of abdominal and chest muscles. Lying flat reduces the expansion space of the lungs (abdominal organs shift upward).*

NURSING DIAGNOSES	OUTCOME CRITERIA	INTERVENTIONS
5 High Risk for Impaired Skin Integrity *r.t. decreased mobility and maceration secondary to urinary drainage*	• Demonstrates skin integrity free of open areas, ulcerations, or pressure spots	• Inspect pressure point areas with position changes • Perform frequent skin assessments noting changes in skin condition • Reposition at least q2h while in bed • ROM exercises q2h while awake • Encourage early ambulation • Provide skin care and back rubs as needed • Keep dressings dry, change frequently if needed; note characteristics of drainage in contact with skin • Utilize stoma drainage bags for tubes with large amounts of drainage • Provide adequate nutrition to maintain positive nitrogen balance • Consult with enterostomal/skin care clinician

RATIONALE: *Pressure on given area can impair skin integrity as a result of hypoxia. Maceration is a mechanism by which tissue is softened by prolonged moisture thereby weakening cells and eroding epidermis. Anabolism is necessary for healing and maintenance of muscle mass (positive nitrogen balance).*

SURGICAL

OTHER LESS COMMON NURSING DIAGNOSES: *Knowledge Deficit; Fear; Altered Nutrition: Less than body requirements; Fluid Volume Excess or Deficit; Altered Urinary Elimination; Altered Cardiopulmonary Tissue Perfusion; Body Image Disturbance*

ESSENTIAL DISCHARGE CRITERIA

• Maintains balanced I&O

• Exhibits no s/s of infection

• Controls pain with oral analgesia

VAGINAL PLASTIC SURGERY

NURSING DIAGNOSES	OUTCOME CRITERIA	INTERVENTIONS

See Care Plan: "Postoperative Care" in General Section

---

1 High Risk for Fluid Volume Deficit

r.t. hemorrhage

- Demonstrates normal circulating volume
  - VS, BP WNL
  - no pallor, cyanosis
  - balanced I&O
  - electrolytes WNL

- Assess and support circulating volume
  - assess VS per post-op routine
  - assess skin color and temperature
  - monitor I&O
  - monitor lab values, report to physician as indicated

RATIONALE: *VS and lab values are accurate indicators of low blood volume.*

---

2 High Risk for Infection

r.t. immuno-suppression, debilitating disease, poor hygiene, and surgical wound

- Has no odors or drainage around or through wound

- Assess wound status, documenting amount and description of drainage

- Exhibits normal VS, BP

- Monitor temperature at least q24h and notify physician if > 38.5°C (101°F)
- Reassess need for indwelling urinary catheter daily

- Shows normal CBC
- Shows negative cultures

- Monitor lab values (cultures, sensitivities, CBC); notify physician as indicated

RATIONALE: *These measures monitor and prevent wound/nosocomial infections.*

---

3 Altered Sexuality Patterns

r.t. altered body functions or structures

- Discusses sexual concerns and alternatives, alone or with partner

- Provide specific information to patient and partner regarding limitations, correct myths, and misinformation
- Address stress, fear, and sexual concerns of partner and examine relationship with sexual partner
- Examine concerns regarding sexuality and adequacy of sexual function
- Assess level of comfort in discussing topic alone or with partner: provide opportunity for both

NURSING DIAGNOSES	OUTCOME CRITERIA	INTERVENTIONS
		• Invite appropriate health professional referral

RATIONALE: *Effective coping reduces stress response and fosters learning and appropriate perceptions.*

---

4 Pain (acute)
r.t. surgical intervention

• Reports comfort following analgesia

• Collaborate with physician to establish regular schedule administration of parenteral/oral narcotics

• Administer narcotic analgesia as appropriate

• Reports/displays reasonable comfort

• Use a flow sheet to monitor pain [location, intensity, duration, effect of narcotic(s), and comfort measure(s)]

• Identifies medication or activity that reduces or aggravates discomfort

• Provide patient/family with verbal/written accurate information about narcotic analgesics

---

• Alternates periods of activity and rest

• Assist with nonpharmacologic pain control methods (relaxation, music, imagery)

RATIONALE: *The patient achieves satisfaction with progress as pain is controlled.*

SURGICAL

> **OTHER LESS COMMON NURSING DIAGNOSES:**
> *High Risk for Peripheral Neurovascular Dysfunction; Impaired Gas Exchange*

ESSENTIAL DISCHARGE CRITERIA

• Achieves fluid and electrolyte balance

• Is free from infection

• Controls pain with oral analgesia

• Verbalizes sexual concerns and alternatives

VEIN LIGATION AND STRIPPING

NURSING DIAGNOSES	OUTCOME CRITERIA	INTERVENTIONS

See Care Plan: "Postoperative Care" in General Section

1 Knowledge Deficit

r.t. lack of knowledge about disorder and its treatment

- Discusses anatomy and pathophysiology of disease
- Makes realistic statements about expected course of recovery, prognosis

- Explain chronicity of disease and possibility of varices returning

---

- Demonstrates knowledge of lifestyle modifications that will help prevent or relieve acute episodes

- Instruct about promoting venous return and preventing venous stasis
  - avoid sitting or standing for long periods of time
  - change positions frequently
  - do not sit with legs crossed
  - elevate legs when sitting
  - do not wear constrictive garments such as girdles or garters
  - wear elastic support stockings
  - sleep with foot of bed elevated 6-8 in

- Participates in foot/leg care activities

- Explain need for careful foot and leg care
  - no rubbing or massaging of extremities
  - precautions against injury to extremities

- Patient/family discuss relaxation, activity, diet

- Explain need to maintain ideal body weight
- Discuss importance of exercise program such as walking, swimming, or bicycling

---

RATIONALE: *Prevention of venous stasis is essential to maintain comfort and function.*

---

2 Altered Peripheral Tissue Perfusion

r.t. inadequate venous return

- Demonstrates improved peripheral circulation
  - palpable peripheral pulses
  - warm extremities
  - color WNL
  - decrease in peripheral edema

- Check extremities hourly for color, movement, sensation, temperature, presence of edema and pedal pulses; notify physician of any change
- Encourage deep breathing
- Elevate patient's legs above heart level as ordered
- Instruct to not gatch knee

NURSING DIAGNOSES	OUTCOME CRITERIA	INTERVENTIONS
		• Assist with brief periods of ambulation
		• Increase patient's walking periods as ordered
		• Instruct patient to avoid sitting or standing in one position
		• Inform patient to exercise calf muscles while in bed by dorsiflexing and plantarflexing feet
		• Apply individually measured elastic hose from toes to groin
		• Apply hose while patient is supine
		• Leave elastic hose in place 24 h as ordered
		• Remove once q8h for short period and reapply
		RATIONALE: *Deep breathing promotes venous return to right side of heart. Elevation and compression of extremities prevents development of venous stasis and edema.*
3 Pain *r.t. surgical incision*	• Verbalizes/displays freedom from pain	• Evaluate source of pain - postoperative pain - site infection pain - constrictive dressings - bleeding • Monitor VS per post-op routine • Encourage to change positions or elevate legs for comfort
	• Reports comfort following administration of analgesia	• Administer analgesics as ordered
		RATIONALE: *Giving analgesics and positioning decrease venous pressure an promote comfort.*

SURGICAL

> **OTHER LESS COMMON NURSING DIAGNOSES:**
> *High Risk for Impaired Skin Integrity; Body Image Disturbance*

ESSENTIAL DISCHARGE CRITERIA

- Demonstrates improved peripheral tissue perfusion
- Controls pain with oral analgesia

- Verbalizes knowledge regarding self-care to minimize recurrence of varicosities

APPENDIXES

CONTENTS

APPENDIX A: ABBREVIATIONS

Abbreviations used in this book

AAO	alert, awake, and oriented (to person, place, and time)
ABG(s)	arterial blood gases
ACS/NCI	American Cancer Society/National Cancer Institute
ADL	activities of daily living
AIDS	acquired immunodeficiency syndrome
ARDS	adult respiratory distress syndrome
ARF	acute renal failure
Baso	basophils
BID	twice daily
BP	blood pressure
bpm	beats per minute
BUN	blood urea nitrogen
C	centigrade
Ca	calcium
CAD	coronary artery disease
C&S	culture and sensitivity
CBC	complete blood count
cc	cubic centimeter
CCU	critical care unit
CHF	congestive heart failure
Cl	chloride
cm	centimeter
CMS	circulation, movement, sensation
CNS	central nervous system
CO₂	carbon dioxide
COHb	Carboxyl hemoglobin
CPK	creatine phosphokinase
CPM	continuous passive motion
CRF	chronic renal failure
CRT	capillary refill time
CSF	cerebrospinal fluid
CT	chest tube
CVA	cerebral vascular accident
CVP	central venous pressure
d	day
D/C	discharge
DIC	disseminated intravascular coagulation

DM	diabetes mellitus
DVT	deep venous thrombosis
ECG	electrocardiogram/graph
EEG	electroencephalograph
Eos	eosinophils
ESWL	extracorporeal shock wave lithotripsy
EU	Ehrlich units
F	fahrenheit
F&E	fluids and electrolytes
FSP	fibrin split products
g	gram
GGT	glutamyl transpeptidase
GI	gastrointestinal
h	hour
H	hydrogen
H&H	hemoglobin and hematocrit
Hb	hemoglobin
Hct	hematocrit
Hg	mercury
HHNK	hyperglycemic hyperosmolar nonketotic coma
HIV	human immunodeficiency virus
H₂O	water
HOB	head of bed
hpf	high power field
HR	heart rate
HS	hour of sleep
I&O	intake and output
IBW	ideal body weight
ICP	intracranial pressure
ICU	intensive care unit
IM	intramuscular
IPPB	intermittent positive pressure breathing
IU	international units
IV	intravenous
IVF	intravenous fluids
IVP	intravenous pyelogram
JVD	jugular vein distention

K	potassium
kg	kilogram
L	liter
lab	laboratory
L/d	liter(s) per day
LDH	lactic (acid) dehydrogenase
LOC	level of consciousness
mEq	milliequivalent
MI	myocardinal infarction
min	minutes
mL	milliliters
mmHg	millimeters of mercury
mm	millimeters
mm³	cubic millimeters
Mono	monocytes
MSW	medical social worker
Na	sodium
ND	nursing diagnosis
neuro	neurologic, neurology
NG	nasogastric
NGT	nasogastric tube
NPO	nothing by mouth
N/S	normal saline
NSAID	nonsteroidal anti-inflammatory drug
N/V	nausea and/or vomiting
O₂	oxygen
OG	orogastric
O₂Hb	oxygenated hemoglobin
O₂ sat	oxygen saturation
OT	occupational therapy
OTC	over the counter
P	pulse
PA	pulmonary artery
PaO₂	partial arterial pressure, oxygen
PaCO₂	partial arterial pressure, carbon dioxide
Pap	Papanicolaou test
PCA	patient controlled analgesia
PCP	primary care provider

PCWP	pulmonary capillary wedge pressure	**RBC**	red blood cells	**TCDB**	turn, cough, deep breathe
PE	pulmonary embolism	**REEDA**	redness, edema, ecchymosis, drainage, approximated	TCO_2	total carbon dioxide
PERL	pupils equal and reactive to light	**ROM**	range of motion	**TENS**	transcutaneous electrical nerve stimulation
PERRLA	pupils equal, round, react to light, and accommodation	**RR**	respiratory rate	**THb**	total hemoglobin
		r.t.	related to	**tid**	three times daily
pg	picogram	**RTC**	round the clock	**TPN**	total parenteral nutrition
pH	measure of acidity			**TPR**	temperature, pulse, and respiration
PO, po	orally, by mouth	SaO_2	saturated oxygen		
PO_2	partial pressure of oxygen	**SCDs**	sequential compression devices	**TUR**	transurethral resection
PRBC	packed red blood cells	**SCU**	special care unit		
prn	when necessary	**sec**	seconds	**U**	units
PT	prothrombin time	**SGPT**	serum glutamic pyruvic transaminase	**UA**	urinalysis
PT	physical therapy	**SGOT**	serum glutamic oxalacetic transaminase	μg	microgram
PTT	partial thromboplastin			**URI**	upper respiratory infection
PVD	peripheral vascular disease	**SL**	sublingual	**UTI**	urinary tract infection
		SOB	shortness of breath		
q	every	**sp. gr.**	specific gravity	**VS**	vital signs
qd	every day	**SQ**	subcutaneous		
qh	every hour	**s/s**	signs and symptoms	**WBC**	white blood cells
qid	four times daily	**ST-T**	specific segement of ECG tracing	**WNL**	within normal limits
qod	every other day			**WNR**	within normal range
qs	as much as will suffice				
				x	times, frequency

APPENDIX B: NORMAL VALUES

This appendix is organized in the way that test results are commonly grouped by laboratories.

BLOOD
HEMATOLOGY

DIFFERENTIAL BLOOD COUNT
BLOOD COAGULATION

BLOOD GASES
URINALYSIS

URINE (output)
VITAL SIGNS

BLOOD

TEST	REFERENCE RANGE
Albumin	3.5-5.0 g/dL
BUN	9-20 mg/dL
Calcium	8.5-10.5 mg/dL
Chloride	95-109 mEq/L
Cholesterol	100-199 mg/dL
CO_2	24-32 mEq/L
CPK	20-230 IU/L
Creatinine clearance	F 81-134 mL/min
	M 88-146 mL/min
Creatinine	0.7-1.4 mg/dL
GGT	3-60 IU/L
Glucose	65-110 mg/dL
Iron	35-200 µg/dL
LDH	100-225 IU/L
Potassium	3.5-5.2 mEq/L
SGOT	7-40 IU/L
SGPT	0-45 IU/L
Sodium	135-145 mEq/L
Total Protein	6.0-8.0 g/dL
Triglycerides	10-190 mg/dL
Valproic acid	Therapeutic 50-100 µg/mL

HEMATOLOGY

TEST	REFERENCE RANGE
Hb	M 14-18 g/dL
	F 12-16 g/dL
Hct	M 42-52%
	F 37-47%
MCH	26-34 pg
MCHC	32-36%
MCV	80-99/u^3
Platelet count	150,000-400,000/mm^3
RBC	M 4.7-6.1 M/mm^3
	F 4.2-5.4 M/mm^3
WBC	4.5-11.1 K/mm^3

DIFFERENTIAL BLOOD COUNT

TEST	%	ABSOLUTE
Bands	0-11	< 10% of total differential
Baso	0-2	0-0.2
Eos	0-3	0-0.5
Left shift		RBC morph
Lymphs	21-45	1-4.8
Mono	2-9	0-0.8
Neutrophils	42-77	1.8-7.7
Reticulocytes	0.5-1.5%	
Sed rate west	M 0-15	
	F 0-20	

BLOOD COAGULATION

TEST	REFERENCE RANGE
Bleeding time	2.5-9.5 min
D-Dimer	< 0.5 mg/dL
Fibrinogen	200-400 mg/dL
PT	10.8-12.6 sec
PTT	24-34 sec

BLOOD GASES

TEST	REFERENCE RANGE
B.E.	-2 to 2
CO Hb	0.0-9.0% (tHb)
O_2 ct	15-23 (Vol %)
O_2 Hb	94-100%
$PaCO_2$	34-46 mmHg
pH	7.35-7.45
PO_2	75-100 mmHg
SaO_2	91.9-98.5%
T Hb	12.0-18.0 (G%)
TCO_2	23-27 mm/L

URINALYSIS

TEST	REFERENCE RANGE
Bacteria	0-2+
Bilirubin	negative
Blood	negative
Casts	cast per hpf
Clarity	clear
Color	amber
Crystals	present
Epithelial cells	few
Glucose	negative g/dL
Ketones	negative
Leukocyte esterase	negative
Mucus	few
pH	5-8 U
Protein	negative
RBC	0-2 # hpf
Sp. gr.	1.003-1.035 U
Urobilinogen	0-4 EU/24 h
WBC	0-4 # hpf

URINE

TEST	REFERENCE RANGE
Output	50-60 mL/h

VITAL SIGNS

TEST	REFERENCE RANGE	
Blood pressure		
diastolic	60-90	(older adults 70-90)
systolic	95-140	(older adults 140-160)
Pulse	60-100 bpm	
Respiration	12-20 breaths/minute	
Temperature		
core	36.5-37.6°C (97.7-99.7°F)	
oral	0.5°C (0.9°F) lower than rectal	
rectal	0.1°C (0.2-1.2°F) higher than oral	

SOURCE: Oregon Medical Laboratories, Eugene, Oregon.

APPENDIX C: DEFINITIONS, CARE PLAN TOPICS

GENERAL

Casting: The application of hard structures such as plaster (gypsum); used to immobilize musculoskeletal tissues following injury or surgery.

Confusion: A disturbed state of consciousness characterized by disorientation, hallucinations, agitation, and/or impaired perception, reasoning, and memory.

Death and Dying: Dying is the process of life coming to an end. Death is the state of permanent cessation of all vital functions. A grieving process for patient and family usually accompanies death and dying.

Education for Discharge: Training the patient/family to care for patient after discharge; various situations are addressed in the subsections of this care plan.

Geriatric Patient, Hospitalized: An older individual whose hospitalization is complicated by the biologic, psychological, and sociological changes of aging.

Immobility: The inability to move independently because of bed rest or reduced function; immobility can lead to further medical complications.

Pain Management: Interventions for an individual who experiences and reports/demonstrates the presence of severe discomfort or an uncomfortable sensation.

Parenteral Nutrition: The intravenous administration of carbohydrates, proteins, fats, vitamins, minerals, and trace elements.

Postoperative Care: General nursing care for the adult following surgical intervention.

Pressure Ulcers: Local areas of infarcted soft tissue that occur when the pressure applied to the skin over time is greater than the capillary pressure.

Traction: The application of force to the skin, muscles, and bones to aid in reduction of fractures, hold reduced bones in alignment for healing, relieve muscle spasms and pain, and relieve pressure on peripheral spinal nerves.

Urinary Elimination, Altered: The state in which the individual experiences a disturbance in urine elimination.

MEDICAL

Adult Respiratory Distress Syndrome: Respiratory failure characterized by increased capillary permeability that produces lungs that are wet, heavy, stiff, hemorrhagic, and unable to diffuse oxygen.

Alcoholism, Acute Phase: Alcohol withdrawal delirium that follows sudden cessation of prolonged alcohol intake, producing tremors, nervousness, delirium tremens, and increased mortality.

Alzheimer's Disease: A chronic neurologic disorder characterized by progressive degeneration of neurons in the cerebral cortex and portions of the subcortical structures.

Anemia, Pernicious: A progressive anemia caused by a lack of the intrinsic factor needed to absorb Vitamin B_{12}.

Anemia, Sickle Cell, Acute Crisis: A severe, incurable anemia that occurs in people who are homozygous for hemoglobin S; hypoxia and elevated blood viscosity contribute to the crisis of more sickling and infarctions.

Arthritis: Inflammation of one or more joints of the body.

Asthma: A respiratory condition characterized by bronchospasm, bronchoconstriction, wheezing, and recurrent attacks of dyspnea.

Cancer, Advanced: Growth of abnormal cells has produced extensive destruction of healthy tissues.

Cerebrovascular Accident: The cerebral vessels are occluded by an embolus or cerebrovascular hemorrhage, resulting in ischemia of the related area.

Chemical Dependency: Intermittent or chronic use of stimulants or depressants resulting in alterations in mental and physiological function.

Cholecystitis, Cholelithiasis: Acute or chronic inflammation of the gallbladder with gall stones.

Chronic Obstructive Pulmonary Disease: A group of diseases that includes bronchitis, emphysema, and bronchiectasis.

Cirrhosis of the Liver: A chronic degenerative disease of the liver in which diffuse destruction of hepatic parenchymal cells has occurred, ultimately leading to liver failure.

Colitis, Ulcerative: A chronic mucosal inflammatory disease limited to the colon and rectum.

Congestive Heart Failure: A state in which the cardiac output is inadequate to meet the body's metabolic needs.

Deep Venous Thrombosis: An abnormal vascular condition in which a thrombus develops within a deep vein.

Diabetes Mellitus: A chronic disorder characterized by disturbances in carbohydrate, protein, and fat metabolism as a result of insufficient insulin.

Disseminated Intravascular Coagulation: This syndrome is a bleeding disorder resulting from an increased tendency of the blood to clot.

Gastrointestinal Bleeding: Hemorrhage of the gastrointestinal tract, often secondary to gastritis and peptic ulcer disease, producing blood in vomitus and stools.

HIV/AIDS: Acquired Immune Deficiency Syndrome includes the final stages of a wide range of health problems caused by the human immunodeficiency virus (HIV).

Intestinal Inflammation: Inflammation of the mucous membranes of the gastrointestinal tract.

Intestinal Obstruction: A mechanical or functional obstruction occurring when the contents of the intestines fail to propel forward through the bowel.

Leukemia, Acute Phase: Characterized by uncontrolled proliferation of leukocyte precursors in blood, bone marrow, and reticuloendothelial tissues.

Meningitis, Bacterial or Viral: Involves inflammation of the meninges.

Multiple Myeloma: A malignant condition in which a clone of transformed plasma cells proliferates in bone marrow, resulting in bone marrow disruption.

Multiple Sclerosis: A progressive, degenerative disease that affects the myelin sheath and conducting pathway of the central nervous system.

Myocardial Infarction: A life-threatening condition characterized by the permanent formation of necrosis in the myocardium from a lack of oxygen.

Pancreatitis: Acute or chronic inflammation of the pancreas.

Parkinson's Disease: A movement disorder involving the basal ganglia and substantia nigra, characterized by resting tremors, rigidity, and bradykinesia.

Pneumonia: An inflammatory process of the lungs classified by area involved and/or causative agent.

Pneumothorax: An accumulation of air or fluid in the pleural cavity resulting in lung collapse.

Pulmonary Embolism: Result of a thrombus breaking loose from an attachment and blocking a branch of the pulmonary artery.

Renal Calculi: Kidney stones; urolithiasis, a deposition of crystalline substances excreted in the urine.

Renal Failure, Acute: A sudden, severe impairment of renal function, causing an acute uremic episode.

Renal Failure, Chronic: A slow, insidious, irreversible impairment of renal function in which uremia usually develops slowly.

Rib Fractures: Ribs broken usually from direct, blunt chest trauma (uncomplicated, does not include hemo- or pneumothorax).

Seizure Disorders: Sudden and violent involuntary motor movements of a group of skeletal muscles; generally are transitory and often involve disturbances in LOC and motor-sensory and/or autonomic functions.

Shock: A pathologic condition characterized by abnormal cellular metabolism as a result of inadequate oxygen delivery to body tissues or inadequate usage of oxygen by the body.

Subarachnoid Hemorrhage: Bleeding occurring in the subarachnoid space as a result of trauma, hypertension, aneurysm leakage, or a congenital arteriovenous malformation of the brain.

Tuberculosis: A chronic, acute, or subacute infectious disease caused by the tubercle bacillus, *Mycobacterium tuberculosis,* most commonly affecting the alveolar structures of the lung.

Venous Insufficiency (Leg Ulcers): A disease state resulting from the reflux or obstruction of superficial or deep venous valves in the legs.

Wound Infection: Skin trauma characterized by an infected, draining ulcer and related tissue destruction.

SURGICAL

Adrenalectomy: Unilateral or bilateral removal of the adrenal gland.

Amputation: Removal of a body part, unintentionally, as in an accident, or intentionally, as by surgery.

Appendectomy: Surgical removal of the vermiform appendix.

Arthroplasty, Total Joint Replacement: The reconstruction or repair of one or both sides, parts, or specific tissues within a joint, such as a hip or knee.

Burns and Grafts: Burns are physical insults to epithelial tissues from injuries inflicted on the skin. Grafts involve the surgical placement of skin to re-establish skin integrity in wounds that cannot heal via processes of epithelialization and contraction.

Cardiac Surgery: Surgical procedure to provide palliative or restorative function of the heart and/or cardiovascular system.

Cholecystectomy: Surgical removal of the gallbladder.

Cholelithiasis, Lithotripsy: Gallstones removed by a machine that emits shock waves to crush them.

Colon Resection: Surgical reconstruction of the colon to remove a diseased portion; may include colostomy formation; may require one or more stages.

Facial Fractures: Traumatic injury to the facial bones, most commonly involving nasal fractures; injury typically resulting from a sporting accident or an assault.

Femoropopliteal Bypass: Surgical bypass of an obstructed segment of the femoropopliteal artery, using prosthetic materials or an autogenous artery or vein.

Femur Fracture: A break of the femur, usually the lower two thirds, resulting from trauma.

Gastric Resection, Gastrostomy: Partial or total removal of the stomach with anastomosis of the remaining segment to the duodenum or jejunum with or without the creation of an opening into the stomach for feeding.

Hiatal Hernia Repair: Surgical correction of a displaced lower esophagus and possibly stomach above the diaphragm.

Hip Pin: Surgical implantation of metallic devices to immobilize or repair a traumatized hip fracture.

Hysterectomy: Surgical removal of the uterus through an abdominal incision or through the vagina.

Laparotomy: A surgical incision into the abdominal wall.

Laryngectomy (Total or Partial): Total or partial surgical removal of the larynx, usually due to cancer.

Mammoplasty: Plastic surgery of the breast.

Mastectomy: Surgical removal of a breast.

Nasal Surgery: Surgery to relieve nasal obstruction or trauma by removal of cartilage and bone; reconstruction of the nasal septum or external nose; or removal of polyps from the nose.

Neck Surgery, Radical: Surgical removal of the submandibular salivary gland, sternocleidomastoid muscle, internal jugular vein, and spinal accessory nerve.

Nephrectomy: Surgical removal of a kidney.

Pelvic Fracture: A traumatic break to the pelvic bone typically resulting from a motor vehicle accident or fall.

Portal Shunt: A surgical bypass shunting procedure in which a portion of the portal vein blood flow is diverted from the liver. This procedure is used for portal hypertension and esophageal varices.

Prostatectomy, TUR: Surgical rem the prostate gland performed by ins a resectoscope through the urethra

Rectal Surgery: Surgical excisi fistula tracts, partial division of or removal of hemorrhoidal ma

Retinal Detachment: Surgical repair to a retinal hole or tear; procedure places the retina in contact with underlying structures; accompanying vitreous bleeding is corrected by surgical removal of the vitreous.

Shoulder Separation: A traumatic injury to the shoulder, such as an injury resulting from a fall on an outstretched arm.

Splenectomy: Surgical removal of the spleen, for example, as a result of trauma or hypersplenism.

Thoracotomy: A surgical incision into the chest wall.

Thyroidectomy: Surgical removal of all or part of the thyroid gland.

Ureteral Lithotripsy: Kidney stones removed by a machine that emits shock waves to crush them.

Ureterolithotomy: Surgical removal of a stone from a ureter.

Vaginal Plastic Surgery: Vaginal reconstructive surgery, such as following removal of the vagina.

Vein Ligation and Stripping: Stripping of the saphenous veins through small incisions at the groin, knee, and ankle.

APPENDIX D: NANDA NURSING DIAGNOSES

This list represents the NANDA nursing diagnoses approved for clinical use and testing (1992).[1]

Pattern 1: Exchanging

1.1.2.1.*	Altered +**Nutrition**: More than body requirements
1.1.2.2.	Altered **Nutrition**: Less than body requirements
1.1.2.3.	Altered **Nutrition**: Potential for more than body requirements
1.2.1.1.	High Risk for **Infection**
1.2.2.1.	High Risk for Altered **Body Temperature**
1.2.2.2.	Hypothermia
1.2.2.3.	Hyperthermia
1.2.2.4.	Ineffective **Thermoregulation**
1.2.3.1.	**Dysreflexia**
1.3.1.1.	**Constipation**
1.3.1.1.1.	Perceived **Constipation**
1.3.1.1.2.	Colonic **Constipation**
1.3.1.2.	**Diarrhea**
1.3.1.3.	**Bowel** Incontinence
1.3.2.	Altered **Urinary** Elimination
1.3.2.1.1.	Stress Incontinence **(Urinary)**
1.3.2.1.2.	Reflex Incontinence **(Urinary)**
1.3.2.1.3.	Urge Incontinence **(Urinary)**
1.3.2.1.4.	Functional Incontinence **(Urinary)**
1.3.2.1.5.	Total Incontinence **(Urinary)**
1.3.2.2.	**Urinary** Retention
1.4.1.1.	Altered **Tissue Perfusion** (Specify Type) (Renal, cerebral, cardiopulmonary, gastrointestinal, peripheral)
1.4.1.2.1.	**Fluid** Volume Excess
1.4.1.2.2.1.	**Fluid** Volume Deficit
1.4.1.2.2.2.	High Risk for **Fluid** Volume Deficit
1.4.2.1.	Decreased **Cardiac** Output
1.5.1.1.	Impaired **Gas** Exchange
1.5.1.2.	Ineffective **Airway** Clearance
1.5.1.3.1.	Inability to Sustain Spontaneous **Ventilation**
1.5.1.3.2.	Dysfunctional **Ventilatory** Weaning Response (DVWR)
1.6.1.	High Risk for **Injury**
1.6.1.1.	High Risk for **Suffocation**
1.6.1.2.	High Risk for **Poisoning**
1.6.1.3.	High Risk for **Trauma**
1.6.1.4.	High Risk for **Aspiration**
1.6.1.5	High Risk for **Disuse Syndrome**
1.6.2.	Altered **Protection**
1.6.2.1.	Impaired **Tissue Integrity**
1.6.2.1.1.	Altered **Oral** Mucous Membrane
1.6.2.1.2.1.	Impaired **Skin** Integrity
1.6.2.1.2.2.	High Risk for Impaired **Skin** Integrity

Pattern 2: Communicating

2.1.1.1.	Impaired Verbal **Communication**

Pattern 3: Relating

3.1.1.	Impaired **Social Interaction**
3.1.2.	**Social Isolation**
3.2.1.	Altered **Role** Performance
3.2.1.1.1.	Altered **Parenting**
3.2.1.1.2.	High Risk for Altered **Parenting**
3.2.1.2.1.	**Sexual** Dysfunction
3.2.2.	Altered **Family** Processes
3.2.2.1.	**Caregiver** Role Strain
3.2.2.2.	High Risk for **Caregiver** Role Strain
3.2.3.1.	**Parental** Role Conflict
3.3.	Altered **Sexuality** Patterns

Pattern 4: Valuing

4.1.1.	**Spiritual Distress** (Distress of the Human Spirit)

Pattern 5: Choosing

5.1.1.1.	Ineffective Individual **Coping**
5.1.1.1.1.	Impaired **Adjustment**
5.1.1.1.2.	Defensive **Coping**
5.1.1.1.3.	Ineffective **Denial**
5.1.2.1.1.	Ineffective Family **Coping**: Disabling
5.1.2.1.2.	Ineffective Family **Coping**: Compromised
5.1.2.2.	Family **Coping**: Potential for Growth
5.2.1.	Ineffective Management of **Therapeutic** Regimen (Individuals)
5.2.1.1.	**Noncompliance** (Specify)
5.3.1.1	**Decisional** Conflict (Specify)
5.4.	**Health** Seeking Behaviors (Specify)

Pattern 6: Moving

6.1.1.1.	Impaired Physical **Mobility**
6.1.1.1.1.	High Risk for **Peripheral Neurovascular** Dysfunction
6.1.1.2.	**Activity** Intolerance
6.1.1.2.1.	**Fatigue**
6.1.1.3.	High Risk for **Activity** Intolerance
6.2.1.	**Sleep** Pattern Disturbance
6.3.1.1.	**Diversional** Activity Deficit
6.4.1.1.	Impaired **Home Maintenance** Management
6.4.2.	Altered **Health Maintenance**
6.5.1.	Feeding **Self-Care Deficit**
6.5.1.1.	Impaired **Swallowing**
6.5.1.2.	Ineffective **Breastfeeding**
6.5.1.2.1.	Interrupted **Breastfeeding**
6.5.1.3.	Effective **Breastfeeding**
6.5.1.4.	Ineffective **Infant** Feeding Pattern
6.5.2.	Bathing/Hygiene **Self-Care Deficit**
6.5.3.	Dressing/Grooming **Self-Care Deficit**
6.5.4.	Toileting **Self-Care Deficit**
6.6.	Altered **Growth** and Development
6.7.	**Relocation** Stress Syndrome

Pattern 7: Perceiving

7.1.1.	**Body Image** Disturbance
7.1.2.	**Self-Esteem** Disturbance
7.1.2.1.	Chronic Low **Self-Esteem**
7.1.2.2.	Situational Low **Self-Esteem**
7.1.3.	**Personal** Identity Disturbance
7.2.	**Sensory/Perceptual** Alterations (Specify) (Visual, auditory, kinesthetic, gustatory, tactile, olfactory)
7.2.1.1.	**Unilateral** Neglect
7.3.1.	**Hopelessness**
7.3.2.	**Powerlessness**

Pattern 8: Knowing

8.1.1.	**Knowledge** Deficit (Specify)
8.3.	Altered **Thought** Processes
9.1.1.	**Pain**
9.1.1.1.	Chronic **Pain**
9.2.1.1.	Dysfunctional **Grieving**
9.2.1.2	Anticipatory Grieving
9.2.2.	High Risk for **Violence**: Self-directed or directed at others
9.2.2.1.	High Risk for **Self-Mutilation**
9.2.3.	**Post-Trauma** Response
9.2.3.1.	**Rape-Trauma** Syndrome
9.2.3.1.1.	**Rape-Trauma Syndrome**: Compound Reaction
9.2.3.1.2.	**Rape-Trauma Syndrome**: Silent Reaction
9.3.1.	**Anxiety**
9.3.2.	**Fear**

* Numbers refer to location in *NAND Nursing Diagnoses: Definitions and Classifications 1992-1993.*

+ Bold type indicates alphabetical in Appendix E.

NANDA DX

APPENDIX E: DEFINITIONS, NURSING DIAGNOSES

This appendix includes only the definitions and defining characteristics of those nursing diagnoses that are used in this book.

Abridged from NANDA Nursing Diagnoses: Definitions and Classification, 1992

ACTIVITY INTOLERANCE A state in which an individual has insufficient physiological or psychological energy to endure or complete required or desired daily activities. **Defining Characteristics:** Verbal report of fatigue or weakness; abnormal heart rate or blood pressure response to activity; exertional discomfort or dyspnea; electrocardiographic changes reflecting arrhythmias or ischemia.

ACTIVITY INTOLERANCE, HIGH RISK FOR A state in which an individual is at risk of experiencing insufficient physiological or psychological energy to endure or complete required or desired daily activities. **Defining Characteristics:** *Presence of risk factors such as:* History of previous intolerance; deconditioned status; presence of circulatory/respiratory problems; inexperience with the activity.

AIRWAY CLEARANCE, INEFFECTIVE A state in which an individual is unable to clear secretions or obstructions from the respiratory tract to maintain airway patency. **Defining Characteristics:** Abnormal breath sounds (rales [crackles], rhonchi [wheezes]); changes in rate or depth of respiration; tachypnea; cough, effective/ineffective, with or without sputum, cyanosis; dyspnea.

ANXIETY A vague uneasy feeling whose source is often nonspecific or unknown to the individual. **Defining Characteristics:** *Subjective:* Increased tension; apprehension; painful and persistent increased helplessness; uncertainty; fearful; scared; regretful; overexcited; rattled; distressed; jittery; feelings of inadequacy; shakiness; fear of unspecific consequences; expressed concerns regarding change in life events; worried; anxious. *Objective:* Sympathetic stimulation-cardiovascular excitation, superficial vasoconstriction, pupil dilation; restlessness; insomnia; glancing about; poor eye contact; trembling/hand tremors; extraneous movement (foot shuffling, hand/arm movements); facial tension; voice quivering; focus "self"; increased wariness; increased perspiration.

ASPIRATION: HIGH RISK FOR The state in which an individual is at risk for entry of gastrointestinal secretions, oropharyngeal secretions, and solids or fluids into tracheobronchial passages.

Defining Characteristics: *Presence of risk factors such as:* Reduced level of consciousness; depressed cough and gag reflexes; presence of tracheostomy or endotracheal tube; incomplete lower esophageal sphincter; gastrointestinal tubes; tube feedings; medication administration; situations hindering elevation of upper body; increased intragastric pressure; increased gastric residual; decreased gastrointestinal motility; delayed gastric emptying; impaired swallowing; facial/oral/neck surgery or trauma; wired jaws.

BODY IMAGE DISTURBANCE Disruption in the way one perceives one's body image. **Defining Characteristics:** A or B must be present to justify the diagnosis of Body Image Disturbance. **A** = verbal response to actual or perceived change in structure and/or function. **B** = nonverbal response to actual or perceived change in structure and/or function. The following clinical manifestations may be used to validate the presence of A or B. *Objective:* Missing body part; actual change in structure and/or function; not looking at body part; not touching body part; hiding or overexposing body part (intentional or unintentional); trauma to nonfunctioning part; change in social involvement; change in ability to estimate spatial relationship of body to environment. *Subjective:* Verbalization of: change in lifestyle; fear of rejection or of reaction by others; focus on past strength, function, or appearance; negative feelings about body; feelings of helplessness, hopelessness, or powerlessness; preoccupations with change or loss; emphasis on remaining strengths, heightened achievement; extension of body boundary to incorporate environmental objects; personalization of part or loss by name; depersonalization of part or loss by impersonal pronouns; refusal to verify actual change.

BODY TEMPERATURE, ALTERED: HIGH RISK FOR The state in which the individual is at risk for failure to maintain body temperature within normal range. **Defining Characteristics:** *Presence of risk factors such as:* Extremes of age; extremes of weight; exposure to cold/cool or warm/hot environments; dehydration; inactivity or vigorous activity; medications causing vasoconstriction/vasodilation; altered metabolic rate; sedation; inappropriate clothing for environmental

temperature; illness or trauma affecting temperature regulation.

BOWEL INCONTINENCE A state in which an individual experiences a change in normal bowel habits characterized by involuntary passage of stool. **Defining Characteristics:** Involuntary passage of stool.

BREATHING PATTERN, INEFFECTIVE The state in which an individual's inhalation and/or exhalation pattern does not enable adequate pulmonary inflation or emptying. **Defining Characteristics:** Dyspnea, shortness of breath, tachypnea, fremitus, abnormal arterial blood gas, cyanosis, cough, nasal flaring, respiratory depth changes, assumption of 3-point position, pursed-lip breathing/prolonged expiratory phase, increased anteroposterior diameter, use of accessory muscles, altered chest excursion.

CARDIAC OUTPUT, DECREASED A state in which the blood pumped by an individual's heart is sufficiently reduced that it is inadequate to meet the needs of the body's tissues. **Defining Characteristics:** Variations in blood pressure readings, arrhythmias; fatigue; jugular vein distention; color changes, skin and mucous membranes; oliguria; decreased peripheral pulses; cold clammy skin; rales; dyspnea, orthopnea; restlessness. **Other Possible Characteristics:** Change in mental status; shortness of breath; syncope; vertigo; edema; cough; frothy sputum; gallop rhythm; weakness.

COMMUNICATION, IMPAIRED, VERBAL The state in which an individual experiences a decreased or absent ability to use or understand language in human interaction. **Defining Characteristics:** Unable to speak dominant language; speaks or verbalizes with difficulty; does not or cannot speak; stuttering; slurring; difficulty forming words or sentences; difficulty expressing thought verbally; inappropriate verbalization; dyspnea; disorientation.

CONSTIPATION A state in which an individual experiences a change in normal bowel habits characterized by a decrease in frequency and/or passage of hard, dry stools. **Defining Characteristics:** Decreased activity level; frequency less than usual pattern; hard, formed stools; palpable mass; reported feeling of pressure or fullness in rectum; straining at stool. **Other Possible Characteristics:** Abdominal pain; appetite impairment; back pain; headache; interference with daily living; use of laxatives.

CONSTIPATION, COLONIC The state in which an individual's pattern of elimination is characterized by hard, dry stool which results from a delay in passage of food residue. **Defining Characteristics:** *Major:* Decreased frequency; hard, dry stool; straining at stool; painful defecation; abdominal distention; palpable mass. *Minor:* Rectal pressure; headache; appetite impairment; abdominal pain.

COPING, FAMILY: POTENTIAL FOR GROWTH Effective management of adaptive tasks by family member involved with the client's health challenge, family member exhibits desire and readiness for enhanced health and growth in regard to self and in relation to the client. **Defining Characteristics:** Family member attempts to describe growth impact of crisis on his or her own values, priorities, goals, or relationships; family member is moving in direction of lifestyle which supports and monitors health and the maturational processes; audits and negotiates treatment programs; generally chooses experiences which optimize wellness; individual expresses interest in making contact on a one-to-one basis or on a mutual-aid group basis with another person who has experienced a similar situation.

COPING, INEFFECTIVE, FAMILY: COMPROMISED A usually supportive primary person (family member or close friend) provides insufficient, ineffective, or compromised support, comfort, assistance, or encouragement which may be needed by the client to manage or master adaptive tasks related to his or her health challenge. **Defining Characteristics:** *Subjective:* Client expresses or confirms a concern or complaint about significant other's response to his or her health problem; significant person describes preoccupation with personal reaction (fear, anticipatory grief, guilt, anxiety) to client's illness, disability, or other situational or developmental crises; significant person describes or confirms an inadequate understanding or knowledge base which interferes with effective assistance or supportive behaviors. *Objective:* Significant person attempts assistive or supportive behaviors with less than

satisfactory results; significant person withdraws or enters into limited or temporary personal communication with the client at the time of need; significant person displays protective behavior disproportionate (too little or too much) to the client's abilities or need for autonomy.

COPING, INEFFECTIVE, FAMILY: DISABLING Behavior of significant person (family member or other primary person) that disables his or her own capacities and the client's capacities to effectively address tasks essential to either person's adaptation to the health challenge. **Defining Characteristics:** Neglectful care of the client in regard to basic human needs and/or illness treatment; distortion of reality regarding the client's health problem, including extreme denial about its existence or severity; intolerance; rejection; abandonment; desertion; carrying on usual routines while disregarding client's needs; psychosomaticism; takes on illness signs of client; decisions and actions by family that are detrimental to economic or social well-being; agitation; depression; aggression, hostility; impaired restructuring of a meaningful life for self; impaired individualization; prolonged overconcern for client; neglectful relationships with other family members; client's development of helpless, inactive dependence.

COPING, INEFFECTIVE (INDIVIDUAL) Impairment of adaptive behaviors and problem-solving abilities of a person in meeting life's demands and roles. **Defining Characteristics:** Verbalization of inability to cope or inability to ask for help; inability to meet role expectations; inability to meet basic needs; inability to problem-solve; alteration in societal participation; destructive behavior toward self or others; inappropriate use of defense mechanisms; change in usual communication patterns; verbal manipulation; high illness rate; high rate of accidents.

DIARRHEA A state in which an individual experiences a change in normal bowel habits characterized by the frequent passage of loose, fluid, unformed stools. **Defining Characteristics:** Abdominal pain; cramping; increased frequency; increased frequency of bowel sounds; loose, liquid stools; urgency. **Other Possible Characteristics:** Change in color.

DISUSE SYNDROME: HIGH RISK FOR A state in which an individual is at risk for deterioration of body systems as

the result of prescribed or unavoidable musculoskeletal inactivity. **Defining Characteristics:** *Presence of risk factors such as:* Paralysis; mechanical immobilization; prescribed immobilization; severe pain; altered level of consciousness.

FAMILY PROCESSES, ALTERED The state in which a family that normally functions effectively experiences a dysfunction. **Defining Characteristics:** Family system unable to meet physical needs of its members; family system unable to meet emotional, security, or spiritual needs of its members; parents do not demonstrate respect for each other's views on childrearing practices; inability to express/accept wide range of feelings; inability to express/accept feelings of members; inability of the family members to relate to each other for mutual growth and maturation; uninvolved in community activities; unable to accept/receive help appropriately; rigidity in function and roles; a family not demonstrating respect for individuality and autonomy of its members; family unable to adapt to change/deal with traumatic experience constructively; family failing to accomplish current/past developmental task; unhealthy family decision-making process; failure to send and receive clear messages; inappropriate boundary maintenance; inappropriate/poorly communicated family rules, rituals, symbols; unexamined family myths; inappropriate level and direction of energy.

FATIGUE An overwhelming sustained sense of exhaustion and decreased capacity for physical and mental work. **Defining Characteristics:** *Major:* Verbalization of an unremitting and/or overwhelming lack of energy; inability to maintain usual routines. *Minor:* Perceived need for additional energy to accomplish routine tasks; increase in physical complaints; emotionally labile or irritable; impaired ability to concentrate; decreased performance; lethargic or listless; disinterest in surroundings/introspection; decreased libido; accident prone.

FEAR Feeling of dread related to an identifiable source which the person validates. **Defining Characteristics:** Ability to identify object of fear.

FLUID VOLUME DEFICIT The st[...] which an individual experiences vas[...] cellular, or intracellular dehydratio[...] **Defining Characteristics:** Char[...] urine output; change in urine concentration; sudden weight los[...] decreased venous filling;

hemoconcentration; change in serum sodium. **Other Possible Characteristics:** Hypotension; thirst; increased pulse rate; decreased skin turgor; decreased pulse volume/pressure; change in mental state; increased body temperature; dry skin; dry mucous membranes; weakness.

FLUID VOLUME DEFICIT: HIGH RISK FOR The state in which an individual is at risk of experiencing vascular, cellular, or intracellular dehydration. **Defining Characteristics:** *Presence of risk factors such as:* Extremes of age; extremes of weight; excessive losses through normal routes, e.g., diarrhea; loss of fluid through abnormal routes, e.g., indwelling tubes; deviations affecting access to or intake or absorption of fluids, e.g., physical immobility; factors influencing fluid needs, e.g., hypermetabolic state; knowledge deficiency related to fluid volume; medications, e.g., diuretics.

FLUID VOLUME EXCESS The state in which an individual experiences increased fluid retention and edema. **Defining Characteristics:** Edema; effusion; anasarca; weight gain; shortness of breath, orthopnea; intake greater than output; S/3 heart sound; pulmonary congestion (chest x-ray); abnormal breath sounds, rales (crackles); change in respiratory pattern; change in mental status; decreased hemoglobin and hematocrit; blood pressure changes; central venous pressure changes; pulmonary artery pressure changes; jugular vein distention; positive hepatojugular reflex; oliguria; specific gravity changes, azotemia, altered electrolytes; restlessness and anxiety.

GAS EXCHANGE, IMPAIRED The state in which the individual experiences a decreased passage of oxygen and/or carbon dioxide between the alveoli of the lungs and the vascular system. **Defining Characteristics:** Confusion; somnolence; restlessness; irritability; inability to move secretions; hypercapnea; hypoxia.

GRIEVING, ANTICIPATORY Potential loss of significant object*; expression of distress at potential loss; denial of potential loss; guilt; anger; sorrow; choked feelings; changes in eating habits; alterations in sleep patterns; alterations in activity level; altered libido; altered communication patterns.

GRIEVING, DYSFUNCTIONAL Verbal expression of distress at loss*; denial of loss; expression of guilt; expression of

unresolved issues; anger; sadness; crying; difficulty in expressing loss; alteration in eating habits, sleep or dream patterns, activity level, libido; idealization of lost object; reliving of past experiences; interference with life functioning; developmental regression; labile affect; alterations in concentration and/or pursuits of tasks.

* Object loss is used in the broadest sense; objects may include people, possessions, a job, status, home, ideals, parts and processes of the body.

HEALTH MAINTENANCE, ALTERED Inability to identify, manage and/or seek out help to maintain health. **Defining Characteristics:** Demonstrated lack of knowledge regarding basic health practices; demonstrated lack of adaptive behaviors to internal/external environmental changes; reported or observed inability to take responsibility for meeting basic health practices in any or all functional pattern areas; history of lack of health-seeking behavior; expressed interest in improving health behaviors; reported or observed lack of equipment; financial and/or other resources; reported or observed impairment of personal support systems.

HOME MAINTENANCE MANAGEMENT, IMPAIRED Inability to independently maintain a safe, growth-promoting immediate environment. **Defining Characteristics:** *Subjective:* Household members express difficulty in maintaining their home in a comfortable fashion; household request assistance with home maintenance; household members describe outstanding debts or financial crises. Objective: Disorderly surroundings; unwashed or unavailable cooking equipment, clothes, or linen; accumulation of dirt, food wastes, or hygienic wastes; offensive odors; inappropriate household temperature; overtaxed, exhausted, or anxious family members; lack of necessary equipment or aids; presence of vermin or rodents; repeated hygienic disorders, infestations, or infections.

HYPERTHERMIA A state in which an individual's body temperature is elevated above his/her normal range. **Defining Characteristics:** *Major:* Increase in body temperature above normal range. *Minor:* Flushed skin, warm to touch; increased respiratory rate; tachycardia; seizures/convulsions.

HYPOTHERMIA The state in which an individual's body temperature is reduced

below normal range. **Defining Characteristics**: *Major:* Reduction in body temperature below normal range; shivering (mild); cool skin; pallor (moderate). *Minor:* Show capillary refill; tachycardia; cyanotic nail beds; hypertension; piloerection.

INFECTION: HIGH RISK FOR The state in which an individual is at increased risk for being invaded by pathogenic organisms. **Defining Characteristics:** *Presence of risk factors such as:* Inadequate primary defenses (broken skin, traumatized tissue, decrease in ciliary action, stasis of body fluids, change in pH secretions, altered peristalsis); inadequate secondary defenses (e.g., decreased hemoglobin, leukopenia, suppressed inflammatory response) and immunosuppression; inadequate acquired immunity; tissue destruction and increased environmental exposure; chronic disease; invasive procedures; malnutrition; pharmaceutical agents; trauma; rupture of amniotic membranes; insufficient knowledge to avoid exposure to pathogens.

INJURY: HIGH RISK FOR A state in which the individual is at risk of injury as a result of environmental conditions interacting with the individual's adaptive and defensive resources. **Defining Characteristics:** *Presence of risk factors such as: Internal:* Biochemical, regulatory function (sensory dysfunction, integrative dysfunction, effector dysfunction, tissue hypoxia); malnutrition; autoimmune; abnormal blood profile (leukocytosis/ leukopenia, altered clotting factors, thrombocytopenia, sickle cell, thalassemia, decreased hemoglobin); physical (broken skin, altered mobility); developmental age (physiological, psychosocial); psychological (affective, orientation). *External:* Biological (immunization level of community, microorganism); chemical (pollutants, poisons, drugs, pharmaceutical agents, alcohol, caffeine, nicotine, preservatives, cosmetics, and dyes); nutrients (vitamins, food types); physical (design, structure, and arrangement of community, building, and/or equipment); mode of transport/transportation; people/provider (nosocomial agents, staffing patterns; cognitive, affective, and psychomotor factors).

KNOWLEDGE DEFICIT (SPECIFY) Defining Characteristics: Verbalization of problem; inaccurate follow-through of instruction; inaccurate performance of test; inappropriate or exaggerated behaviors, e.g., hysterical, hostile, agitated, apathetic.

MOBILITY, IMPAIRED PHYSICAL A state in which the individual experiences a limitation of ability for independent physical movement. **Defining Characteristics:** Inability to purposefully move within the physical environment, including bed mobility, transfer, and ambulation; reluctance to attempt movement; limited range of motion; decreased muscle strength, control, and/or mass; imposed restrictions of movement, including mechanical, medical protocol; impaired coordination.

+*SUGGESTED FUNCTIONAL LEVEL CLASSIFICATION*
0 = completely independent
1 = requires use of equipment or device
2 = requires help from another person, for assistance, supervision, or teaching
3 = requires help from another person and equipment device
4 = dependent, does not participate in activity.
+Code adapted from E. Jones, et al. *Patient Classification for Long-Term Care: Users' Manual*, HEW, Publication No. HRA-74-3107, November 1974.

NUTRITION, ALTERED: LESS THAN BODY REQUIREMENTS The state in which an individual experiences an intake of nutrients insufficient to meet metabolic needs. **Defining Characteristics:** Loss of weight with or without adequate food intake; reported inadequate food intake less than RDA (recommended daily allowance); weakness of muscles required for swallowing or mastication; body weight 20% or more under ideal; reported or evident of lack of food; aversion to eating; lack of interest in food; reported altered taste sensation; satiety immediately after ingesting food; abdominal pain with or without pathology; sore, inflamed buccal cavity; capillary fragility; abdominal cramping; diarrhea and/or steatorrhea; hyperactive bowel sounds; perceived inability to ingest food; pale conjunctival and mucous membranes; poor muscle tone; excessive loss of hair; lack of information, misinformation; misconceptions.

NUTRITION, ALTERED: MORE THAN BODY REQUIREMENTS: The state in which an individual is experiencing an intake of nutrients which exceeds metabolic needs. **Defining Characteristics:** Weight 10% over ideal for height and frame; weight 20%* over ideal for height and frame; triceps skin fold greater than 15 mm in men, 25 mm in women; sedentary activity level. Reported or observed dysfunctional eating pattern: pairing food with other activities;

concentrating food intake at the end of day; eating in response to external cues such as time of day, social situation; eating in response to internal cues other than hunger, e.g., anxiety.

*Critical

ORAL MUCOUS MEMBRANE, ALTERED The state in which an individual experiences disruptions in the tissue layers of the oral cavity. **Defining Characteristics:** Oral pain/discomfort; coated tongue; xerostomia (dry mouth); stomatitis; oral lesions or ulcers; lack of or decreased salivation; leukoplakia; edema; hyperemia; oral plaque; desquamation; vesicles; hemorrhagic gingivitis, carious teeth; halitosis.

PAIN [Acute] A state in which an individual experiences and reports the presence of severe discomfort or an uncomfortable sensation. **Defining Characteristics:** *Subjective:* Describes or communicates (verbal or coded) pain. *Objective:* Guarding behavior, protective; self-focusing; narrowed focus (altered time perception, withdrawal from social contact, impaired thought process); distraction behavior (moaning, crying, pacing, seeking out other people and/or activities, restlessness); facial mask of pain (eyes lack luster, "beaten look", fixed or scattered movement, grimace); alteration in muscle tone (may span from listless to rigid); autonomic responses not seen in chronic stable pain (diaphoresis, blood pressure, and pulse change, pupillary dilation, increased or decreased respiratory rate).

PAIN, CHRONIC A state in which the individual experiences pain that continues for more than six months in duration. **Defining Characteristics:** *Major:* Verbal report or observed evidence of pain experienced for more than 6 months. *Minor:* Fear of re-injury; physical and social withdrawal; altered ability to continue previous activities; anorexia; weight changes; changes in sleep patterns; facial mask; guarded movement.

POWERLESSNESS Perception that one's own action will not significantly affect an outcome; a perceived lack of control over a current situation or immediate happening. **Defining Characteristics:** *Severe:* Verbal expressions of having no control or influence over situation or its outcome; verbal expressions of having no control over self-care; depression over physical deterioration which occurs despite patient compliance with regimens; apathy.

Moderate: Nonparticipation in care or decision-making when opportunities are provided; expressions of dissatisfaction and frustration over inability to perform previous tasks and/or activities; does not monitor progress; expression of doubt regarding role performance; reluctance to express true feelings; fearing alienation from caregivers; passivity; inability to seek information regarding care; dependence on others that may result in irritability, resentment, anger, and guilt; does not defend self-care practices when challenged. *Low:* Expressions of uncertainty about fluctuating energy levels; passivity.

PROTECTION, ALTERED The state in which an individual experiences a decrease in the ability to guard the self from internal or external threats such as illness or injury. **Defining Characteristics:** *Major:* Deficient immunity; impaired healing; altered clotting; maladaptive stress response; neurosensory alteration. *Minor:* Chilling; perspiring; dyspnea; cough; itching; restlessness; insomnia; fatigue; anorexia; weakness; immobility; disorientation; pressure sores.

RELOCATION STRESS SYNDROME Physiological and/or psychosocial disturbances as a result of transfer from one environment to another. **Defining Characteristics:** *Major:* Change in environment/location; anxiety; apprehension; increased confusion (elderly population); depression; loneliness. *Minor:* Verbalization of unwillingness to relocate; sleep disturbance; change in eating habits; dependency; gastrointestinal disturbances; increased verbalization of needs; insecurity; lack of trust; restlessness; sad affect; unfavorable comparison of post/pre-transfer staff; verbalization of being concerned/upset about transfer, vigilance; weight change; withdrawal.

ROLE PERFORMANCE, ALTERED Disruption in the way one perceives one's role performance. **Defining Characteristics:** Change in self-perception of role; denial of role; change in other's perception of role; conflict in roles; change in physical capacity to resume role; lack of knowledge of role; change in usual patterns of responsibility.

SELF-CARE DEFICIT(S): ADL A state in which the individual experiences an impaired ability to perform or complete one or more of the following activities for oneself:
BATHING/HYGIENE, Defining Characteristics: Inability to wash body or body parts; inability to obtain or get to

water source; inability to regulate temperature or flow.

DRESSING/GROOMING, Defining Characteristics: Impaired ability to put on or take off necessary items of clothing; impaired ability to obtain or replace articles of clothing; impaired ability to fasten clothing; inability to maintain appearance at a satisfactory level.
FEEDING, Defining Characteristics: Inability to bring food from a receptacle to one's mouth.
TOILETING, Defining Characteristics: Unable to get to toilet or commode; unable to sit on or rise from toilet or commode; unable to manipulate clothing for toileting; unable to carry out proper toilet hygiene; unable to flush toilet or commode.

Note: See suggested *Functional Level Classification* under diagnosis MOBILITY, IMPAIRED PHYSICAL.

SELF-ESTEEM DISTURBANCE
Negative self-evaluation of capabilities, or negative feelings about self or own capabilities, which may be directly or indirectly expressed. **Defining Characteristics:** Self negating verbalizations; expressions of shame/guilt; evaluates self as unable to deal with events; rationalizes away/rejects positive feedback and exaggerates negative feedback about self; hesitant to try new things/situations; denial of problems obvious to others; projection of blame/responsibility for problems; rationalizing personal failures; hypersensitive to slight or criticism; grandiosity.

SENSORY/PERCEPTUAL ALTERATIONS: VISUAL, AUDITORY, KINESTHETIC, GUSTATORY, TACTILE, OLFACTORY (SPECIFY) A state in which an individual experiences a change in the amount or patterning of oncoming stimuli accompanied by a diminished, exaggerated, distorted, or impaired response to such stimuli.
Defining Characteristics: Disoriented in time, in place, or with persons; altered abstraction; altered conceptualization; change in problem-solving abilities; reported or measured change in sensory acuity; change in behavior pattern; anxiety; apathy; change in usual response to stimuli; indication of body-image alteration; restlessness; irritability; altered communication patterns. **Other Possible Characteristics:** Complaints of fatigue; alteration in posture; change in muscular tension; inappropriate responses; hallucinations.

SEXUALITY PATTERNS, ALTERED
The state in which an individual expresses concern regarding his/her sexuality.
Defining Characteristics: *Major:* Reported difficulties, limitations, or changes in sexual behaviors or activities.

SKIN INTEGRITY, IMPAIRED A state in which the individual's skin is adversely altered. **Defining Characteristics:** Disruption of skin surface; destruction of skin layers; invasion of body structures.

SKIN INTEGRITY, IMPAIRED: HIGH RISK FOR A state in which the individual's skin is at risk of being adversely altered. **Defining Characteristics:** *Presence of risk factors such as: External (environmental):* Hypo- or hyperthermia; chemical substance; mechanical factors (shearing forces, pressure, restraint); radiation; physical immobilization; excretions/secretions; humidity. *Internal (somatic):* Medication; alterations in nutritional state (obesity, emaciation); altered metabolic state; altered circulation; altered sensation; altered pigmentation; skeletal prominence; developmental factors; alterations in skin turgor (change in elasticity); psychogenic; immunologic.

SLEEP PATTERN DISTURBANCE
Disruption of sleep time causes discomfort or interferes with desired lifestyle.
Defining Characteristics: Verbal complaints of difficulty falling asleep; awakening earlier or later than desired; interrupted sleep; verbal complaints of not feeling well-rested; changes in behavior and performance (increasing irritability, restlessness, disorientation, lethargy, listlessness); physical signs (mild fleeting nystagmus, slight hand tremor, ptosis of eyelid, expressionless face, dark circles under eyes, frequent yawning, changes in posture); thick speech with mispronunciation and incorrect words.

SOCIAL INTERACTION, IMPAIRED:
The state in which an individual participates in an insufficient or excessive quantity or ineffective quality of social exchange. **Defining Characteristics:** *Major:* Verbalized or observed discomfort in social situations; verbalized or observed inability to receive or communicate a satisfying sense of belonging, caring, interest, or shared history; observed use of unsuccessful social interaction behaviors; dysfunctional interaction with peers, family, and/or others. Minor: Family report of change of style or pattern of interaction.

SOCIAL ISOLATION Aloneness experienced by the individual and perceived as imposed by others and as a negative or threatened state. **Defining Characteristics:** *Objective:* Absence of family, friends, or other supportive significant other(s); sad, dull affect; inappropriate or immature interests/activities for development age/stage; uncommunicative, withdrawn, no eye contact; preoccupation with own thoughts, repetitive, meaningless actions; projects hostility in voice, behavior; seeks to be alone or to exist in subculture; shows behavior unaccepted by dominant cultural group; evidence of physical/mental handicap or altered state of wellness. *Subjective:* Expresses feelings of aloneness imposed by others; expresses feelings of rejection; experiences feelings of difference from others; lacks significant purpose in life; unable to meet expectations of others; shows insecurity in public; expresses values acceptable to the subculture but unacceptable to the dominant cultural group; expresses interests inappropriate to developmental age/state.

SPIRITUAL DISTRESS (DISTRESS OF THE HUMAN SPIRIT) Disruption in the life principle that pervades a person's entire being and that integrates and transcends one's biological and psychosocial nature. **Defining Characteristics:** Expresses concern with meaning of life/death and/or belief systems; expresses anger toward deity; questions meaning of suffering; questions meaning of own existence; verbalizes inner conflict about beliefs; questions moral/ethical implications of therapeutic regimen; gallows humor; verbalizes concern about relationship with deity; unable to participate in usual religious practices; seeks spiritual assistance; displacement of anger toward religious representatives; description of nightmares/sleep disturbances; alteration in behavior/mood evidenced by anger, crying, withdrawal, preoccupation, anxiety, hostility, apathy, and so forth.

SWALLOWING, IMPAIRED The state in which an individual has decreased ability to voluntarily pass fluids and/or solids from the mouth to the stomach. **Defining Characteristics:** *Major:* Observed evidence of difficulty in swallowing, e.g., stasis of food in oral cavity, coughing/choking. *Minor:* Evidence of aspiration.

THERAPEUTIC REGIMEN MANAGEMENT (INDIVIDUAL), INEFFECTIVE A pattern of regulating and integrating into daily living a program for treatment of illness and the sequelae of illness that is unsatisfactory for meeting specific health goals. **Defining Characteristics:** *Major:* Choices of daily living ineffective for meeting the goals of a treatment or prevention program. *Minor:* Acceleration (expected or unexpected) of illness symptoms; verbalized desire to manage the treatment of illness and prevention of sequelae; verbalized difficulty with regulation/integration of one or more prescribed regimens for treatment of illness and its effects or prevention of complications; verbalized that did not take action to include treatment regimens in daily routines; verbalized that did not take action to reduce risk factors for progression of illness and sequelae.

THERMOREGULATION, INEFFECTIVE The state in which the individual's temperature fluctuates between hypothermia and hyperthermia. **Defining Characteristics:** Fluctuations in body temperature above or below the normal range. See also characteristics present in hypothermia and hyperthermia.

THOUGHT PROCESSES, ALTERED A state in which an individual experiences a disruption in cognitive operations and activities. **Defining Characteristics:** Accurate interpretation of environment; cognitive dissonance; distractibility; memory deficit/problems; egocentricity; hyper- or hypovigilance. **Other Possible Characteristics:** Inappropriate or nonreality-based thinking.

TISSUE INTEGRITY, IMPAIRED A state in which an individual experiences damage to mucous membrane, corneal, integumentary or subcutaneous tissue. **Defining Characteristics:** *Major:* Damaged or destroyed tissue (cornea, mucous membrane, integumentary, or subcutaneous).

TISSUE PERFUSION, ALTERED: RENAL, CEREBRAL, CARDIOPULMONARY, GASTROINTESTINAL, PERIPHERAL (SPECIFY TYPE) The state in which an individual experiences a decrease in nutrition and oxygenation at the cellular level due to a deficit in capillary blood supply. **Defining Characteristics:** Skin temperature: cold in extremities. Skin color: dependent, blue or purple and pale on elevation; color does not return on lowering of leg; diminished arterial pulsations. Skin quality: shining; lack of lanugo; slow healing of lesions; gangrene; slow-growing, dry, brittle nails. Other: claudication; blood pressure changes in extremities; bruits.

URINARY ELIMINATION, ALTERED The state in which the individual experiences a disturbance in urine elimination. **Defining Characteristics:** Dysuria; frequency; hesitancy; incontinence; nocturia; retention; urgency.

URINARY INCONTINENCE, FUNCTIONAL The state in which an individual experiences an involuntary, unpredictable passage of urine. **Defining Characteristics:** Urge to void or bladder contractions sufficiently strong to result in loss of urine before reaching an appropriate receptacle.

URINARY INCONTINENCE, REFLEX The state in which an individual experiences an involuntary loss of urine, occurring at somewhat predictable intervals when a specific bladder volume is reached. **Defining Characteristics:** No awareness of bladder filling; no urge to void or feelings of bladder fullness; uninhabited bladder contraction/spasm at regular intervals.

URINARY INCONTINENCE, STRESS The state in which an individual experiences a loss of urine of less than 50 mL occurring with increased abdominal pressure. **Defining Characteristics:** *Major:* Reported or observed dribbling with increased abdominal pressure. *Minor:* Urinary urgency; urinary frequency (more often than every two hours).

URINARY INCONTINENCE, TOTAL The state in which an individual experiences a continuous and unpredictable loss of urine. **Defining Characteristics:** *Major:* Constant flow of urine occurs at unpredictable times without distention or uninhibited bladder contractions/spasm; unsuccessful incontinence refractory treatments; nocturia. *Minor:* Lack of perineal or bladder filling awareness; unawareness of incontinence.

URINARY INCONTINENCE, URGE The state in which an individual experiences involuntary passage of urine occurring soon after a strong sense of urgency to void. **Defining Characteristics:** *Major:* Urinary urgency; frequency (voiding more often than every two hours); bladder contracture/spasm. *Minor:* Nocturia (more than two times per night); voiding in small amounts (less than 100 mL) or in large amounts (more than 550 mL); inability to reach toilet in time.

URINARY RETENTION The state in which the individual experiences incomplete emptying of the bladder. **Defining Characteristics:** *Major:* Bladder distention; small, frequent voiding or absence of urine output. *Minor:* Sensation of bladder fullness; dribbling; residual urine; dysuria; overflow incontinence.

VIOLENCE, HIGH RISK: SELF DIRECTED OR DIRECTED AT OTHERS A state in which an individual experiences behaviors that can be physically harmful either to the self or others. **Defining Characteristics:** *Presence of risk factors such as: Body Language:* Clenched fists, tense facial expression, rigid posture, tautness indicating effort to control. *Hostile threatening verbalizations:* Boasting to or prior abuse of others; increased motor activity (pacing, excitement, irritability, agitation). *Overt and aggressive acts:* Goal-directed destruction of objects in environment; possession of destructive means (gun, knife, weapon); rage; self-destructive behavior, active aggressive suicidal acts; suspicion of others, paranoid ideation; delusion, hallucinations; substance abuse/withdrawal. **Other Possible Characteristics:** Increasing anxiety levels; fear of self or others; inability to verbalize feelings; repetition of verbalizations (continued complaints, requests, and demands); anger; provocative behavior (argumentative, dissatisfied, overreactive, hypersensitive); vulnerable self-esteem; depression.

DX DEFINITIONS

BIBLIOGRAPHY

Ackley, Betty J., and Gail B. Ladwig: *Nursing Diagnosis Handbook: A Guide to Planning Care*, C. V. Mosby Company, St. Louis, 1993.

Agency for Health Care Policy and Research: *Clinical Practice Guidelines: Acute Pain Management*, U.S. Department of Health and Human Services, Washington D.C., 1992.

Alfaro, R.: *Applying Nursing Diagnosis and Nursing Process: A Step-by-Step Guide*, 2d ed., J. B. Lippincott Company, Philadelphia, 1990.

Alspach, JoAnn Grif (Ed.): *Core Curriculum for Critical Care Nursing*, 4th ed., W. B. Saunders Company, Philadelphia, 1991.

Alvarez, O., J. Rozint, and D. Wiseman: "Moist Environment: Matching the Dressing to the Wound," *Wounds 1*(1), 1989, pp. 35-51.

Amenta, M., and N. Bohnot: *Nursing Care of the Terminally Ill*, Little, Brown, and Company, Boston, 1986.

American Diabetes Association: "National Standards for Diabetes Patient Education and American Diabetes Association Review Criteria," *Diabetes Care 14*(suppl. 2), March 1991, pp. 76-81.

_____: "Standards of Medical Care for Patients with Diabetes Mellitus," *Diabetes Care 14*(suppl. 2), March 1991, pp. 10-13.

American Pain Society: *Principles of Analgesia Use in Treatment of Acute Pain and Chronic Cancer Pain*, American Pain Society, Skokie, Illinois, 1989.

Baird, Susan, Michelle Donehower, Valerie Stalsbroten, and Terri Ades (Eds.): *A Cancer Source Book for Nurses*, 6th ed., The American Cancer Society, Atlanta, 1991.

Barry, Patricia D.: *Psychosocial Nursing Assessment and Intervention*, J. B. Lippincott Company, Philadelphia, 1989.

Bass, J. B. (Ed.): "The Medical Clinics of North America," *Tuberculosis 77*(6), November 1993, n.p.

Baxter, C., and P. Mertz: "Wound Assessment and Categorization," in William Eaglestein, Charles Baxter, and Patricia Mertz (Eds.), *New Directions in Wound Healing*, E. R.

Squibb and Sons, Princeton, New Jersey, 1990.

Beare, Patricia G., and Judith L. Myers: *Principles and Practice of Adult Health Nursing*, C. V. Mosby Company, St. Louis, 1990.

Beck, C., R. Rawlins, and S. Williams: *Mental Health: Psychiatric Nursing*, C. V. Mosby Company, St. Louis, 1988.

Beeson, Paul, Walsh McDermott, and James Wyngaarden: *Textbook of Medicine*, 15th ed., W. B. Saunders Company, Philadelphia, 1979.

Bensimon, Hector: *Urologic Surgery*, McGraw-Hill, Inc., New York, 1991.

Berkow, R., and A. Fletcher: *The Merck Manual*, 15th ed., Merck Sharp and Dohme International Laboratories, New Jersey, 1987.

Black, J., and E. Matassarin-Jacobs: *Luckman and Sorensen's Medical-Surgical Nursing: A Psychophysiologic Approach*, 4th ed., W. B. Saunders Company, Philadelphia, 1993.

Blandy, J. P., and R. G. Notley: *Transurethral Resection*, 3d ed., Butterworth Heinemann, Ltd., London, 1993.

Boback, Irene M., and Margaret Duncan Jensen: *Maternity and Gynecologic Care*, 5th ed., C. V. Mosby Company, St. Louis, 1992.

Boyda, Ellen K.: *Respiratory Problems: RN Nursing Assessment Series 5*, Medical Economics Books, 1985.

Brown, R., and G. Preminger: "Changing Surgical Aspects of Urinary Stone Disease," *Surgical Clinics of North America 68*(5), October 1988, pp. 1085-1101.

Brunner, Lillian Sholtis, and Doris Smith Suddarth: *The Lippincott Manual of Nursing Practice*, 4th ed., J. B. Lippincott Company, Philadelphia, 1986.

_____: *The Lippincott Manual of Nursing Practice*, 7th ed., J. B. Lippincott Company, Philadelphia, 1992.

Bulechek, Gloria M., and Joanne C. McCloskey: *Nursing Interventions: Essential Nursing Treatments*, 2d ed., W. B. Saunders Company, Philadelphia, 1992.

Burnside, Irene M.: *Nursing and the Aged*, 3d ed., C. V. Mosby Company, St. Louis, 1988.

Burrell, L.: *Adult Nursing in Hospital and Community Settings*, Appleton and Lange, Norwalk, Conn., 1992.

Cahill, Matthew: *Nursing Process in Clinical Practice*, Springhouse Corporation, Springhouse, Pennsylvania, 1993.

Caine, R., and P. Bufalino: *Nursing Care Planning Guides for Adults*, Williams & Wilkins Publishing Company, Baltimore, 1987.

_____: *Nursing Care Planning Guides for Adults*, 2d ed., Williams & Wilkins Publishing Company, Baltimore, 1991.

Carini, G., and J. Birmingham: *Traction Made Easy*, McGraw-Hill Book Company, New York, 1980.

Carnevali, D., and M. Patrick: *Nursing Management for the Elderly*, 3d ed., J. B. Lippincott Company, Philadelphia, 1993.

_____ and M. Thomas: *Diagnostic Reasoning and Treatment Decision Making in Nursing*, J. B. Lippincott Company, Philadelphia, 1993.

Carpenito, Lynda Juall: *Nursing Care Plans and Documentation*, J. B. Lippincott Company, Philadelphia, 1991.

_____: *Nursing Care Plans and Documentation*, J. B. Lippincott Company, Philadelphia, 1993.

_____: *Nursing Diagnosis: Application to Clinical Practice, 1989-90*, 3d ed., J. B. Lippincott Company, Philadelphia, 1989.

_____: *Nursing Diagnosis: Application to Clinical Practice, 1989-90*, 4th ed., J. B. Lippincott Company, Philadelphia, 1992.

_____: *Nursing Diagnosis: Application to Clinical Practice*, 5th ed., J. B. Lippincott Company, Philadelphia, 1993.

Carroll-Johnson, Rose Mary (Ed.) *North American Nursing Diagnosis Association Classification of Nursing Diagnoses: Proceedings of the Ninth Conference*, J. B. Lippincott Company, Philadelphia, 1991.

Cerrato, P.: "Kidney Stones Don't Have to Recur," *RN 55*(6), 1992, pp. 63-64.

Chipps, E., N. Clanin, and V. Campbell: *Neurological Disorders*, C. V. Mosby Company, St. Louis, 1992.

Chopra, S., and R. May: *Pathophysiology of Gastrointestinal Diseases*, Little, Brown, and Company, Boston, 1989.

Clark, Cheryl: "Nursing Care for Multiple Sclerosis," *Orthopaedic Nursing*, January-February 1991, pp. 21-34.

Clark, Jane C., and Rose F. McGee: *Oncology Nursing Society Core Curriculum for Oncology Nursing*, 2d ed., W. B. Saunders Company, Philadelphia, 1992.

Clochesy, J., C. Breu, S. Cardin, E. Rudy, and A. Whittake: *Critical Care Nursing*, W. B. Saunders Company, Philadelphia, 1993.

Coleman, D. A.: "RN Master Care Plan: When a Patient Requires Isolation," *RN* 47(9), pp. 59-60.

Cooke, Dorothy M.: "Inflammatory Bowel Disease: Primary Health Care Management of Ulcerative Colitis and Crohn's Disease," *Nurse Practitioner*, August 1991, pp. 27-39.

Cooper, Diane: "Challenge of Open Wound Assessment in the Home Setting," *Progressions: Developments in Ostomy and Wound Care 2(3)*, 1990, pp. 11-18.

_____: "Wound Assessment and Evaluation," in Ruth A. Bryant (Ed.), *Acute and Chronic Wounds: Nursing Management*, Mosby Year Book, St. Louis, 1992.

Corney, Joslyn: "The Care of the Patient Undergoing Surgery for Gynecological Cancer: The Need for Information, Emotional Support and Counseling," *Journal of Advanced Nursing 17*, 1992, pp. 667-671.

Covington, Holly: "Nursing Care of Patients with Alcoholic Liver Disease," *Critical Care Nurse*, June 1993, pp. 47-57.

Cox, Helen, Mittie Hinz, Mary Lubno, Susan Newfield, Nancy Ridenour, Mary Slater, and Kathryn Sridaromont: *Clinical Applications of Nursing Diagnosis: Adult, Child, Women's Psychiatric, Gerontic and Home Health Considerations*, 2d ed., F. A. Davis Company, Philadelphia, 1993.

Crow, Susan: "Infection Control Perspectives," in Diane Krasner (Ed.), *Chronic Wound Care*, Health

Management Publications, King of Prussia, Pennsylvania, 1991.

Davis, Crystal: "Nursing Care of Total Parenteral Nutrition," in Josef E. Fischer (Ed.), *Total Parenteral Nutrition*, Little, Brown, and Company, Boston, 1991.

Deglin, Judith Hopfer, and April Hazard Vallerand: *Davis's Drug Guide for Nurses*, F. A. Davis Company, Philadelphia, 1991.

Doenges, Marilynn E., and Mary Frances Moorhouse: *Application of Nursing Process and Nursing Diagnosis: An Interactive Text*, F. A. Davis Company, Philadelphia, 1992.

_____: *Nurse's Pocket Guide: Nursing Diagnoses with Interventions*, 4th ed., F. A. Davis Company, Philadelphia, 1993.

_____: *Nursing Diagnoses with Interventions*, C. V. Mosby Company, St. Louis, 1988.

_____: *Nursing Diagnoses with Interventions*, 4th ed., F. A. Davis Company, Philadelphia, 1993.

_____: *Nursing Care Plans: Guidelines for Planning and Documenting Patient Care*, 3d ed., F. A. Davis Company, Philadelphia, 1993.

Dolan, J.: *Critical Care Nursing: Clinical Management Through the Nursing Process*, F. A. Davis Company, Philadelphia, 1991.

Doughty, D. B.: "Principles of Wound Healing and Wound Management," in Ruth A. Bryant (Ed.), *Acute and Chronic Wounds: Nursing Management*, Mosby Year Book Company, St. Louis, 1992.

_____: "The Process of Wound Healing: A Nursing Perspective," *Progressions: Developments in Ostomy and Wound Care 2(3)*, 1990, pp. 3-12.

_____ and D. B. Jackson: *Gastrointestinal Disorders*, C. V. Mosby Company, St. Louis, 1993.

"Downtime Final Report Form," Oregon Medical Laboratories, Eugene, Oregon, n.d.

Ebersole, P., and P. Hess: *Toward Healthy Aging: Human Needs and Nursing Response*, 2d ed., C. V. Mosby Company, St. Louis, 1985.

_____: *Toward Healthy Aging: Human Needs and Nursing Response*, 3d ed.,

Mosby Year Book Company, St. Louis, 1985.

Eliopoulos, Charlotte: *Gerontological Nursing*, 3d ed., J. B. Lippincott Company, Philadelphia, 1993.

Engram, Barbara: *Medical-Surgical Nursing Care Plans*, Delmar, Albany, New York, 1993.

Esberger, K., and S. Hughes: *Nursing Care of the Aged*, Appleton and Lange, Norwalk, Conn., 1987.

Ferguson, R. S., and N. B. Wairath: *Nurse Review: A Clinical Update System: Volume I: Gastrointestinal Problems*, Springhouse Corporation, Springhouse, Penna., 1986.

Forzeman, Joy, and Carol Bowdoin: *Decision Making in Medical-Surgical Nursing*, B. C. Decker, Philadelphia, 1990.

Fowler, Jackson E.: *Manual of Urologic Surgery*, Little, Brown, and Company, Boston, 1990.

_____: *Urologic Surgery*, Little, Brown, and Company, Boston, 1992.

Gardner, T. W., and D. E. Shoch: *Handbook of Ophthalmology: A Practical Guide*, Appleton and Lange, Norwalk, Connecticut, 1987.

Gettrust, Kathy V., and Paula D. Brabec: *Nursing Diagnosis in Clinical Practice: Guides for Care Planning*, Delmar Publishers, Incorporated, Albany, New York, 1992.

Gordon, Marjory: *Manual of Nursing Diagnosis, 1993-1994*, C. V. Mosby Company, St. Louis, 1993.

Gulanick, Meg, Audrey Klopp, and Sue Galanes: *Nursing Care Plans: Nursing Diagnosis and Intervention*, C. V. Mosby Company, St. Louis, 1986.

Graves, K. W., L. B. Noel, D. B. Knight, S. G. Lessans, and K. J. Judy: *The Johns Hopkins Hospital Surgical Nursing Care Guidelines*, Appleton and Lange, Norwalk, Connecticut, 1988.

Groenwald, S., M. Frogge, M. Goodman, and C. Yarbro: *Cancer Nursing: Principles and Practice*, 3d ed., Jones and Bartlett Publishers, Incorporated, Boston, 1993.

Gulanick, M., A. Klopp, S. Galanes, D. Gradishar, and M. Puzas: *Nursing Care Plans: Nursing Diagnosis and Intervention*, 2d ed., C. V. Mosby Company, St. Louis, 1990.

BIBLIOGRAPHY

Holloway, Nancy M.: *Medical Surgical Care Plans*, Springhouse Corporation, Springhouse, Pennsylvania, 1988.

_____: *Medical Surgical Care Plans*, Springhouse Corporation, Springhouse, Pennsylvania, 1993.

Hudak, C. M., B. M. Guilo, and J. L. Benz: *Critical Care Nursing: A Holistic Approach*, J. B. Lippincott Company, Philadelphia, 1990.

Ignatavicius, Donna D., and Marilyn Varner Bayne: *Medical-Surgical Nursing: A Nursing Process Approach*, W. B. Saunders Company, Philadelphia, 1991.

Jaffe, M.: *Geriatric Nursing Care Plans*, Skidmore-Roth Publishing, El Paso, Texas, 1991.

Jervis, Carolyn: *Physical Examination and Health Assessment*, W. B. Saunders Company, Philadelphia, 1992.

Joachim, Gloria: "Inflammatory Bowel Disease: Effects on Lifestyle," *Journal of Advanced Nursing*, December 1987, pp. 483-487.

Johnson, Brenda Crispell, Consuelo Certula Dungca, Sara Jeanne Wells, and Denise Hoffmeister: *Standards for Critical Care*, 3d ed., C. V. Mosby Company, St. Louis, 1988.

Joint Commission on the Accreditatation of Health Care Organizations: 1994 Accreditation Manual for Hospitals, Vol III, "Scoring Guidelines," The Joint Commission on the Accreditation of Health Care Organizations, Oakbrook Terrace, Ill, 1993, page 5.

Jones, Dorothy, Claire Ford Dunbar, and Mary Marmoll Jerovic: *Medical-Surgical Nursing: A Conceptual Approach*, McGraw-Hill Book Company, New York, 1978.

Katelaris, P. H., and D. B. Jones: "Fulminant Hepatic Failure," *Medicine Clinics of North America*, 1989, pp. 955-970.

Kelly, B., and S. Mahon: "Nursing Care of the Patient With Multiple Sclerosis," *Rehabilitation Nursing*, September-October 1988, pp. 238-242.

Kim, Mi Ja, Gertrude K. McFarland, and Audrey M. McLane: *Pocket Guide to Nursing Diagnoses*, 3d ed., Mosby Year Book Company, St. Louis, 1989.

_____: *Pocket Guide to Nursing, Diagnoses*, 4th ed., Mosby Year Book Company, St. Louis, 1991.

_____: *Pocket Guide to Nursing, Diagnoses*, 5th ed., Mosby Year Book Company, St. Louis, 1993.

Kinash, Rose G.: "IBD: Implications for Patients, Challenges for Nurses," *Rehabilitation Nursing*, March-April 1987, pp. 69, 82-89.

_____, Donald G. Fischer, Bryan E. Lukie, and Tracey L. Carr: "Coping Patterns and Related Characteristics in Patients with IBD," *Rehabilitation Nursing*, January-February 1993, pp. 12-19.

Klopp, A., and S. Galores: *Nursing Care Plans, Nursing Diagnosis and Interventions*, C. V. Mosby Company, St. Louis, 1986.

Kucharski, Sandra: "Fulminant Hepatic Failure," *Critical Care Nursing Clinics of North America*, March 1993, pp. 141-150.

Kuhn, Rebecca C. (Ed.): *Outcome Standards for Nursing Care of the Critically Ill*, American Association of Critical-Care Nurses, Laguna Niguel, 1990.

Krumberger, Joanne M.: "Gastrointestinal Disorders," in Marguerite Kinney, Donna R. Packa, and Sandra B. Dunbar (Eds.), *AACN's Clinical Reference for Critical-Care Nursing*, 2d ed., C. V. Mosby Company, St. Louis, 1993.

_____: "Gastrointestinal Disorders," in Jeanette Hartshorn, Marilyn Lamborn, and Mary Lou Noll (Eds.), *Introduction to Critical Care Nursing*, W. B. Saunders Company, Philadelphia, 1993.

Lawer, Judith: "Maxillofacial Trauma," *Nursing Clinics of North America* 21(4), 1986, pp. 611-628.

Lewis, Sharon M., and Idolia C. Collier: *Medical-Surgical Nursing: Assessment and Management of Clinical Problems*, 3d ed., C. V. Mosby Company, St. Louis, 1992.

Lockhart, J., J. Troff, and L. Artrim: "Total Laryngectomy and Radical Neck Dissection," *AORN* 55(2), 1992, pp. 458-479.

London, F.: "Nursing Diagnoses and Caring for Patients with Sickle Cell Disease," *Advancing Clinical Care*, September-October 1990, pp. 12-16.

Long, Barbara C., and Wilma J. Phipps: *Medical-Surgical Nursing: A Nursing Process Approach*, 2d ed., C. V. Mosby Company, St. Louis, 1989.

_____ and Virginia L. Cassmeyer: *Medical-Surgical Nursing: A Nursing Process Approach*, 3d ed., C. V. Mosby Company, St. Louis, 1993.

Loxley, Cynthia Ruth, and Sheila Sparks Cress: *The Pocket Guide to Clinical Nursing Process for an Adult Medical-Surgical Client*, The Miller Press, New York, 1983.

Luckman, J., and K. Sorensen: *Medical-Surgical Nursing: A Psychophysiologic Approach*, W. B. Saunders Company, Philadelphia, 1980.

McCaffery, M., and A. Beebe: *Pain: Clinical Manual for Nursing Practice*, C. V. Mosby Company, St. Louis, 1989.

McCloskey, J. C., and G. M. Bulechek: *Nursing Interventions Classifications*, C. V. Mosby Company, St. Louis, 1992.

McFarland, G., and E. McFarlane: *Nursing Diagnoses and Intervention*, C. V. Mosby Company, St. Louis, 1989.

_____ and E. Walsh: *Nursing Diagnoses and Process in Psychiatric Health*, J. B. Lippincott Company, Philadelphia, 1986.

McMahon, Edith: *Diseases*, Springhouse Corporation, Springhouse, Pennsylvania, 1993.

Maimonides Medical Center, Department of Nursing: *Nursing Standards of Practice for the Patient with a CVA*, Maimonides Medical Center, Brooklyn, New York, 1993.

Marvis, Carolyn: *Physical Examination and Health Assessment*, W. B. Saunders Company, Philadelphia, 1992.

Matteson, M., and E. McConnell: *Gerontological Nursing: Concepts and Practice*, Harcourt-Brace-Jovanovich, Philadelphia, 1988.

Mayers, Marlene: *Clinical Care Plans: Medical Nursing*, Markham-McKenzie Publishers, Eugene, Oregon, 1989.

_____: *Clinical Care Plans: Orthopedic and Neurologic Nursing*, Markham-McKenzie Publishers, Eugene, Oregon, 1989.

_____: *Clinical Care Plans: Pediatric Nursing*, Markham-McKenzie Publishers, Eugene, Oregon, 1989.

_____: *Clinical Care Plans: Surgical Nursing*, Markham-McKenzie Publishers, Eugene, Oregon, 1989.

Michael Reese Hospital, Department of Nursing: *Nursing Care Plans: Nursing Diagnosis and Intervention*, C. V. Mosby Company, Chicago, 1986.

Moorhouse, Mary F., Alice C. Geissler, and Marilynn E. Doenges: *Critical Care Plans: Guidelines for Advanced Medical-Surgical Care*, F. A. Davis Company, Philadelphia, 1991.

Mosby's Manual for Urological Nursing, C. V. Mosby Company, St. Louis, 1982.

Mudge-Grout, Christine L.: *Immunologic Disorders*, C. V. Mosby Company, St. Louis, 1992.

Murphy, L. C.: "Establishing and Clarifying the Etiologies and Characteristics of the Nursing Diagnosis Alterations in Nutrition: Less Than Body Requirements," in Rose Mary Carroll-Johnson (Ed.), *Proceedings of the Eighth Conference*, NANDA, J. B. Lippincott Company, Philadelphia, 1988.

Myers, D.: *Exploring Psychology*, Worth Publishers, New York, 1990.

National Association of Orthopedic Nurses: *Guidelines for Orthopedic Nursing*, NAON, New Jersey, 1992.

Neal, M., M. Pacquette, and M. Mirch: *Nursing Diagnosis Care Plans for Diagnosis-Related Groups*, Jones and Bartlett Publishers, Boston, 1990.

Neel, Carol J., and Mark B. Wallerstein: *A Pocket Guide for Medical-Surgical Nursing*, Brachy Communications Company, Maryland, 1985.

Neurologic Disorders: Nurses' Clinical Library, Springhouse Corporation, Springhouse, Pennsylvania, 1984.

Newman, D. K., and D. A. Smith: *Geriatric Care Plans*, Springhouse Corporation, Springhouse, Pennsylvania, 1991.

North American Nursing Association: *NANDA Nursing Diagnoses: Definitions and Classifications 1992-93*, North American Nursing Association, St. Louis, 1992.

_____: *Taxonomy 1992-93*, J. B. Lippincott Company, Philadelphia, 1992.

Nurses Clinical Library: Respiratory Disorders, Springhouse Corporation, Springhouse, Pennsylvania, 1984.

Olson, Edith: "Hazards of Immobility," *American Journal of Nursing*, April 1967, pp. 780-797.

Ondruseh, Robin Spangler: "Cholecystectomy: An Update," *RN*, January 1993, pp. 28-32.

Palandri, Mary K., and Catherine Rollman Sorrentino: *Handbook for Luckmann and Sorensen's Medical Surgical Nursing: A Psychophysiologic Approach*, 4th ed., W. B. Saunders Company, Philadelphia, 1993.

Panel for the Prediction and Prevention of Pressure Ulcers in Adults: *Pressure Ulcers in Adults: Prediction and Prevention*, Clinical Practice Guideline, Number 3, AHRCPR Publication No. 92-0047, Agency for Health Care Policy and Research Public Health Service, U.S. Department of Health and Human Services, Rockville, Maryland, May 1992.

Patrick, M., S. Woods, R. Craven, J. Rokosky, and P. Bruno: *Medical-Surgical Nursing: Pathophysiological Concepts*, 2d ed., J. B. Lippincott Company, Philadelphia, 1991.

Phipps, Wilma J., Barbara C. Long, and Nancy Fugate Woods: *Medical-Surgical Nursing: Concepts and Clinical Practice*, 3d ed., C. V. Mosby Company, St. Louis, 1987.

_____ and Virginia L. Cassmeyer: *Medical-Surgical Nursing: Concepts and Clinical Practice*, 4th ed., Mosby Year Book Company, St. Louis, 1991.

Pires, M., and A. Muller: "Detection and Management of Early Tissue Pressure Indicators: A Pictoral Essay," *Progressions: Developments in Ostomy and Wound Care* 3(3), 1991, pp. 3-11.

Porth, Carol Mattson: *Pathophysiology: Concepts of Altered Health States*, 3d ed., J. B. Lippincott Company, Philadelphia, 1990.

Preminger, G.: "Renal Calculi: Pathogenesis, Diagnosis, and Medical Therapy," *Seminars in Nephrology* 12(2), 1992, pp. 200-216.

"Pressure Ulcers in Adults: Prediction and Prevention," *Clinical Practice Guideline #3, Quick Reference Guide for Clinicians # 3*, U.S. Department of Health and Human Services Public Health Service, Washington D.C., n.d.

Quinless, Frances: "Severe Liver Dysfunction: Client Problems and

Nursing Actions," *Focus on Critical Care*, February 1985, pp. 24-32.

Raffensperger, Ellen Baily, Mary Lloyd Musy, and Lynn Claire Marchesseault: *Clinical Nursing Handbook*, J. B. Lippincott Company, Philadelphia, 1986.

Rakel, Robert E.: *Conn's Current Therapy*, W. B. Saunders Company, Philadelphia, 1993.

Reiner, Ann (Ed.): *Manual of Patient Care Standards*, Aspen Publishers, Gaithersburg, Maryland, 1991.

Reishtein, Judith: "Liver Failure: Case Study of a Complex Problem," *Critical Care Nurse*, October 1993, pp. 36-47.

Rivers, R., and N. Williamson: "Sickle Cell Anemia: Complex Disease, Nursing Challenge," *RN*, June 1990, pp. 24-28.

Rombeau, J. L., and M. D. Caldwell: *Clinical Nutrition: Enteral and Tube Feeding*, 2d ed., W. B. Saunders Company, Philadelphia, 1990.

Rowland, Gayle A., Delores A. Marks, and William E. Torres: "The New Gallstone Destroyers and Dissolvers," *American Journal of Nursing*, November 1989, pp. 1473-1476.

Sands, Judith K.: *Clinical Manual of Medical-Surgical Nursing: Concepts and Clinical Practice*, 2d ed., Mosby Year Book Company, St. Louis, 1991.

Sawyer, D., and M. Bruya: "Care of the Patient Having Radical Neck Surgery or Permanent Laryngostomy: A Nursing Diagnostic Approach," *Focus on Critical Care* 17(2), 1990, pp. 166-173.

Seidel, H., J. Ball, J. Dains, and G. Benedict: *Mosby's Guide to Physical Examination*, 2d ed., Mosby Year Book Company, St. Louis, 1991.

Shack, R., and P. Manson: "Traumatic Wounds," in F. Dagher, *Cutaneous Wounds*, Futura Publishing Company, Mt. Kisco, New York, 1985.

Shapiro, Barry A., Ronald A. Harrison, Robert M. Kacmarek, and Roy D. Cane: *Clinical Applications of Respiratory Care*, Year Book Medical Publisher, Chicago, 1985.

Shlafer, M.: *The Nurse, Pharmacology, and Drug Therapy: A Prototype Approach*, Addison-Wesley Company, Redwood City, California, 1993.

BIBLIOGRAPHY

Sholtis, Brunner L., and G. S. Suddarth: *The Lippincott Manual of Nursing Practice*, J. B. Lippincott Company, Philadelphia, 1986.

Simmons, Michelle A.: "Using the Nursing Process in Treating Inflammatory Bowel Disease," *Nursing Clinics of North America*, March 1984, pp. 11-25.

Smeltzer, Suzanne C., and Brenda G. Bare: *Brunner and Suddarth's Textbook of Medical-Surgical Nursing*, 7th ed., J. B. Lippincott Company, Philadelphia, 1992.

Smith, R. B., and R. M. Ehrlich: *Complications of Urologic Surgery: Prevention and Management*, 2d ed., W. B. Saunders Company, Philadelphia, 1990.

Sparks, Sheila M., and Cynthia M. Taylor: *Nursing Diagnosis Reference Manual*, Springhouse Corporation, Springhouse, Pennsylvania, 1987.

_____: *Nursing Diagnosis Reference Manual*, 2d ed., Springhouse Corporation, Springhouse, Pennsylvania, 1993.

Spratto, George R., and Adrienne L. Woods: *RN Magazine's NDR-94: Nurses' Drug Reference*, Delmar Publishers, Incorporated, Albany, New York, 1994.

Stead, W. W.: *Understanding Tuberculosis Today*, 8th ed., Central Press, Incorporated, Milwaukee, Wisconsin, 1992.

Stephenson, C. A.: *Clinical Manual of Gerontological Nursing*, Mosby Year Book Company, St. Louis, 1992.

Stotts, Nancy A., Kathleen A. Fitzgerald, and Karen R. Williams: "Care of the Patient Critically Ill with Inflammatory Bowel Disease," *Nursing Clinics of North America*, March 1984, pp. 61-69.

Stuart, G., and S. Sundeen: *Principles and Practice of Psychiatric Nursing*, 4th ed., Mosby Year Book Company, St. Louis, 1991.

Suitor, C. W., and M. F. Crowley: *Nutrition: Principles and Application of Health Promotion*, 2d ed., J. B. Lippincott Company, Philadelphia, 1984.

Swearington, Pamela L. (Ed.): *Pocket Guide to Medical-Surgical Nursing*, Mosby Year Book Company, St. Louis, 1992.

Taylor, C., C. Lillis, and P. LeMore: *Fundamentals of Nursing: The Art and Science of Nursing Care*, 2d ed., J. B. Lippincott Company, Philadelphia, 1993.

_____ and S. Sparks: *Nursing Diagnosis Cards*, 7th ed., Springhouse Corporation, Springhouse, Pennsylvania, 1993.

Thompson, June M., Gertrude K. McFarland, Jane E. Hirsch, and Susan M. Tucker: *Clinical Nursing*, C. V. Mosby Company, St. Louis, 1986.

_____: *Mosby's Clinical Nursing*, 3d ed., C. V. Mosby Company, St. Louis, 1993.

"Traction Programmed Instruction," *American Journal of Nursing*, October 1979, pp. 1771-1798.

Tucker, Susan Martin, Mary M. Canobbio, Eleanor Vargo Paquette, and Marjorie Fyfe Wells: *Patient Care Standards*, 4th ed., C. V. Mosby Company, St. Louis, 1988.

_____: *Patient Care Standards: Nursing*, C. V. Mosby Company, St. Louis, 1992.

_____: *Patient Care Standards: Nursing Process, Diagnosis, and Outcome*, Mosby Year Book Company, St. Louis, 1992.

Turner-Beatty, M., M. Grotewiel, and S. Fosha-Solezal: "Biochemical and Histologic Changes Due to Moisturization during Wound Healing," *Wounds* 2(4), 1990, pp. 156-161.

Ulrich, S. P., S. W. Canole, and S. A. Wendell: *Nursing Care Planning Guides: A Nursing Diagnosis Approach*, W. B. Saunders Company, Philadelphia, 1990.

Urden, L., J. Davie, and L. Thelan: *Essentials of Critical Care Nursing*, Mosby Year Book Company, St. Louis, 1992.

"Urinary Incontinence in Adults," *Clinical Practice Guideline, Quick Reference Guide for Clinicians*, U.S. Department of Health and Human Services Public Health Service, Washington D.C., n.d.

Vogt, Gordon: *Mosby's Manual of Neurological Care*, C. V. Mosby Company, St. Louis, 1985.

Wade, Jacqueline: *Comprehensive Respiratory Care*, C. V. Mosby Company, St. Louis, 1989.

Wesovick, Bonnie: *Standards of Nursing Care: A Model for Clinical Practice*, J. B. Lippincott Company, Philadelphia, 1990.

Williams, S. R.: *Nutrition and Diet Therapy*, 7th ed., C. V. Mosby Company, St. Louis, 1993.

Williamson, Marvel L.: "Sexual Adjustment after Hysterectomy," *Journal of Obstetric, Gynecologic, and Neonatal Nursing* 21(1), January/February 1992, pp. 42-47.

Williamson, Verdell: "Amputation of the Lower Extremity: An Overview," *Orthopaedic Nursing* 2(2), 1991, pp. 55-65.

Wilson, H., and C. Kniesl: *Psychiatric Nursing*, 4th ed., Addison-Wesley Nursing, Redwood City, California, 1992.

Wold, Gloria: *Basic Geriatric Nursing*, C. V. Mosby Company, St. Louis, 1993.